By the same authors

The Melatonin Miracle

THE

Superhormone Promise

NATURE'S ANTIDOTE TO AGING

WILLIAM REGELSON, M.D., AND CAROL COLMAN

Foreword by Walter Pierpaoli, M.D., Ph.D.

SIMON & SCHUSTER

SIMON & SCHUSTER
Rockefeller Center
1230 Avenue of the Americas
New York, NY 10020

SIMON & SCHUSTER and colophon are registered trademarks
of Simon & Schuster Inc.

Designed by Irving Perkins Assoc.

Manufactured in the United States of America

1   3   5   7   9   10   8   6   4   2

Library of Congress Cataloging-in-Publication Data is available.

ISBN 0-684-83011-6

The ideas, procedures, and suggestions contained in this book are not intended to replace the services of a trained health professional. All matters regarding your health require medical supervision. If you have any preexisting medical conditions, you should consult your physician before adopting the suggestions and procedures in this book. Any applications of the treatments set forth in this book are at the reader's discretion. If you are taking prescription medication on a regular basis, please check with your physician before using any of the hormones described in this book. In some cases, some of the hormones may enhance the effect of certain types of medication, so you may need to reduce your dosages accordingly.

The names of some individuals in
this book have been changed.

The author gratefully acknowledges permission from Mary Ann Liebert, Inc., Publishers to reprint "DHEA (Dehydroepiandrosterone)—A Pleiotropic Steroid. How Can One Steroid Do So Much?" from *Advances in Anti-Aging Medicine*, v. I, ed. by Ronald M. Klatz, New York: Mary Ann Liebert, Inc., Publishers, 1996.

Acknowledgments

WE WOULD LIKE to thank all the researchers in the United States and throughout the world, who so willingly shared information and exchanged ideas, and from whose work we all benefit.

Much thanks to Laurie Bernstein, a terrific editor whose dedication, unique vision, and hard work has made this book a reality. Special thanks to Annie Hughes, a tireless worker who can always be counted on to get the job done, no matter how difficult. We are very grateful to Ted Landry and Gypsy da Silva for going that extra mile. Thanks also to Barbara Lowenstein, Bill's agent, and Richard Curtis, Carol's agent, who have been there for this and all other projects. Also, Eva Gross, Bill's secretary for over twenty years.

In addition, Bill acknowledges the contribution of the Fund for Integrative Biomedical Research (FIBER), a nonprofit foundation that stimulated research in the biology of aging (1980–85). It was organized by Don Yarborough and Senator Alan Cranston, and acted as an interdisciplinary catalyst, an Institute without walls, that saw the debility and dependency of aging as a problem that could be solved. Thanks to FIBER, Bill was able to develop a creative collaboration with Walter Pierpaoli, Norman Applezweig and other scientists who saw aging as a syndrome, a programmed event, and not a random collection of degenerative diseases. Bill also wishes to make special mention of his good friend Mohammed Kalimi, who made Bill's participation in DHEA research possible. Arthur Schwartz acted as a catalyst to focus our attention on DHEA, which led to its dramatic recognition. The late Vernon Riley was the first to show the antistress role of DHEA but did not live to see its elaboration. J. B. Hamilton, Bill's professor of anatomy, first called Bill's attention to the role of reproductive hormones as a factor in aging when Bill was a student. Finally, Bill acknowledges his friend Paul Gallop, whose efforts will move us beyond hormonal replacement to restoration of the fundamental center of the physiology of aging, which begins with the loss of mitochondrial integrity and energy loss, and to Paul Glenn, who has faithfully supported aging research.

To Michael and Josh, whose love and support can be counted on always.
—CC

To our parents and our delightful Family.
—WR

Contents

PART V
The Age-Reversing Superhormone

PART VI
Making the Superhormone Promise Work for You

Foreword

How MANY TIMES have you heard someone make a birthday toast with the wish that the person "live to be 120, and I hope to be around to celebrate with you."

Countless times, no doubt. And countless times you have probably thought of this as nothing more than a good humored toast.

I ask you to reconsider.

In point of fact *we all should aspire to live to be 120!*

Science has actually demonstrated that we humans have the capacity to live twelve decades. The reason that we almost never achieve this full life span is that we have not known how to stop the aging process, which leaves us vulnerable to diseases that rob us of our strength—and ultimately of our full life expectancy.

I am not referring to the process by which we accumulate years and suffer normal wear and tear. That is merely the passage of time. Rather, I am referring to aging for what it really is: a disease process.

As the body ages, there is a breaking down of bodily systems that makes us more susceptible to disease. Disease, in turn, causes the body to age, and the cycle repeats. There is, however, a way to intervene and interrupt this aging → disease → aging cycle. The downward spiral of physical and mental decline that we have come to accept as a natural part of growing older is not our inescapable destiny. This fate is not something that we have to accept. On the contrary, there is nothing natural about growing weaker with each passing year! And the joyous news is that it is no longer necessary.

If you have read *The Melatonin Miracle,* the book that I wrote with Dr. William Regelson and Carol Colman, who have now written *The Superhormone Promise,* you know that one of my foremost goals—and one that I share with Bill and Carol—is to encourage a basic shift in the way we view aging. I want people to recognize that the progressive deterioration that occurs in our adult years and that makes us increasingly vulnerable to disease can be forestalled permanently by treating the underlying disease, which is aging itself. My hope is that the general public and medical professionals will come to understand that the most effective solution to aging, as with any disease, is prevention.

The Melatonin Miracle opened our eyes to the fact that maintaining the strength and function of our body systems is the key to breaking the aging → disease → aging cycle. *The Melatonin Miracle* showed us that, by keeping our body systems in a youthful state, we can prevent the debility and illness that have come to embody the aging process.

The promise of superhormones is that they each have their own unique role in the prevention, as well as in the treatment, of the diseases of aging and the disease we call aging.

I think no one is better qualified to convey this life-affirming message than Bill, a brilliant oncologist, researcher, and teacher, who is largely responsible for bringing anti-aging research to the forefront in the United States. He is also one of the first scientists to recognize and study the power of the hormone dehydroepiandrosterone, or DHEA, which is a major focus of this book. I can think of no better collaborator for him than Carol, who has made an art of translating the most complex scientific and technical information into the most readable and understandable prose.

Candidly, I do not know whether I respect Bill most for the depth and breadth of his knowledge or for his generosity of spirit.

Bill is a medical oncologist who also works in the fields of microbiology and biomedical engineering. As an undergraduate at the University of North Carolina, he became interested in physiology and embryology (the study of life in its earliest stages). After graduating from Downstate Medical College of the State University of New York, he did his post-graduate medical training at the famed Memorial Sloan-Kettering Cancer Research Institute, where he was one of the earliest researchers in the field of cancer chemotherapy and immunotherapy. Bill continued his research at Buffalo's Roswell Park Memorial Institute, the oldest cancer research center in the nation, and he later joined the faculty of the Medical College of Virginia at Virginia Commonwealth University.

Bill has often said that his interest in the biology of aging is a natural outgrowth of his efforts to control cancer because, although cancer can strike anyone at any time, it is primarily a disease of aging. In other words, our risk of getting cancer increases significantly as we age. Many years of research and treating patients led Bill to the conclusion that the way to prevent cancer was to prevent the physical deterioration that occurs in our bodies as we age. If we can remain in the youthful state, we can keep our bodies youthful and strong, and we can make ourselves less vulnerable to cancer and to other diseases as well.

Nearly two decades ago, Bill organized the Fund for Integrative Biomedical Research (FIBER), which he describes as an "institute without walls." FIBER was devoted to encouraging and funding innovative research in the field of aging. Bill's goal was to promote interdisciplinary programs of research and provide seed money to scientists who had novel ideas to pursue, in order to help them get the recognition that they needed in order to secure additional funding from traditional sources. The hope was to foster a spirit of cooperation and partnership among scientists. Especially when funding is scarce, scientists sometimes become secretive and overly protective of their turf, and this serves no one's interests, the public's least of all. FIBER's goal was to buck that trend and encourage a freer exchange of ideas among scientists. I was one of the researchers FIBER brought to the United States in 1979 and 1980. I am particularly indebted to FIBER for that opportunity because not only did it enable me to become fast friends with Bill, but also I met another scientist whom Bill and I both hold in tremendous regard, the late Dr. Vernon Riley, whose innovative work documenting the lethal effects of stress is reported in the chapter on DHEA. Vernon died prematurely, and Bill and I both miss him as both a friend and a colleague.

After spending time with Bill, I was so impressed with his work that I invited him to work with me on the research that eventually led to the discovery of the body's aging clock, the center in the brain that controls the aging process, and revealed to us the role of melatonin, its chemical messenger.

Bill's interest in anti-aging research inspired him twenty years ago to take up the study of DHEA. His instincts about DHEA have now been fully validated. DHEA has been shown to protect against cancer and heart disease, improve memory, enhance mood, and improve sexual function in men. Interestingly, at the time we were working on *The Melatonin Miracle,* Bill told me, with some sadness, that he feared that it would be years before the public would be able to benefit from DHEA in the same way that it would be benefiting from melatonin because DHEA was, at that time, available only by prescription. This is no longer the case, as DHEA has just become available over the counter. I should like to think that this welcome

event is due at least in small part to the heightened interest in anti-
aging research and the power and promise of superhormones that
The Melatonin Miracle inspired.

And thus inspired I close with a toast, secure in the knowledge
that after reading *The Superhormone Promise* you will surely understand that my toast is more than a fond wish, but an attainable goal.

I wish you health and long life, and I expect to join you for your
120th birthday celebration.

WALTER PIERPAOLI, M.D., PH.D.
Interbion Foundation for Basic
    Biomedical Research
Bellinzona, Switzerland
August 1996

Introduction: The Superhormone Revolution

The Antidote to Aging

PICTURE THIS.

It's your thirtieth college reunion. You're having lunch with your former roommate. You recall that at your last reunion he looked worn-out and flabby, dragged himself from event to event, and never stopped complaining about how tired he was. But today he looks better than he's looked in years. His muscles are taut, his posture is perfect, and you'd swear he has more hair on his head and fewer wrinkles on his face. You're picking at iceberg lettuce while he's enjoying a generous portion of pasta and wondering out loud what to have for dessert. You mention that you haven't been able to eat that way in years. If you did, you think to yourself, you'd weigh three hundred pounds. No matter how much you exercise these days, you're still putting on weight and losing muscle tone.

Your roommate tells you that he and his wife have just returned from a romantic week in the Caribbean, scuba diving and water-skiing. You used to do that, but, wow, you think, if you tried to do that today, you'd kill yourself. Listening to him brings home acutely the realization that you can't seem to do a lot of the things you used to do. You can't keep up with the young turks at the office, you don't enjoy playing sports anymore, and as far as romance is concerned . . . well, you've just sort of lost your appetite. Then your roommate tells you that he has signed up to organize the fortieth class reunion, and he asks (between bites of chocolate cream pie) whether you think he should hold the event at a ski chalet in Biarritz or at some out-of-the-way resort in Morocco where folks could go hot-air ballooning over the Sahara. You've been thinking that there's something wrong with this picture, and suddenly you realize precisely what it is: While you've been growing older, your roommate seems inexplicably to be growing younger.

"So I finally asked him," says Jeff Miller, whose name has been changed but whose true story is the basis of this vignette, " 'What's going on here? I watch my diet. I exercise. But I look and feel like hell. What are you doing that I'm not?' "

Then Jeff's college roommate, a biochemist, took out his pen and drew a graph on a paper napkin. He plotted out a series of curved lines that, he said, represented certain hormones, the levels of which fall off as we age. Hormones, he explained, are chemical messengers in the body that tell our cells what to do. Hormones regulate virtually every body function, from the manufacture and organization of thoughts in our brains to the beating of our hearts. Moreover, hormones play a major role in keeping us healthy and youthful.

Then came the kicker. He told me that his doctor had prescribed hormone supplements and that this, he believed, was why he was looking, feeling, and functioning better than he had in years and why he could say with utter confidence that he was going to live to be 120.

As amazing as it all sounded, Jeff saw clearly that whatever it was his roommate was doing, it was working. As he considered it, Jeff realized he had two choices. "I could have gone back to my own doctor, but every time I tried to tell him how I no longer felt like myself and could no longer do the things that I used to enjoy doing, he always replied, 'Well, Jeff old boy, what you are experiencing is perfectly normal for a man your age.' So I decided on the spot to do something different."

Jeff went to his roommate's doctor and asked him to run a blood test to get a reading of his current hormone levels. The test results revealed why Jeff was feeling so worn-out and run-down. As is the case for most people his age, his levels of nearly all the key hormones were low, down to nearly half of what they were when he was in his youthful prime. In other words, Jeff's body had already begun its descent into old age, and like an airplane leaking fuel, it had only one place to go . . . with Jeff along for the ride.

But this doctor was throwing him a parachute, and Jeff grabbed for it. The doctor prescribed a "hormone cocktail," a combination of hormone supplements specifically tailored to meet Jeff's particular needs. The supplements were designed to boost Jeff's hormones back to their youthful levels.

Jeff describes the results of taking these hormone supplements as nothing short of miraculous. "Within six months my weight was under control and body fat was down from 26 percent to 13 percent. I've actually regained my muscle tone, and my skin looks and feels smooth and young. I work hard and exercise three days a week, and I have energy to spare. I feel as though I've been given my life back."

Jeff, grinning, says he and his wife, who also began taking hormone supplements, are now planning a second honeymoon next month. And he tells me with an even bigger grin that he's just signed up to plan his class's fiftieth reunion.

Welcome to the Superhormone Revolution

Jeff's story is typical of what is being reported from tens of thousands of men and women who are part of a revolutionary change in how we practice medicine and, more important, a revolutionary change in how we live and how we age. It is a revolution that started because people are beginning to realize that they no longer have to accept the conventional wisdom that from middle age on their health and their mind and their looks must deteriorate. They no longer have to accept as "normal" that as the years pass, they must grow increasingly sick, grow frail, and grow disabled. The superhormone revolution is the culmination of research efforts over years from some of the most distinguished medical and scientific research centers in the country, from Harvard to Stanford, from Johns Hopkins to the University of Washington. What scientists are discovering (myself included) is how the ebb and flow of these hormones—we call them the *superhormones* to distinguish them from the other hormones that pulse through our body—do the work that determines how, and how rapidly, we age.

The Superhormone Revolution not only has rendered stunning results in leading research laboratories but, even more exciting, has entered another stage and is already in force in thousands of doctors' offices from coast to coast. Knowledgeable, well-trained physicians have come to realize that the traditional approach of simply attempting to treat the individual symptoms of aging as they arise is insufficient. These physicians have rightly concluded that simply advising patients to lower their expectations with every passing year is not practicing "good medicine." These physicians recognize that now, for the first time, science has the tools to extend life while also enhancing the quality of life by preventing and even reversing the ravages of aging. These physicians realize that there is absolutely no reason that we cannot live to be 90, 100, 110, and perhaps even to our potential maximum life span of 120, in strong, healthy bodies.

(Scientists know that attaining the age of 120 is theoretically possible for everyone, because some men and women have done so.) These physicians are truly practicing preventive medicine and are in the process of creating a new paradigm of what aging is all about. These physicians and their patients understand that it is now possible, even as the years pass, for us to "grow young" in bodies that are strong, healthy, and vigorous.

The Melatonin Miracle marked the opening salvo in the Superhormone Revolution. In that groundbreaking book, my good friend and coauthor, Dr. Walter Pierpaoli, and I introduced readers to the radical concept that the downward spiral we had come to accept as part of the normal aging process is neither normal nor inevitable. We explained that by taking supplements of the hormone melatonin we can actually slow down and reverse the aging process.

In *The Superhormone Promise* this story continues with more good news about cutting-edge discoveries in the field of age reversal and how they can change all of our lives. In *The Superhormone Promise* I will tell you not only about new findings concerning the miraculous power of melatonin but also about the other key superhormones that decline as we age and that, like melatonin, need to be replenished in order for us to grow younger, even as we age chronologically.

At the heart of the superhormone story is the discovery of the body's aging clock, a tiny gland called the pineal, located in the brain; it is the mechanism that controls how and when we age. The pineal gland produces the superhormone melatonin, which acts as the orchestra leader of all the other superhormones and also transmits information from the pineal to the rest of the body. At a certain point, usually around age forty-five to fifty, melatonin levels start to significantly decline; this in turn sends a signal to the rest of the superhormones and to the other body systems that we have crossed the threshold, and the aging process begins. Not only has the aging clock sent out the signal to let the body begin to run down, but the clock itself begins to wear down as a result of the diminished melatonin levels. Indeed, the downward spiral that we have come to associate with normal aging is a direct consequence of the breakdown of the body's aging clock. The good news is that we believe it is possible to reset the aging clock and to slow down and even reverse the aging process by restoring our superhormone levels to their youthful peaks.

When we speak of an aging clock, we do not mean a clock that merely passively marks the passage of time. Rather, it is a mechanism that actively regulates how well and how quickly we age by transmitting "timed" messages throughout our bodies, triggering specific changes at key developmental moments throughout our lives. For example, between the ages of ten and fourteen, the aging clock strikes puberty, at which time a signal is transmitted from the pineal gland via melatonin that tells our bodies it is time to start pumping the superhormones that control our growth and sexual development. During our young adult years, the clock ticks on mightily, signaling to virtually every cell in our body the message that we are young, strong, and in our physical prime. Then when we reach our forties or early fifties, for most of us the aging clock strikes midlife, at which time the clock itself begins to run down. As a result, our melatonin levels begin to decline, which signals the rest of the body that it is time to begin the body's descent into "old age." In other words, a signal is sent out that we are past our prime, and the way this signal is carried throughout our body is through the decline in the production of superhormones. As a result of this signal, we begin to wind down. We become ever more vulnerable to the diseases of aging—or, perhaps more accurately, to the disease of aging. We now have the tools and the knowledge to change all that.

But to understand the science of the Superhormone Revolution, you first need to understand the reason that Mother Nature would have us age in the first place—or why our aging clocks have been programmed to run down. From nature's point of view, all creatures on earth, from the simplest one-celled organisms to human beings, have one job: to reproduce. In order for any species to survive, it has to pass on its genetic material to its young. In order to reproduce, our bodies need to be healthy and strong, not merely for a matter of months, in order to conceive and to carry our progeny to term, but for many years thereafter, in order to care for and ensure the survival of our offspring.

When those years have passed and we have finished our reproductive and nurturing tasks, we become, in Mother Nature's eyes, expendable.

Mother Nature doesn't care that we may want to nurture our grandchildren. Mother Nature doesn't care that we may want to start a new career or enjoy our retirement. Mother Nature doesn't care that we want to travel or perfect our golf swing or do volunteer work or write novels or do all the things that we postponed doing in order to earn a living and raise and care for our children. As far as Mother Nature is concerned, once we are no longer capable of—or necessary for—the propagation of the species, there is no reason to keep us fit and strong.

Of course, we humans have been blessed with extraordinary brains, and our brains have enabled us to overcome many of life's challenges. So while less intelligent species may have no choice but to "roll over" and let nature call the shots, we humans, fortunately, have other ideas.

Nature's Blueprint

Since the earliest days of recorded history, man has been looking for the fountain of youth, the elixir that would erase the ravages of time and stop the aging process. The irony is that all along the answer was inside us. As you will see, nature has provided each of us with our own personal blueprint for age reversal, and it is written in our hormones—to be exact, our superhormones.

Superhormones control virtually all our bodily functions, including our reproductive and immune systems and our metabolism. At any moment in time there are scores of hormones coursing through our bloodstream. Most of these hormones have a single task to perform. However, I have identified the eight superhormones that have far more broad-ranging and profound effects on many different body systems. The superhormones actually determine how we age by controlling our overall physical and mental health. Superhormones are what I call the true *biomarkers* of aging; that is, they are a true reflection of the aging process itself. As the levels of these superhormones decline, so do we, physically and mentally. The loss of these precious superhormones saps us of our energy and vitality, and shaves decades off our lives. By restoring these superhormones to their youthful levels, it is possible to restore our youthful zeal and energy, and to strengthen and bolster both our bodies and our minds.

In addition to melatonin, the names of some of the other superhormones may already be familiar to you. These include *estrogen, progesterone,* and *testosterone.* You may be surprised to find these familiar hormones on the list of superhormones. Don't be. Although we have been aware of the existence of these hormones for decades, we remained completely in the dark about the most important role they play within our bodies. Only now do we know that these are superhormones, and are aware of their profound influence on our lives. You may not yet have heard about some of the superhormones, such as *dehydroepiandrosterone* (DHEA for short), *pregnenolone, human growth hormone,* and *thyroid hormone*. These new kids on the block, the superhormones that have recently attracted the attention of medical researchers because of their remarkable attributes, may not be well known by the general public. I will share the latest findings on all these superhormones with you, and I can assure you that you will soon understand why they are causing such excitement in the scientific community.

Youth Equals Resilience

To help you understand what happens to us when levels of superhormones decline, I want you to do an exercise. Think about what your body was like when you were in your twenties or thirties. Chances are you were in the physical prime of your life. Your heart was strong. Your immune system was efficient. Your brain was sharp. Your muscles were firm. You were at your sexual peak. The ravages of disease were most likely not a concern for you during those years. Why? Because such degenerative diseases as heart disease, cancer, and arthritis do not generally strike in youth; they are the diseases of aging. The simple fact is, we can resist disease far better in our youth when our bodies are in their prime. It is no mere coincidence that when we are in the so-called prime of our lives, our levels of these superhormones are at their adult peaks. In the subsequent years, their levels gradually decline. By the time we reach our forties and fifties, the effect of that decline becomes palpable for the first time. It is apparent in slight changes in how we look and how we feel. Despite our best efforts to exercise and eat well, we get fatter and flabbier; our sex drive declines; and we notice that we tire more easily and are more vulnerable to disease. In sum, our bodies and our brains begin the decline that we have learned to accept as normal aging.

To me, what is so striking about the aging process is that the same challenges we can defeat so easily in our twenties and thirties and even our forties become increasingly difficult in our later years. Think about it. Throughout our lives we are bombarded with "stressors" that require a quick reaction on the part of our different body systems. When I use the word "stressor," I am referring not only to emotional stress, such as a tension-filled day at work, but also the constant environmental challenges that confront us daily and to which we must marshal a response. For example, when we are exposed to a virus or bacteria or to a cancer-causing agent, as we are daily, our immune systems must mount an immediate attack to ward off the invader before it can cause illness. In addition to these challenges, we are also faced daily with routine physical challenges; for example, when we have to run quickly to catch a bus or train, our hearts must pump blood faster so that we have extra oxygen to energize our cells. When we are confronted with a challenging mental task, we need our brains to work rapidly and efficiently so that we can solve the problem. When we are injured, we need the cells of our bodies to repair themselves quickly so that we can begin to heal. What I have described are the kinds of occurrences or "stressors" that confront us each and every day of our lives.

When we are young and our superhormones are at their youthful peaks, our bodies have the resilience to withstand the continual challenges of everyday living. We bounce back quickly from each of these daily stressors, renewed and ready to face the next. As we age, however, these hits become harder to absorb, and the challenges become more difficult to withstand. The stressors that we could easily have handled when our bodies were at their youthful peak begin to wear us down and take their toll. When the aging clock begins to wear out, the organ systems that we rely on—our hearts, our immune system, in some cases even our brains—also begin to wear out, leaving us more vulnerable to the stressors that used to pose no threat. In a very real sense, we lose the ability we had in youth to rise to the challenges and to bounce back from them. It is a loss of resilience that defines us as old.

We believe that the aging process—the loss of youthful resilience —is not a normal life event but a disease in and of itself. Very simply, it is caused by the decline in our superhormones. Ordinarily, when you think of disease, you think of isolated ailments such as cancer or heart disease or arthritis, each caused by a separate entity. I have worked as a clinical oncologist for more than thirty years, and I, too, used to think of diseases as separate and unrelated occurrences. Yet, through my work as a cancer researcher, I eventually became aware of the fact that in many cases what had originally appeared to be separate diseases actually had a common origin. These isolated diseases were actually mere symptoms of an underlying disease, and that "disease" is the aging process itself.

Let me explain what I mean. As a cancer researcher I have tested many new drugs over the years. One common technique that I would use involved implanting a cancerous tumor in an animal and then administering a new drug to see how well the animal responded. I knew better than to implant a tumor into a young animal because I knew from experience that the young animal's immune system would be strong enough to resist the tumor with or without the drug I was testing, and the animal would remain cancer free. If I implanted the same tumor into an old animal, however, it would quickly succumb to the disease. As I tell you this, you are probably thinking, "Aha! Why is the young animal protected from cancer, and why does the old animal so easily and predictably fall prey? Someone ought to research this!" Well, this question may seem obvious now, but back when I was doing my early work, no one (myself included) thought to ask it. Why? I think we overlooked it because we were all so convinced that the cure for cancer would be in the form of a "magic bullet" that one of us would develop in our laboratories. Thus, it never even dawned on us that Mother Nature might have already provided us with the answer. After decades of looking for the cure for cancer and never finding it, I realized that I was focusing on the wrong end of the problem. The internal environment of the young animals enabled them to fight off a stressor (in this case cancer) that was defeating the old animal. It finally occurred to me that to learn how to defeat cancer we would have to learn why young animals are resistant to the disease and why old animals are prone to succumb to it. It struck me that the answer to cancer, and to all the other diseases that had become synonymous with normal aging, was to cure the underlying condition that allows disease to take hold in the first place. The answer had in fact been staring us in the face all along. The underlying condition that makes us susceptible to cancer and other degenerative diseases is a systematic breakdown in the workings of our body systems—and particularly the immune system—and the breakdown is part and parcel of the process we call aging. Yet what we consider normal aging is itself the underlying disease that opens us up to a host of ravages that leave us increasingly debilitated. This revelation sparked my interest in the aging process itself and eventually in the role that the superhormones play in reversing it.

As will be explained in *The Superhormone Promise,* by restoring these superhormones to more youthful levels, we can eliminate and in some cases reverse many of the symptoms that we have come to associate with old age. We can regain the youthful resilience that enables us to cope gracefully with the stressors that challenge us every day.

I want to make it clear that I am not suggesting that with superhormones we can stay permanently at age nineteen, twenty-nine, or even thirty-nine. The years will still pass. The difference is that with superhormones we can stop the precipitous decline that occurs after midlife. Simply put, this means that the transition from our fifties to our sixties and seventies, and even from our eighties to our nineties and one hundreds can be as uneventful as the transition from our twenties to our thirties and forties. There will be no sudden falling off in our physical or mental health; we will stay resilient.

Nor am I suggesting that you pump your body full of chemicals that are unnatural or unnecessary. Our aim is to simply replenish the hormones that already occur naturally in your body and boost them back up to the appropriate, medically sound levels necessary to maintain youthful health and vigor.

Each of the superhormones has its own unique role in the body, but the secret to their life-affirming and age-reversing capacity is the way they work together, producing a synergistic effect. The underlying principle of my program is not to boost any single superhormone to an artificially high level but rather restore the youthful balance among key superhormones so that they continue to work together as well and as effectively as they do when we are younger. *When taken in combinations tailored to your particular needs, the superhormones are a juggernaut against the aging process.* Which superhormones you need to replenish depends on your blood levels as well as how you feel. That is why the key to *the superhormone promise* is an individualized cocktail; it's tailored to each person's particular needs. Not only will individuals vary, but each person's needs will vary over time so that adjustments to the superhormone cocktail will have to be made periodically.

This book will explain how to make the superhormone revolution work for you, and it will also examine each of the eight superhormones and how they work together to stop and reverse the aging process. But first, here is a brief overview of the eight superhormones.

DHEA   I consider DHEA the superstar of the superhormones. It not only works its wonders inside the body by rejuvenating virtually every organ system, but it actually makes you look, feel, and think better. At one time DHEA was difficult to obtain because it was sold by prescription only and was stocked only by a handful of pharmacies. Yet now, for the first time, it is sold over the counter at pharmacies and health food stores. You will notice the chapter on DHEA is extensive, and the reason is that there is so much to say about this remarkable hormone. Five years ago I edited a scholarly book on DHEA for the scientific community, and one of the reasons I have written *The Superhormone Promise* is to share some of this exciting news with the general public as well. I have spent more than twenty years researching DHEA and prescribing it to patients; and for the last ten years I have been taking it myself along with melatonin. My wife, Sylvia, has taken it for nearly eighteen years. From my own personal experience with DHEA I can attest that the benefits can be felt almost immediately. It restores energy, improves mood, increases sex drive, enhances memory, relieves stress, reduces body fat, and even makes your skin softer and your hair shinier. It is also a potent cancer fighter and has some amazing strengthening effects on the immune system. I think that just about every adult age forty-five or older can benefit from taking DHEA.

Pregnenolone This is the smart superhormone that enhances your brain function. Chances are you've never heard of this superhormone, but back in the 1940s, pregnenolone was given to factory workers to enhance their performance on the job. More recent studies show this superhormone has a positive effect on learning and concentration.

Testosterone This is the superhormone for sex and strength, controlling sex drive in both men and women. My prediction is that testosterone for midlife men will soon be as common as estrogen is for women. About one-third of all men will experience a significant midlife decline in testosterone that can affect their physical and emotional health. Studies have shown that restoring testosterone to youthful levels combats depression, enhances sex drive, preserves muscle strength, and protects against heart disease, the number one killer of middle-aged men. Although testosterone is known as the male sex hormone, testosterone is definitely not for men only. Women also produce testosterone, and they experience a dramatic decline in levels of this hormone after menopause, which also can result in depression and loss of sex drive. A tiny amount of testosterone included in hormone cocktails for women can make a huge difference in how a woman looks, loves, and lives.

Estrogen I consider estrogen in some ways the "mother" of the superhormone revolution because it has been used longer than any of the other superhormones, and in a very real sense it served as the original model for what we now see taking shape in the form of the superhormone revolution. For more than thirty years women have been taking estrogen once they reach menopause, so that today some 10 million women use estrogen, and it is the most widely prescribed drug in the United States. Since the early days of estrogen replacement therapy, we have learned a great deal about this superhormone. We have discovered that estrogen is far more than a cure for hot flashes; it is a superhormone with amazing anti-aging powers. Estrogen can have a profound effect on both a woman's body and mind. Estrogen makes women smarter and sharper, and protects against Alzheimer's disease. It has also been shown to significantly reduce the risk of heart disease in women. Estrogen is a potent antioxidant and can prevent osteoporosis and colon cancer. In the chapter on estrogen, I will also be telling you about the availability of new "smart" forms of estrogen that may actually protect against cancer.

Progesterone This is the "feel-good" superhormone for women. Progesterone is a natural mood elevator; it is the superhormone that is produced in very high quantities during pregnancy to enhance a woman's sense of well-being and is now being included by more and more women in their estrogen therapy. Natural progesterone creams are sold over the counter in health food stores and pharmacies, and natural progesterone capsules are available by prescription to treat menopausal symptoms and other health problems that arise during midlife. In women, progesterone is also used in conjunction with estrogen to prevent uterine cancer and bone loss. Some studies suggest that natural progesterone may offer the benefits of estrogen without the remote cancer risks sometimes associated with conventional estrogen.

Thyroid hormone This is the energizing superhormone, providing energy to virtually every part of the body that is essential for maintaining the "youthful state." Like the other superhormones, thyroid levels decline dramatically with age, and at least one out of every ten women and one out of every twenty men past age fifty has signs of thyroid deficiency. Indeed, many of the symptoms that we have come to associate with normal aging, such as poor immune function, sluggishness, and the inability to maintain body heat, are actually caused by a deficiency of thyroid hormone.

Human growth hormone   Some of the most promising research surfacing is with human growth hormone, the "restorative" superhormone that makes children grow. In adults, this superhormone builds up what time has broken down. Human growth hormone not only makes people feel younger, but it also makes them look younger. It strengthens bone and muscle, and reduces body fat. Growth hormone may prove to be the ultimate "fixer" for the breakdown in organ systems that occurs once the disease of aging takes hold of the body. Growth hormone has been used successfully to treat kidney failure, and it may forestall the need for dialysis in some patients. Recently, researchers found that growth hormone can reverse cardiomyopathy, a severe and potentially fatal heart condition. At present, one drawback of human growth hormone is the cost; it is very expensive. New drugs are currently being tested, however, that are designed to stimulate the body's own production of human growth hormone; these drugs are appropriately called *growth-hormone-releasing factors*. Researchers predict that by the year 2005, everyone over the age of fifty will be taking a pill to stimulate the body's own production of growth hormone.

Melatonin   The story of the melatonin miracle continues with some exciting new chapters. The superhormone that started the revolution not only extends life and reverses aging but also strengthens the immune system, increases our resistance to cancer and other diseases, is a safe, nonaddictive sleep aid, lowers cholesterol, relieves stress, and cures jet lag. The latest studies suggest that melatonin can restore youthful patterns of sex hormones in older animals, and they also confirm that it is a potent antioxidant.

What is especially important and exciting about superhormones is that they can be tailored to the individual: Each superhormone cocktail can be *targeted* or customized to suit your body. *Your* individual hormone cocktail should be designed to replace what *you* are lacking, and the dose should be based on whatever it takes to restore *your* youthful function. Not every superhormone is for every body at all times. Superhormone levels vary widely from person to person, and while some of us may experience a dramatic falloff in one key hormone, others may not and therefore do not need to replace it.

It's also important to keep in mind that from time to time our levels of hormones may change, and so will our needs. For example, a woman who is forty-five may require melatonin and DHEA, but will not need to include estrogen or progesterone in her hormone cocktail until she reaches menopause. Even then she may find, as some women do, that DHEA makes it unnecessary to use estrogen. A fifty-year-old man who is taking DHEA may not require testosterone, because in men DHEA produces many of the same benefits as testosterone. Later in this book I will explain how to obtain the right superhormone prescription for your particular needs.

I am not advocating the practice of medicine by number. Test results alone do not determine treatment; how a patient feels is of equal importance and may reveal important information not indicated by test results. For example, some men with borderline low testosterone levels may be "normal" according to the textbook but may be experiencing symptoms that point to a testosterone deficiency. Despite what the numbers say, you and your doctor need to discuss your physical and emotional state and determine from there your personal superhormone ℞. You and your doctor also need to review the specific effects of each hormone so that you can choose the program that will be of greatest benefit to you.

Although four of the superhormones can be purchased over the counter, I strongly recommend working with your doctor to determine the superhormone prescription for several important reasons. For one thing, anyone who takes any medication on a regular basis, whether it is aspirin, melatonin, or DHEA, should be monitored. With all medications, from aspirin to antacid, you want to keep track of how your body is responding to the medication. This is particularly important if you are already taking medication for a chronic condition. Some superhormones may interact with medication, and your physician needs to consider this when the two of you design your personal ℞. For example, melatonin often succeeds in lowering high blood pressure, and many individuals are therefore able to cut back on their blood pressure medicine. In some cases, people taking DHEA will find that they no longer need to take cholesterol-lowering medications, or if they are diabetic, their insulin needs may change. Both you and your physician need to be aware of these or any other changes occurring in your body that may require changing the dose of your other medications or altering your hormone regimen.

I also recommend that you try to work with the doctor you already have, who knows you, and with whom you presumably have a good rapport. I understand that the concept of targeted superhormones is new and that many doctors may still be unaware of its benefits. For that reason I am also including a detailed bibliography for physicians (or lay people) who want to learn more about this fascinating field. If your physician seems resistant to learning about superhormones or is not interested in working with you, you should consult the section of this book called "Resources" for a directory of organizations that will help you find a doctor in your area.

I believe that the superhormone revolution is the most exciting medical breakthrough to come about in decades, and the implications of this revolution are enormous. For the first time we no longer have to be helpless and hapless victims as the aging process leaves us vulnerable to illness and debility. For the first time we have the knowledge and the power to "stop the clock" and stop and reverse the downward spiral. For the first time, with superhormones, we can prevent the diseases of aging from taking hold of our bodies. The discovery of superhormones does not mean, however, that we can forget about the other health routines we follow to take care of ourselves. As powerful as superhormones are at giving us a second chance at youthful fitness and health, we cannot abuse our bodies, smoke, eat a bad diet, use harmful drugs, abuse alcohol, or practice unsafe sex and expect any amount of medication to save us. Superhormones can effect miraculous results, *but we need to work with them, not against them.* The food we eat, our lifestyles, and our health habits can make a profound difference in helping to maintain youthful superhormone levels and in making our hormone cocktail work more effectively at keeping us at our youthful prime no matter what our age.

There will no doubt be naysayers, scientists and lay people alike, who will protest that intervening in the aging process is somehow unnatural and that we should leave well enough alone and let nature take its course. Nor would it be surprising if critics resorted to that tired old argument. Since the dawn of modern medicine, innovators have been told to let nature take its course, and the history of medicine is replete with dramatic examples of this. As hard as it is to believe it today, it is a historical fact that when anesthesia was first introduced in the nineteenth century, there was a great outcry against its use, and physicians were among its most vocal opponents. These people believed that man was fated to suffer pain, and they were positively scandalized at the thought of eliminating the agony of surgery. Until the discovery of antibiotics and vaccines, it was commonly believed that the only way to deal with infection was to "let nature take its course." We now know that this is certainly not true, and that anesthesia, antibiotics, and vaccines have saved millions of lives. Standing by to let nature take its course often results in suffering and premature death. I do not consider this natural.

The discovery of anesthesia, vaccines, and antibiotics have not only proved to be true lifesavers but have changed our expectations about how medicine should be practiced. For example, it would be unthinkable today for a patient to undergo a painful surgical procedure without the benefit of anesthesia. Parents would find it equally unacceptable to have their child treated by a pediatrician who did not stock vaccines and administer them at the appropriate times. Nor would any physician worth his salt send a patient home with bacterial pneumonia without prescribing a regimen of antibiotics. In the same way that these medical breakthroughs affected the practice of medicine, I believe the superhormone revolution will similarly change our expectations about the way physicians should treat us once we reach middle age.

Let me give you a vivid example of what I mean and how I believe the superhormone revolution will impact the way that medicine is normally practiced. If a doctor today were to discover that one of his young patients had an elevated level of blood sugar, a condition that can cause diabetes and lead to heart disease, he would undoubtedly prescribe immediate treatment. At the very least, the young patient would probably be placed on a diet, given medication, and instructed to exercise regularly. In contrast, if a sixty- or seventy-year-old patient had exactly the same blood sugar levels, his physician would more than likely shrug it off as nothing more than a sign of age, and the older patient would be sent home empty-handed. Frankly, I think that this attitude is archaic, as archaic as a physician not prescribing an antibiotic to treat a serious infection, or using anesthesia to eliminate the pain of surgery. It should not matter how old a patient is; if high blood sugar levels are unhealthy for a twenty-year-old, they are certainly more dangerous for an older person who is at even greater risk of developing serious diseases that can be caused by this condition. Thanks to the superhormone revolution, it will be simply unacceptable for a doctor to assume that once a patient has reached a certain chronological age, it is somehow acceptable for that patient's body systems to go out of whack, and to assume that what is abnormal in younger patients is somehow "normal" in older patients. Because we can now prevent the disease and the disability associated with aging, it will be unthinkable for a physician to tell a patient that he or she needs to accept the ravages of degenerative diseases as "normal."

Our new vision of life in our upper decades will feature healthy, strong, active men and women who are still in their prime. Patients will demand that their doctors use the tools that are now available to rewind the aging clock and restore the body back to its youthful peak.

Some will argue that we should not try to interfere with the aging process; instead, we should be happy to grow old gracefully. By gracefully they mean that we should lie down and accept our fate and take it on the chin, that we should be willing to grow weak and frail, lose our mental capacity, and ultimately become dependent on others. Let me tell you that there is nothing graceful about growing old gracefully. I am seventy-one years old and look and feel as if I am twenty years younger. If I was not practicing what I preach, if I were not taking superhormones, I could not do what I do. I would not be able to teach and practice medicine on a full-time basis, write, lecture, and find the time and energy to enjoy myself and my six beautiful grandchildren. To me it is quite natural to desire to live a long, full life, feeling and looking young and strong. To my mind it is quite natural to desire to live longer so that I can continue to make a positive contribution to this world.

Based on my research in the field over the last twenty years, it is my belief that it is possible for people to live well past 100 and eventually achieve the maximum life span of 120. I am not talking about lives confined to wheelchairs or nursing homes. I am talking about living as strong, healthy, productive citizens inhabiting well-functioning bodies capped by well-functioning minds.

The Superhormone Revolution is important not only for the quality of our individual survival but for the very survival of our nation. Think about it. The fastest-growing segment of the U.S. population consists of men and women ages seventy-five and over. By the year 2030, 52 million Americans will be over the age of seventy. We are already buckling under the cost of caring for the old and infirm. In fact, a recent government study concluded that if the present trend continued, the medicare trust fund would bust by the time the baby boomers began cashing in their benefits. We as a nation cannot afford indefinitely to foot the bill for a growing debilitated and dependent population, nor can we as a nation turn our backs on people who need help. We must do more to provide for a youthful quality of survival, and that is why it is imperative that the medical profession change its focus from treating the diseases of aging to treating what I believe is the ultimate disease, aging itself. We must do more to enable people to live out their longer lives in health and vitality, and that is why the superhormone revolution is becoming ever more critical.

My reason for writing this book is first and foremost to inform you about the superhormone revolution, but I also want to stimulate interest in the scientific research community. Here is the reason: Hormones are natural substances and, with few exceptions, cannot be patented. As a result, there is little incentive for drug companies to fund research on hormones that are already widely available and inexpensive. It costs hundreds of millions of dollars to bring a new drug to market through the standard FDA-approval route, so it is hard to blame the pharmaceutical companies for their unwillingness to invest in a drug from which they will probably not be able to recoup their investment. I am hoping that consumer demand will force the government to fund some of the studies that the drug companies will not. For those who wonder why I am writing this book now and why I don't wait until all the studies are done and all the results are in and the FDA has approved each and every hormone for each and every use, here is my answer: I can't afford to wait that long, and neither can most of you. It will be decades before all these events occur, if indeed they ever do. I can't afford to wait until the middle of the twenty-first century for the slow-moving bureaucracy to give the official nod to what is already working to reverse aging by restoring superhormones to their youthful peaks. If I had followed this philosophy, I would not be where I am now. I would not have the same strength and vigor, and could not possibly maintain my active life. I feel an obligation to share the superhormone story with you, and to give you and your doctor the information you need to begin your own age reversal program.

Moreover, I personally feel that it is unfair for scientists and researchers to keep the superhormone revolution to themselves and deny the public this lifesaving information. As mentioned earlier, I have been taking DHEA and melatonin for years. Many other researchers in the field have also been self-prescribing their own hormone cocktails. It seems to me that you, the public, have a right to information so that you can make an informed choice about superhormones. It would be wrong, in my opinion, to withhold information that can not only extend life but can enhance the quality of your life.

Finally, I believe that this book is relevant for people of all ages. Whether you are age forty or eighty, you can benefit from superhormones, although naturally the benefits will be felt differently at different ages. If you are in your thirties, the time is ripe to begin thinking and gathering information about your hormones, learning about the options, and planning ahead. If you are between the ages of forty and forty-five, it's time to have your hormone levels tested, to develop a baseline, and to begin charting your program.

Most of all, it is my hope that this book will forever change your view of the aging process and your expectations of what life will be like for you and the people you love in the decades to come. The future has never been brighter, and it is this message of hope that I want to leave you with before you continue with the rest of this book and the rest of your lives. We are truly blessed in that for the first time in history we will be able to live out our days in strength and vitality, unhampered by sickness and debility. With superhormones we have the know-how and the ability to live out our lives the way we want, on our terms.

A Note to Readers

By now, many of you are probably eager to begin learning about how you and your doctor can design your own personal superhormone program. You also undoubtedly have a lot of questions. In the chapters to come, I'll be answering your questions about each of these hormones, but first, here is some background information that is important to have before you read further.

As alluded to earlier, half of the superhormones are currently available over the counter at pharmacies, health food stores, and through mail order. They are melatonin, DHEA, natural progesterone, and pregnenolone.

Melatonin This is sold in various strengths in a variety of forms including tablets, capsules, and a sublingual form that dissolves under the tongue.

DHEA Sold until recently only by prescription, DHEA is now available in capsules and tablets without a prescription in 25 to 50 mg. (milligram) strength and can be purchased at pharmacies, health food stores, and by mail order. Information on how to obtain DHEA from these various sources is given in the Resource section.

Natural progesterone   Available over the counter at pharmacies and health food stores are natural progesterone creams (under 3 percent strength).

Pregnenolone   This hormone has recently become available over the counter and is sold in tablets and capsules of 10 to 50 mg.

DHEA, natural progesterone, and pregnenolone are available in stronger strengths only by prescription.

The remaining superhormones (estrogen, testosterone, thyroid, and human growth hormone) are available by prescription.

Some of the superhormones are marketed under brand names by major pharmaceutical companies and are sent to pharmacists in pre-measured, prepackaged doses. For example, Premarin, the most commonly used estrogen in the United States, is typically sold in tablets of .625 mg. strength, and Provera, the most commonly used synthetic progesterone, is sold in tablets of 2.5 mg. or 5 mg. strength.

Even though DHEA and pregnenolone are now available over the counter, they are also still produced by major pharmaceutical houses and sent in bulk to pharmacies in powdered form. The pharmacists then formulate or "compound" them into capsules, creams, gels, tablets, or even suppositories in various dosages, according to the physician's prescription.

The superhormones can be divided into two categories: natural and synthetic. The term "natural hormone" is actually a misnomer because all hormones sold today are chemically processed in one way or another. What is meant by the term "natural" actually refers to the chemical structure of the hormone. The so-called natural hormones are believed to be closer in chemical structure to the hormones produced by the body than the so-called synthetic hormones. For example, many physicians are now prescribing natural estrogen (estradiol or estriol), which is derived from soy and believed to be in a form that is closer to the estrogen produced in the human body than is Premarin. The use of natural versus synthetic hormones is one of the hottest issues in medicine today and will be discussed at greater length later in this book.

Not every pharmacist has the training or the tools to custom-fill prescriptions, and you may have to check with several in your area before you find a "compounding pharmacist." There are about fifteen hundred compounding pharmacists in the United States. Compounding pharmacies also exist that will fill a prescription by mail. These include the Woman's International Pharmacy in Sun City, Arizona; the Bajamar Women's Health Care Pharmacy in St. Louis, Missouri; and the Medical Center Pharmacy in Fairfax, Virginia. All of these compounding pharmacies fill thousands of prescriptions submitted to them from all over the United States.

For more information on how to find a doctor in your area who uses superhormones or how to buy superhormones, please consult the Resource section at the end of the book.

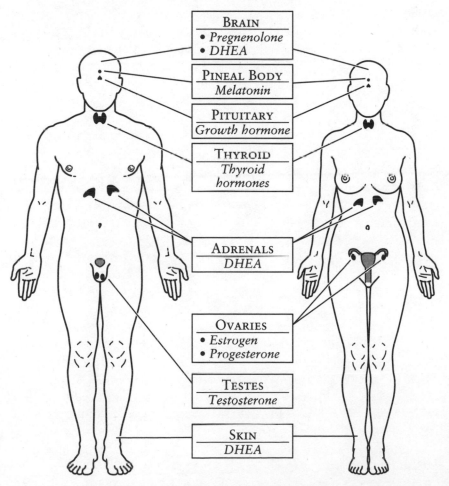

A map of the superhormones and where they are made

PART I

Two Superhormones Capturing the Spotlight

Introduction: DHEA and Pregnenolone

THIS SECTION OF *The Superhormone Promise* is devoted to DHEA and pregnenolone, two superhormones that are now attracting a great deal of attention from the medical/scientific community as well as the general public.

For the past decade, scientists (myself among them) have been studying the promise of DHEA as an anti-aging agent, and now that promise is being realized on a spectacular scale. The dramatic discoveries about DHEA that have been made in laboratories throughout the world have focused attention on it just as it now becomes available over the counter for the first time.

A by-product of our work on DHEA has been the discovery—or I should say "rediscovery"—of the power of another superhormone that is closely related and similar to DHEA. This cousin hormone is called pregnenolone, and it, too, has just become available over the counter. I say rediscover because, as you will see, pregnenolone was used as far back as fifty years ago to improve memory and learning skills, and as a treatment for arthritis. Inspired by the promise of DHEA, researchers are now showing renewed interest in pregnenolone, and the results of early studies are nothing short of amazing. Although as of this writing we do not have the comprehensive data and research about pregnenolone as we do about DHEA, its potential is vast as will become evident to you even from the preliminary research that we do have.

CHAPTER 1

DHEA

SUPERSTAR OF THE SUPERIIORMONES

Energizes
Enhances libido
Restores memory
Rejuvenates the immune system
Tames stress
Fights cancer
Prevents heart disease
Reduces body fat
Therapy for menopause
Helps erase fine wrinkles
Helps dry eye
New hope for lupus sufferers
Heals burns

There are times when I get these momentary flashes of energy and well-being that are reminiscent of when I was in my late teens and early twenties. I just don't remember experiencing that in a very, very long time. I haven't felt this way in decades.

—MONICA R., 44, lawyer, taking
DHEA for three months

I began to notice that I was slowing down. I couldn't do what I used to. I teach second grade, and even after spending the day with twenty very active seven-year-olds, I used to be able to have an active social life after work. At night I would think nothing of going to the movies with friends or going out dancing. But later, I could barely drag myself out of bed in the morning, and it was tough making it through the day. I desperately wanted to feel like I did before. My doctor checked my DHEA level and found that it was very low, so he recommended that I start taking DHEA. Within a month I was back to normal, I had my stamina back. I had enough energy to do what I wanted. I noticed other positive things happening to me. I look better. My skin is softer, and my hair is shinier. I haven't felt or looked this good in years.

—KAREN B., 49, taking DHEA for
one year

I run three miles in the morning, and I go to the gym on my way home from work at least three times a week. I'm still working full-time as a lawyer. I take DHEA and melatonin every day. Most seventy-five-year-olds are walking around stooped over, they've slowed down. I'm really enjoying life. People want to know my secret.

—JOHN G., 75, taking DHEA for six
years

If you had asked me last year what my old age was going to be like, I would have said that by eighty I'd probably be in a nursing home, because that's what happens to most of the people in my family. But if you were to ask me the same question today, I would give you quite a different answer. I'm still going to be banging out my inventions. I'm starting to write music. I'm planning for two to three careers down the road. I expect to be very active in my eighties and nineties, so why not in my hundreds? I've got kids and grandkids. I'm pretty sure that I'll be around for my great-grandkids.

—STEVEN R., 72, taking DHEA for
one year

ASTONISHING AS THESE reports may sound, they are similar to the reports that other doctors and I who have been prescribing DHEA to their patients hear regularly. Patients who are taking DHEA supplements to restore them to youthful levels report that they feel more energetic, generally healthier, and also sexier than they had since youth. They feel this way on the outside, because, inside their bodies, DHEA is actually correcting and reversing much of the deterioration to their organs and body systems—the "wear and tear"—that has been occurring since they reached middle age.

I call DHEA the "superstar" of the superhormones because of its extraordinary effect on both the body and the mind. Within the past decade, researchers (myself included) have discovered some amazing things about this superhormone that not only makes people feel terrific but does some pretty terrific things to virtually every important body system. DHEA rejuvenates the immune system, improves brain function, relieves stress, and may prove to be the most potent anti-cancer drug of all time. What is even more exciting is the fact that DHEA is now being sold over the counter, making this safe and effective superhormone readily available to all.

What is DHEA? DHEA is short for *Dehydroepiandrosterone*. Like estrogen and testosterone, DHEA is a steroid, a type of hormone distinguished from others by its unique chemical structure. Although this may bring to mind the synthetic steroids that you associate with athletes who are trying to "pump muscle," the steroids that are naturally made by our bodies are quite different. DHEA is produced by the adrenal glands (located on the kidneys) as well as by the brain and the skin, and is the most abundant steroid in the human body. In comparison with other hormones, we produce vast quantities of DHEA, but, ironically, until the past decade or so, DHEA was considered a "junk" hormone of little importance. Scientists simply did not know what to make of DHEA since it does not behave like other hormones.

French chemist Etienne-Emile Baulieu is credited with being the first researcher to isolate DHEA from the other steroids. Dr. Baulieu showed that DHEA is made from another superhormone, pregnenolone, and that DHEA is, in turn, converted into estrogen and testosterone in both men and women. Women make more estrogen, and men make more testosterone. What confounded scientists, however, was that unlike estrogen and testosterone, DHEA didn't appear to have any particular job to do in the body. Scientists knew that estrogen regulated the ovaries and that testosterone affected the testes. Scientists also knew that a woman deficient in estrogen, or a man deficient in testosterone, would show specific symptoms; for example, a woman low on estrogen might experience menstrual irregularities, and a man short on testosterone might show signs of decreased sex drive or muscle weakness. But as far as scientists could tell, the body did not appear to respond in any specific way to rising or falling levels of DHEA. Therefore, many scientists concluded that DHEA was merely a precursor to the other hormones, that is, the stuff from which the others were made.

There were, however, other scientists (I among them) who simply could not accept the fact that our bodies would produce in such vast quantities a substance that was of no particular value. We suspected that nature had a purpose for this hormone even if we had not yet been able to figure out what that purpose was. One of those scientists was Dr. Norman Orentreich, the world-renowned dermatologist who is perhaps best known for inventing the hair transplant but who also made a major contribution to our understanding of DHEA. In 1984, Dr. Orentreich was among the first to prove that levels of DHEA drop steadily as we age, suggesting that DHEA may be a "biomarker," or measure, of the aging process itself. Dr. Orentreich's research team showed that between the ages of twenty-five and thirty, our DHEA levels peak, and after that they begin to fall at a rate of about 2 percent per year. He showed us that the rise and fall of our DHEA levels follows a specific pattern. DHEA is found in large amounts in the developing human fetus and it acts on the mother's cervix right before labor to soften the cervix for delivery. (In Japan, doctors give DHEA to mothers-to-be prior to labor to ease delivery.)

The previous chapter referred to an aging clock that not only tracks the passage of time but also disseminates information throughout the body that controls the ebb and flow of all the super-hormones. If you look at the rise and fall of DHEA throughout our lifetimes, you can see dramatic evidence of the aging clock in action. As newborns, we have an extremely high level of DHEA, but within a few days after birth, our DHEA level drops to nearly zero. Then, between the ages of six and eight, we experience the event called "adrenarche" in which our adrenal glands begin to stir and gear up for the onset of puberty. At that same time our DHEA level begins to rise steadily and continues to rise until it peaks at around age twenty. From that point on it declines at a rate of about two percent a year, and we begin to feel the result of this decline in our mid-forties. By eighty our DHEA level is only 15 percent of what it was when we were twenty-five. By ninety we are down to 5 percent. Just before death our level of DHEA can be virtually nonexistent.

I first became interested in DHEA back in 1980 at a scientific meeting on the biology of aging that I had helped organize. A young cancer researcher from Temple University named Arthur G. Schwartz reported on a hormone called DHEA that, he said, had some fascinating properties. He told us that a researcher at a pharmaceutical company had found that when DHEA is added to the food of obese rats, it literally melts away fat. No one knew how it did this. Dr. Schwartz told us about a British cancer researcher who had found

DHEA Sulfate Levels Throughout Life

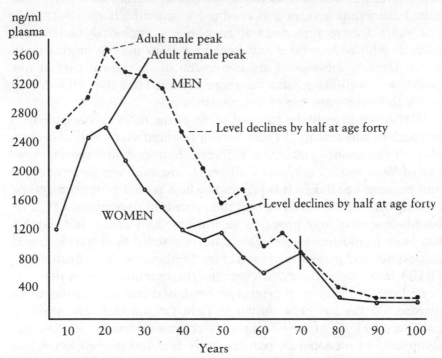

By age forty we produce half of the DHEA-S that we did at age twenty, our adult peak

that the DHEA levels were abnormally low in women with breast cancer. No one knew why. Dr. Schwartz himself had performed some fascinating experiments in which he gave rats a potent carcinogen that normally promoted tumor growth. He found, however, that when he gave the rats an injection of DHEA prior to introducing the carcinogen, they remained cancer free.

As an oncologist who has devoted my career to treating cancer patients after they develop the disease, I was excited by the prospect of a substance that might actually help prevent cancer from occurring in the first place. And as a research scientist who was trying to spark interest in well-grounded scientific aging research, I was also intrigued by the possibility that DHEA might play a pivotal role in the aging process. I set out to learn as much as possible about DHEA, and over the past decade and a half I have devoted a good portion of my career to studying and focusing attention on this truly remarkable superhormone. I have conducted dozens of studies and have published numerous articles and coedited a scientific book on DHEA. For years I have prescribed it to patients, including family and friends, who have needed and benefited from it. The more I learn about DHEA, the more I am convinced of its critical role in our health and well-being, and the more certain I am that DHEA will prove to be the superstar of superhormones.

DHEA is currently the focus of some of the most exciting medical research of this century. Researchers at distinguished medical centers all over the country, including Harvard, Stanford, and the universities of Wisconsin, Utah, and California, are studying the properties and promise of DHEA. It is proving to be a potent protector against cancer, and Arthur Schwartz is in the process of developing a DHEA-based drug that may prove to be the first anti-cancer pill. DHEA has been found to protect against heart disease by lowering blood cholesterol and preventing blood clots. Studies also demonstrate that DHEA improves memory, strengthens the immune system, prevents bone loss, and may even protect us from diabetes and autoimmune disease. DHEA has been shown to fight fatigue and depression; it enhances feelings of well-being and increases strength. It alleviates symptoms of menopause, reduces body fat, and is even known to enhance libido. It is no wonder that researchers worldwide are beginning to treat what had previously been considered a "junk" hormone with newfound respect and sometimes even awe. In this chapter, I will review the results of my own research and the research of others, but first I want to share what I have learned about DHEA from my personal experience with it outside of the laboratory.

I have been taking DHEA for the past ten years, and my wife, Sylvia, has been taking it for sixteen years. What has DHEA done for me? I am seventy-one years old and am fortunate in that I have not experienced the slowing down that has come to typify old age. I teach, treat patients, write, conduct research, and participate in conferences all over the world. I have no plans to retire and feel no need to cut back on my daily activities. In fact, my life has never been fuller. At sixty-nine, my wife has an equally demanding and rewarding schedule. Sylvia is a well-known art collector who specializes in African art and American art pottery. In addition to running her thriving business, she spends a great deal of time with our children and grandchildren. In short, she leads a life that would be regarded as full for a woman of any age. To my knowledge, Sylvia has been taking DHEA for a longer period than anyone else. She is a one-woman "clinical study" who holds the firm conviction that DHEA has improved the quality of her life. In her own words, "DHEA gives you more energy, gives you more ambition, and gives you more get-up-and-go."

What can DHEA do for you? That DHEA gives you energy and makes you feel stronger, more focused, and even happier is, to my mind, a given. Those benefits are at this point already well documented. It is my belief, however, that DHEA's effects are far more profound and far reaching. By taking DHEA you are not only undoing the damage inflicted over time to your body and mind, but you are actually seizing control of the aging process itself. You are no longer a "victim" who is helpless against the ravages of aging, you are the master, in charge, and very much in control. With DHEA, the superstar of superhormones, you, too, will be able to live your life to its fullest, without the fear of having to slow down (unless you want to) or to abandon your dreams and ambitions. With superhormones in general, and DHEA in particular, you will be able to maintain a strong body and a sharp mind throughout your upper decades, into your seventies, eighties, and nineties. You will not experience the slump in energy or vitality that typically begins in middle age and accelerates as we approach "old" age. To me, there is nothing sadder than dreaming dreams and making plans that cannot be fulfilled because of what is, I believe, a preventable slowdown in physical or mental function. The Superhormone Promise is about extending life and maintaining youthful health so that we can live rich and fulfilled lives right up until the last days of life. The Superhormone Promise is about looking back on our lives in contentment, without pangs of sadness and regret over what we could have done or should have done if only our health had held out. The Superhormone Promise is about breaking down the barriers that prevent us from being able to do what we want to do when we want to do it. It is about reinvigorating both the body and the spirit so that we are free to fulfill our potential, regardless of chronological age. DHEA is one of the most powerful tools to help us achieve these life-affirming goals.

Because DHEA is showing such tremendous promise in so many areas, in the pages that follow we will report on each one in some detail.

DHEA: The Energizer

One of the ways that DHEA helps in reversing the downward spiral of "old age" is by helping us regain our youthful energy. Energy is produced from the fuel that keeps our body going, and if we run out of energy, as most of us do, it can severely impair the quality of life. Without energy, we cannot live our lives and achieve our dreams.

Today, tens of thousands of physicians throughout the country are prescribing DHEA to their patients to treat a wide variety of ailments and are embracing the notion that restoring DHEA to its youthful level is a "tonic" to prevent the ravages of aging. In particular, physicians have noted that DHEA is a true fatigue fighter. One of the most common complaints of people middle-aged and beyond is that they do not have the stamina to do what they used to do. Whereas in the past they were able to work and play with equal vigor, now they find, much to their frustration, that they run out of steam long before they would like. They simply don't have the strength or the staying power that they used to.

Fatigue is a complaint often heard by Robert Rountree, a family physician with a thriving practice in Boulder, Colorado. Dr. Rountree is a traditionally trained, highly respected physician who is known for his innovative approach to treating patients. His goal, in his own words, is to "provide affordable, holistic health care to average working people." Dr. Rountree's particular interest is nutritional medicine. He believes that a good diet and a healthy lifestyle are essential for good health. But he also believes in the power of DHEA. When his patients complain of fatigue, in addition to performing a thorough examination and a routine laboratory workup, Dr. Rountree checks their blood level of DHEA. If he finds that the level is low, as he often does, he may prescribe DHEA to restore a youthful level as part of his overall treatment program. "DHEA has a very distinct effect on patients," notes Dr. Rountree. "What patients tell me is that they find themselves doing more things in the course of a day than they did before. They may not feel any different the first week or two, but when they look back after a few months, they realize that something important has happened to them. They have more energy and stamina, and they feel better about themselves. When you ask them if they want to go off DHEA, they say no."

Dr. Rountree was so impressed with the effects of DHEA that he paid it the ultimate compliment: He prescribed it for his own mother,

Dot. Dot is the music director of her local church. Her position requires long hours and unlimited patience. "My job is all encompassing," she explained. "I work day and night. I work with children in the second grade on up to older adults. I have to adapt myself to every age group; it can be very demanding." By the time Dot reached her mid-sixties, she found that she tired easily and lacked the stamina she once enjoyed. Nevertheless, she did not want to quit her job or cut back on her hours. She loved what she was doing and resented the fact that her body was hampering her ability to live an active life. When she explained her dilemma to her son, he suggested that she visit her internist to have her DHEA level checked. When the blood test revealed that her level was low, Dr. Rountree prescribed DHEA. Within a short time Dot felt reinvigorated. "My energy is back, and I can get through the day without feeling exhausted," she reported happily. Dr. Rountree says that he has prescribed DHEA to several hundred patients with similarly positive results.

What is so rewarding to me about Dot's story is that it clearly shows how by taking DHEA she was able to keep on living her life *on her terms*. In other words, she can go on with her busy schedule without skipping a beat and does not have to alter her lifestyle in any way simply because the years are passing. To me, this epitomizes the superhormone revolution. It will enable all of us to live our lives on our terms, unhampered by the conditions that we normally associate with aging.

Although such anecdotal reports about DHEA are important because they give us an impression of how people actually feel when they are taking DHEA, to scientists the gold standard of research is a well-run, objective clinical trial. One such study was recently conducted at the University of San Diego by a group headed by Dr. Samuel S. C. Yen. The study lasted six months. For three months of the study, thirteen men and seventeen women aged forty to seventy took a DHEA supplement sufficient to restore their blood level to that of a young adult. For another three months the participants received a placebo. Neither the researchers nor the subjects knew who was taking DHEA or the placebo at any given time. In other words, the study was what we call "double-blind." The researchers found that when the participants were taking DHEA, they reported a "remarkable increase in perceived physical and psychological well-being for both men and women." In other words, when they were on DHEA, the men and women felt better, a lot better. In particular, Dr. Yen's group found that the men and women on DHEA experienced increased energy and better sleep; they felt more relaxed and were better able to handle stress. Those with a history of arthritic symptoms also reported less joint pain. Moreover, none of the study participants experienced any negative side effects. What is so significant about Dr. Yen's study is that it dramatically shows DHEA does have a true rejuvenating effect in terms of elevating mood and restoring energy. I have no doubt that the superhormone revolution is going to significantly extend life, but what makes it all worthwhile is that we will also have the spirit and the stamina to be productive and to fully enjoy those extra years.

The improvement in mood and the increase in energy levels that people experience on DHEA carries over into many other aspects of life. Many of the people I know who take DHEA use this newfound energy to live their lives with as much gusto as they did when they were younger, and this happy observation leads me to a discussion of yet another wonderful positive effect of DHEA, and that is on the libido.

"Sex Is Better Than Ever"

Some feel that the essence of youth—indeed, the essence of feeling fully alive—is libido. What I call the "youthful state" or the "youthful advantage" is, in reality, the ability to be stimulated and aroused by the environment that surrounds us. That is why I believe remaining sexually vital is often key to remaining youthful. Often the advancing years spell decreased energy and interest in sex, yet this is another area in which DHEA can help turn back the clock.

One of the most constantly repeated comments I hear from patients as well as colleagues and friends who are taking DHEA is that it has renewed their interest in sex. Men, particularly, report that it has revived their sexual interest. Other doctors who prescribe DHEA report that many of their male patients experience an increase in libido and that many older men who did not have morning erections for years suddenly began to experience them after taking DHEA. As one of my friends, a biochemist who uses DHEA, put it, "I feel like I'm twenty again. Sex is better than ever." Needless to say, he has never stopped thanking me for introducing him to DHEA. Neither has his wife. Although women also find that DHEA makes them feel better and more energetic, the heightened libido effect is not as apparent for them, possibly because women do not experience the same pronounced decline in libido that is common for men in their advancing years.

DHEA's effect on male sexual function was documented in the groundbreaking Massachusetts Male Aging Study, which investigated, among other things, sexual function and activity in men aged forty to seventy. The researchers sought to determine whether there was any correlation between health or personality problems and impotence, which is a common condition among middle-aged and older men. At least half of us, at one time or another, experience impotence, which researchers define as "the persistent inability to attain and maintain an erection adequate to permit satisfactory sexual performance." The Massachusetts study demonstrated that the risk of severe or total impotency increases threefold with age. In other words, 5.1 percent of all forty-year-olds compared to 15 percent of all seventy-year-olds complained of complete impotency. The researchers noted that impotency is often associated with underlying medical problems, such as heart disease or high blood pressure, and that impotency is sometimes a side effect of the medications used to treat those conditions. Excess alcohol consumption and cigarette smoking were also shown to be major contributing factors to impotency. One finding, however, particularly caught my eye: Of the seventeen hormones measured in each of the men, only one showed a direct and consistent correlation with impotency: DHEA. As DHEA levels declined, the incidence of impotency increased.

The Massachusetts researchers could not explain why DHEA levels were lower in impotent men. They speculated that falling DHEA levels and impotency might just be two unrelated and coincident characteristics of the aging process. They also theorized that since DHEA appeared to protect against cardiovascular disease, and since heart patients are also prone to impotency, DHEA levels would naturally be lower in heart patients. Their explanations certainly tell part of the story, but other researchers and I believe that DHEA also has a far more direct effect on sexuality. We know that DHEA is converted into testosterone in both men and women, and that testosterone is known to enhance libido in both sexes. This would certainly explain why such men when they take DHEA experience a heightened libido.

Human sexuality, however, is a much more complex process than the simple interaction of hormones. It is a physical and emotional experience in which both the body and the mind play equally critical roles. DHEA enhances feelings of well-being and makes us feel more energetic and happy. It reduces fatigue and depression, two common conditions that have a seriously dampening effect on libido. When it comes to sexuality, I believe that DHEA's effect above the neck is every bit as important, and no less profound, than it is on the rest of the body.

Restoring Memory

Forgetfulness is one of the first signs of aging. It is not uncommon for people in their forties and fifties to begin to complain that their memory isn't what it used to be.

People who take DHEA, however, often remark that it has helped them to "think better." They say that it improves their concentration and enhances their memory. One of my colleagues put it aptly when he said, "Since I've been taking DHEA, it's a lot easier to remember quickly the kinds of things that I would normally forget." The older we are, the more apparent are DHEA's positive effects on mental function.

In a sense, the first human trial that tested the effect of DHEA on memory was performed in 1980 on my mother-in-law, Gussie. This, incidentally, was also the first time I prescribed DHEA for a patient. At eighty, Gussie was suffering from Berger's disease, a particularly cruel vascular disorder that results in blood clots in the small blood vessels, impairing the flow of blood to the legs. Deprived of blood and oxygen, one of Gussie's legs "atrophied," or died, and had to be amputated. After the surgery, Gussie was profoundly depressed and thoroughly confused. This formerly bright and vital woman was unaware of her surroundings, couldn't remember the names of her closest family members, and appeared to be en route to complete senility. Her doctor had written her off, saying that there was little to be done for her, so I decided to try something completely different. I concocted a "cocktail" of drugs which included magnesium, hydergine, and some other vitamins. (At that time hydergine was thought to be a memory-enhancing drug, but subsequent research did not support that belief.) Nothing happened. Then I added DHEA to her daily drug regimen. Within two weeks we saw a dramatic difference. Gussie's thinking was as sharp as ever, and, thankfully, her memory was restored.

Although Gussie's last days were still a struggle, she was relieved and grateful that her mind was functioning well until the day she died. She felt more in control and better able to cope with a situation that was exceedingly difficult for everyone. Since several other substances were also used in Gussie's cocktail, this trial does not offer final proof that DHEA alone was solely responsible for the restoration of Gussie's mind and memory, but I saw strong evidence that it was. Moreover, my belief has been vindicated by several subsequent studies that have shown beyond any doubt whatsoever that DHEA has a direct and profound effect on the brain's ability to process and store information, and those results have now led some researchers to the belief that DHEA may play a major role in preventing the terrible mind- and memory-robbing scourge we call Alzheimer's disease.

Before telling you about those studies, I need to explain a bit about how the brain manages and stores memory. When we are exposed to a new stimuli—that is, when we learn something new—it is "memorized" or recorded by special cells within the brain that form networks interconnected with each other, called neurites. Millions of neurite networks are in constant communication with one another and with other parts of the brain. The more neurites we form, the greater our memory capacity and thus the greater our capacity to learn and store information.

We know from animal studies that when a mouse or a rat or a monkey is raised in a cage by itself without any stimulation, its brain does not form neurite networks and its ability to learn is severely impaired. The same is true for human children, which is why parents are instructed to talk and to read to their children at a young age—even before a child actually understands the words—and to provide sensory stimulation from the earliest days of infancy. Every time we hug an infant, we are helping to build up a working neurite network. It isn't for decoration alone that we intuitively paint children's rooms in bright colors and place mobiles and other toys within their line of sight. We do all this to tweak the formation of these precious neurites.

Don't think, however, that neurite formation is just for the young. Although children do have a greater capacity to build neurite networks, the same process occurs in older people, albeit at a slower rate. This slowdown is why, as we age, many of us find it increasingly difficult to learn new tasks, and some of us also find that our short-term memory is faltering. If we find it difficult to learn a new language or have trouble remembering the names of people we meet at a party, this is due at least partly to the fact that our neurite network is running out faster than we are replacing it.

In light of the important role that neurite formation plays in learning and memory, it will come as no surprise to you that scientists have long searched for a substance that can stimulate the formation of neurites. The good news is that recent studies show DHEA can do just that!

In one groundbreaking study, conducted at the City of Hope Hospital in Duarte, California, by world-renowned scientist Eugene Roberts, DHEA's effect on brain function was tested in two ways. First, Dr. Roberts took tissue cultures of neural (brain) cells from mice, put them in petri dishes to grow, and then added DHEA. He discovered that DHEA stimulated the growth of both axial membranes and the little spikes that interconnect neurons to one another and allow neural cells to communicate with each other. In other words, DHEA helps us "grow" our brain networks by helping us form interconnecting neurites.

In his second study, Dr. Roberts set out to teach old mice new tricks. He put a group of old mice and young mice in a maze in which the animals would receive mild electric shocks if they went in the wrong direction. Younger mice learned their lesson quickly and after a few shocks did not repeat their mistakes. In fact, they even remembered the safe way to navigate the maze long after the training sessions were over. Compared to the younger mice, the older animals did not fare as well. They not only had more difficulty learning but were quick to forget when the lesson was over.

Dr. Roberts then repeated the experiment, but this time he gave each older mouse an injection of DHEA within two minutes after the maze training. After receiving the DHEA, the older mice negotiated the maze with the same ease and agility as the younger mice. What was truly remarkable was that two weeks later, when all the mice were retested, the DHEA-treated mice retained the information as well as the younger mice. This study showed that just one dose of DHEA had a profound and long-term effect on memory in mice. Such astonishing results in animal studies soon attracted the attention of researchers who wanted to know if DHEA could perform similar magic on the brains of humans.

A particularly interesting study was conducted by Dr. Owen M. Wolkowitz of the Department of Psychiatry at the University of California at San Francisco. This small but very fascinating study involved six middle-aged and older patients who suffered from major depression accompanied by memory problems. The patients were given 60 to 90 mg. of oral DHEA every day for four to six weeks. The patients not only showed significant relief from their depression but also experienced significant improvement in memory, particularly in terms of two specific aspects of memory: incidental and semantic. It is important for you to understand what these terms mean. Incidental memory is the ability to recall detail. For example, if you attend a lecture and a day later are asked to describe not what the speaker was talking about, which was probably what you were focusing on, but something less obvious, such as what the speaker was wearing or the color of the walls of the lecture room, you will be calling upon your incidental memory. Semantic memory involves tapping into your brain's database of stored information to give an appropriate response. It is best understood in comparison to what we call episodic memory. For example, if you are asked to recall what you had for breakfast today, you are being asked to use your episodic memory, which remembers what you did or what happened at a particular point in time. But if you are instead asked, "What are some general types of breakfast foods?" you are now being asked to use your semantic memory. You are not required to recall a particular event or incident, but you are required to retrieve stored comparative data.

The reason DHEA's effect on incidental and semantic memory is so fascinating is that these are the first types of memory to deteriorate in patients suffering from Alzheimer's disease. Alzheimer's disease, or "AD" for short, is an irreversible form of dementia characterized by the slow destruction of key areas of the brain that control reasoning and memory. The brains of AD patients are overrun by a type of protein called beta amyloid, which forms characteristic plaques or tangles that some researchers believe may be responsible for the destruction of healthy brain cells.

Some 4 million Americans have AD, including about 10 percent of all people over age sixty-five. The precise cause of AD is unknown, and currently there are no effective treatments. If DHEA helps preserve the type of memory that is lost in AD patients, could DHEA be a useful tool for the treatment of AD? Dr. Wolkowitz's group is currently conducting two studies to determine whether DHEA can affect the outcome of AD. One study, funded by the National Institute on Aging, will involve a group of patients diagnosed with AD. For six months half the group will receive DHEA, and half will get a placebo. Researchers will be looking to see whether members of the DHEA-treated group perform better on psychological tests and whether their quality of life is perceptibly improved.

In another study funded by the Alzheimer's Association, Dr. Wolkowitz will simply follow the progress of thirty AD patients and thirty healthy subjects for eighteen months, tracking their levels of DHEA, DHEA sulfate (DHEA is converted into DHEA sulfate in the body), and cortisol (stress hormone) to see if there is any correlation between each patient's progress and his hormone levels. After twelve and eighteen months, both groups will be given an extensive battery of psychological tests. Researchers will be looking to determine if levels of DHEA in any way predict the course or outcome of AD. Interestingly, some studies have found markedly low levels of DHEA in AD patients, while others have not. Researchers at the University of Wisconsin will be conducting similar studies in memory disorder patients, including patients with early-onset AD and patients over age eighty-five.

Earlier studies using very high doses of DHEA to treat very advanced AD patients were not successful, and for that reason, early research on DHEA and its role in memory was cut short. It is Dr. Wolkowitz's belief, and I agree with him, that these earlier studies were flawed in two ways: First, when it comes to DHEA (or any other hormone for that matter), more is not necessarily more effective. Artificially high doses, in fact, may actually not work as well as lower doses that are more in keeping with the levels of DHEA that are naturally produced by the body, which is why I recommend that people take only the amount necessary to boost their superhormone levels back to their natural, youthful peak. And that is why each individual needs to have his or her superhormone levels checked to see what degree of deficiency needs correction. Giving a patient too high a dose of a hormone such as DHEA can overwhelm the brain cells, overloading the cell's receptors and preventing them from putting the DHEA to good use. Second, giving DHEA to advanced AD patients once the damage has been done may be too late. Dr. Wolkowitz believes that DHEA may play a role in helping to prevent the inception or even the progression of AD but that it cannot reverse the disease once it has taken hold. "I think that it has more of a permissive effect; that is, if there is a neuro toxic degenerative process going on for whatever other reasons, having low DHEA levels could impair the body's natural ability to repair the damage. In other words, if there is some damage going on in the brain, having youthful levels of DHEA could facilitate recovery from the damage or hold the damage in check."

There are several possible ways in which DHEA may protect the brain from the kind of wear and tear that could promote AD. One of these is DHEA's particular ability to protect us from the damaging effects of stress hormones. When we are under stress—whether it is provoked by an argument with a coworker, a traffic tie-up, an illness, or any of life's big and little stressful events—our bodies produce stress hormones called corticosteroids. Corticosteroids can inflict severe damage on many of our organs and body systems, including our brain. Stress, and the resulting flood of corticosteroids, is particularly damaging to older people because, as we age, corticosteroid levels remain higher for longer periods of time than they do in younger people; that is, when we are older and exposed to stress, our bodies are flooded with these harmful stress hormones for longer periods and are more vulnerable to damage. Scientists at McGill University have found that as our stress hormones rise, our ability to perform on attention and memory tests falls. Exposure to stress hormones appears to damage some brain cells in the hippocampus, the portion of the brain responsible for memory and learning. Interestingly, AD patients often display elevated stress hormone levels and, as noted earlier, low DHEA levels. This suggests that as we age and our DHEA levels decline, we become more susceptible to the harmful effects of corticosteroids, including damage to the brain's hippocampus, which may be a factor in, if not the proximate cause, of AD.

This is a tantalizing hypothesis. Should DHEA be used by patients who have been diagnosed with early-stage AD? Since the DHEA/Alzheimer's connection is still being studied, Dr. Wolkowitz believes that making a blanket recommendation of it to AD patients is premature. He says, however, that if physicians are interested in using DHEA for patients with AD, he is willing to talk to doctors on an individual basis about his experiences so that they can determine whether they want to use DHEA for this particular purpose. My personal opinion is that since there are no effective treatments for AD, using DHEA may be both appropriate and reasonable. I also believe that by starting people on DHEA in a timely fashion—that is, at the point when their own natural levels of DHEA and other superhormones begin to recede—we may actually be able to postpone and even prevent the onset of AD in many cases.

I have had great success in using DHEA to treat another condition that produces Alzheimer's-like symptoms in young people, and that is AIDS-related dementia, which is caused by destruction of the central nervous system. One of the cruelest aspects of AIDS is that it can rob victims of their ability to think clearly, and even if they are not physically impaired, they may be too mentally impaired to work or even perform the functions necessary for daily living. I have pre-scribed DHEA to two patients suffering from AIDS-related dementia. Both of these patients were confused, listless, depressed, and lacking energy. Not surprisingly, their DHEA levels were close to zero, and their stress hormone levels were through the roof. Within a short time after they began taking DHEA these patients were restored to their old selves. They were able to think clearly and express their thoughts coherently. One experienced such an astonishing improve-ment in his ability to function that he was able to return to work. Based on my experience, I feel that the physicians of AIDS patients who are suffering from dementia should certainly consider DHEA for their patients.

"The Colds Have Stopped": Rejuvenating the Immune System

I have repeatedly said that DHEA is not merely a feel-good pill, but its effects are experienced by the body on a much deeper and more meaningful level. In particular, DHEA has a remarkable effect on the body's immune system, and I frequently prescribe it as an immune booster. A case in point is a friend and patient of mine, a distin-guished biologist, who was complaining that he was always getting sick. He spends a good deal of time flying to scientific meetings all around the world, breathing recycled, stale airplane air. When he was younger, he was able to resist infection and caught few colds. Recently, however, he found that every time he returned from one of his trips, he would come down with a terrible cold. On his fiftieth birthday, my friend felt torn between limiting his appearances at these important professional meetings by restricting his air travel or resigning himself to chronic respiratory infections. I offered him another option. I recommended that he start taking DHEA. Several months later my friend reported that although he had logged yet another twenty thousand in frequent-flier miles, lo and behold, he had stopped getting sick. "The colds have gone," he told me with a big grin. Always a careful scientist, my-friend-the-distinguished-biologist added, "I won't say that it's due to the DHEA, because I haven't done any studies on it, but I won't say that it's not, either." What is most telling is that my friend plans on continuing to take DHEA indefinitely. Given what I have seen in my own and in others' clinical trials and research with DHEA, I have no reservations about attributing my friend's improved health to his daily dose of DHEA, which has reinvigorated his immune system and given him the strength and stamina to resist infection. I base my view on the fact that some of the most intriguing research on DHEA centers on its role in helping to maintain a strong, youthful immune system. What is important about this research is that it shows precisely how DHEA can prevent senescence, the downward spiral associated with traditional aging, by fortifying our bodies against disease.

Although the connection between the immune system and aging may not seem obvious at first, they are mirror images of each other. The immune system ages as the body ages (and vice versa), and the condition of our immune system is often a reflection of how well or how poorly we are aging. An "old" immune system will leave the body vulnerable to a plethora of ills that not only shorten life but diminish its quality. A strong, youthful immune system helps us stay healthy by protecting us from the countless "enemies" that can wreak havoc on our body systems and accelerate the aging process. Not only is there compelling evidence that DHEA can help us maintain a vigorous immune system, but research has also shown that it can do what was once believed to be impossible: It can take an aging, "broken" immune system and transform it into a young, well-functioning immune system.

To understand the importance of DHEA and its effect on the immune system, you need to know a bit about how the immune system works. The immune system is a collection of specialized cells that protect the body against disease. This is an arduous task. Human beings are just one of the many hundreds of millions of organisms living on this planet, all trying to survive in spite of one another. At any given moment there are countless numbers of viruses, bacteria, and fungi trying to take up residence in your body. Fortunately, a special type of lymphocyte, or white blood cell, in your immune system—the T cell—identifies such unwanted invaders and disarms them before they can cause damage.

There are different kinds of T cells. One type, called a suppressor cell, helps the body differentiate between enemy invaders and the body's own tissue. Suppressor cells are very important cells because they prevent the body from attacking itself. When our suppressor cells fail to function, we become vulnerable to autoimmune diseases such as rheumatoid arthritis and lupus.

Then there are the immune cells that we call NK, for "natural killer," cells. These cells are constantly monitoring our bodies for signs of abnormal cell growth that could result in cancer. When NK cells identify abnormally reproducing cells, they attack them.

Other immune cells, known as macrophages, roam around the bloodstream gobbling up foreign material that crosses their path. Finally, there are also immune cells called follicular dendritic cells (FDCs), which are responsible for long-term immune memory. These cells decline with age and are also among the first to be infected with the AIDS virus. They affect the capacity of still other immune cells, known as B cells, which produce substances called antibodies that attach themselves to invading viruses and bacteria, and kill them. After vanquishing a foe, they remain in our bodies to ambush offending viruses or bacteria should they strike again. This is the principle that explains why we develop immunity against certain diseases. For example, most of us get chicken pox only once in our lives because when we get it, we develop antibodies that will not allow it to take hold again.

As we age, however, some striking changes in the immune system have a profoundly negative effect on our health. Our T cells become sluggish and less effective at weeding out invaders. Thus, we become more prone to pick up a serious cold or flu virus, and more likely to develop pneumonia from what would otherwise be a benign respiratory infection. We call this "immunosenescence." Immunosenescence is why older people are advised to get flu shots during influenza season. A virus that a younger immune system could easily defeat can quickly overtake an older immune system. Our suppressor cells become sloppy and are no longer as efficient at distinguishing between our own tissue and that of invaders. As a result, autoimmune diseases are more common among the elderly. Our antibodies begin to lose their memory and mix up friend and foe, allowing bacteria and viruses to proliferate and, on occasion, attack healthy tissue. Our NK cells, which form our body's anti-cancer surveillance system, begins to fall asleep at the wheel, so to speak, and fails to weed out cancerous growths. Thus, the likelihood that we will develop cancer rises dramatically as we age.

Many of us in the scientific community have come to believe that the age-related decline in immunity is not inevitable and is, in fact, a direct result of the decline in the body's production of superhormones, including DHEA. Of all the superhormones, DHEA may exert the most profound effect on immunity, making it a key player in maintaining health and longevity.

OLD TO YOUNG

Among the very distinguished researchers working on DHEA's role in immune function is Dr. Raymond A. Daynes at the University of Utah School of Medicine. Interestingly, Dr. Daynes says he first encountered DHEA serendipitously about six years ago when he was studying the effects of ultraviolet radiation on the immune system. It was well known at the time that exposure to UV rays was a risk factor for skin cancer and that the immune system was somehow involved. Dr. Daynes and his research group exposed mice to UV rays and then injected tumor cells into them. Under normal conditions the animal's immune system was able to kill the tumor cells before they could kill the host. After the mice were exposed to UV rays, however, the tumor cells grew uncontrollably. Dr. Daynes wondered why the UV-exposed mice were no longer able to detect and weed out the tumors, and he set out to see what had changed within the mouse that could have so radically altered its immune system. The one striking change was that after exposure to UV rays, the mice were producing very high levels of stress hormones. By this time it was well known that stress hormones were able to inhibit immune response— a point that I will come back to and deal with at length later in this chapter—so Dr. Daynes devised an experiment to test whether eliminating the stress hormones from the picture would restore the ability of the UV-exposed animals to restrain tumor growth. In his next study he gave one group of mice a drug that blocks the synthesis or production of stress hormones. Then, as in the first experiment, he exposed the mice to high doses of UV rays and injected them with tumor cells. He discovered something quite astounding: The mice that had been given the drug to block stress hormone production failed to develop tumors. Not only that, these mice actually exhibited a stronger immune response than did the completely normal mice that he had used as a control group!

In other words, he had enhanced their immune systems and had shielded them from the cancer-causing effect of the UV rays.

No one was more surprised by the results than Dr. Daynes. "I sat down and said, 'What the heck have we done?' "

As Dr. Daynes later realized, the explanation was really elegantly simple. When Dr. Daynes gave the mice the drug to block the production of stress hormones, he altered the normal hormonal pathway in the body. Giving the drug was the equivalent of setting up a detour, sending a cascade of chemical reactions down another road. That road led to the increased production of DHEA. Instead of producing stress hormones, which can depress the immune system, the mice were actually producing higher amounts of DHEA, which appeared to have significantly enhanced their immune systems.

Intrigued by his findings, Dr. Daynes performed many experiments using DHEA directly. One particularly fascinating set of experiments showed that "over the hill" immune systems typical of old mice could be rejuvenated by injection or oral ingestion of DHEA sulfate. Animals, including humans, can be immunized against certain viruses by taking, usually by injection, a weakened strain of the virus. The body reacts to the presence of this strain by developing antibodies against it. Later, when the body is exposed to the "real" virus, those antibodies quickly identify, attack, and destroy the virus before it can cause disease. You probably recognize this technique as similar to that used to immunize us against polio, smallpox, and influenza, to cite but a few examples. It is a well-known fact that when an old mouse is vaccinated against a disease-causing bacteria or virus, virtually no immune response is generated. That is, they don't seem to perceive the presence of the strain and don't react by producing antibodies. It is as if their immune systems are just too tired for the vaccination to take. But Dr. Daynes found that when old mice with tired immune systems were given DHEA before being vaccinated against a virus, their immune systems responded strongly and vigorously. Indeed, he discovered that the immune systems of these old mice were largely indistinguishable from those of the younger control mice.

ALL ABOUT CYTOKINES

The great significance of Dr. Daynes's work is that it clearly shows how DHEA can "rescue" an older immune system and rejuvenate it so that it works as well as a young immune system. But why does aging have such a pronounced negative effect on our immune systems? Why is an older immune system so much less effective against infection? Why do older immune systems get "confused" and produce antibodies that attack their own tissue? Why do older immune systems have so much trouble distinguishing friend from foe?

Dr. Daynes and members of his research group made some findings that may help answer these questions. They believe that the answer may reside in hormonelike substances called cytokines, which are produced by immune cells. These molecules are released from immune cells and transmit information to other immune cells. Cytokines govern how our cells respond to a situation. They can spur growth, block growth, trigger a reaction or inhibit one. The army of cells that comprise the immune system "listens" to cytokines; the cells know what normal levels of particular cytokines sound like, and these immune cells do not react unless the cytokines somehow change, thus initiating a response. The cells, according to Dr. Daynes, must know how to discriminate between information and noise. In both animals and humans, we have identified individual cytokines that are known for triggering particular reactions, and even the smallest change in these cytokines can have a profound effect. For reasons that we don't quite understand, some of these key cytokines are altered by aging. The system that transmits signals between the cells somehow breaks down, and the immune cells "hear" and react to unwanted "noises." For example, one cytokine known as IL 6, which is elevated in older humans and animals, is also found in abnormally high levels in people who have autoimmune diseases, osteoporosis, and certain forms of cancer. Some studies have indicated that elevated levels of IL 6 can actually stimulate tumor growth. Notably, all three diseases are more common among the elderly. In addition, as we age, IL 2, the cytokine responsible for stimulating the proliferation of cells that fight disease, goes down, leaving us more vulnerable to infection.

The problem with abnormalities in key cytokines is that they throw the immune system out of whack. They stimulate immune cells to attack the body's own tissue. They can also signal the immune system that it is time to hold back when the body should, in fact, be waging an all-out war against an invader. In other words, cytokine "noise" can distract the immune system from doing its job. Dr. Daynes believes that DHEA rejuvenates immune function by restoring order to these cytokines that are out of control.

When a hormone or drug works as consistently well as DHEA does in animal studies, it strongly suggests that it will be equally effective in humans, but of course the proof is in the pudding. In this context the pudding is human studies, and human studies of the effect of DHEA on the immune system have clearly demonstrated that DHEA supplementation can help restore normal cytokine levels and immune response in patients showing clear cytokine abnormalities. (As will be explained later in more detail, DHEA appears to be an effective treatment for lupus, one of the most common and difficult to treat autoimmune diseases.)

In a study conducted at the University of Tennessee, scientists reported that when postmenopausal women were given DHEA, they showed a rise in cancer-fighting NK cells and a drop in their levels of IL 6 cytokines, the cytokines that have been linked causally to autoimmune and other diseases of aging.

Dr. Omid Khorram, formerly a professor of medicine at the University of California at San Diego and now a member of the University of Wisconsin faculty, found Dr. Daynes's work intriguing and undertook a groundbreaking human study of DHEA and immune function. His is a particularly significant scientific investigation because it is the longest study of the effect of restoring DHEA to youthful levels on otherwise healthy older people. In Dr. Khorram's study, nine healthy older men took DHEA for five months. Dr. Khorram found that DHEA did indeed have a palpable, measurable rejuvenating effect on their aging immune systems. He found that DHEA elevated the men's levels of IGF-1. This is the hormone through which we believe another superhormone, growth hormone, operates. IGF-1 is a powerful immune enhancer in its own right, as will be discussed later. DHEA also normalized the men's levels of cytokine IL 6, the cytokine linked to autoimmune disorders. It increased levels of cytokine IL 2, which is the cytokine responsible for gearing up the immune system to fight unwanted invaders. It stimulated the production of B cells, which produce the antibodies that fight viruses and bacteria, as well as the production of macrophages, the white blood cells that fight infection by "chewing up" infecting organisms. It increased the number and activity of cancer-fighting NK (natural killer) cells, which keep a watchful eye on potential cancerous cells and destroy them before they can grow.

Dr. Khorram found that DHEA clearly restored a "more youthful response pattern" to the immune system of his human subjects. How does it work? Interestingly, Dr. Khorram hypothesizes that DHEA may work its magic on the immune system by virtue of an indirect path. He believes that DHEA is controlling the effect of stress steroid hormones—which, as we saw earlier, have a dampening effect on the immune system. By neutralizing these enemies of the immune system, DHEA indirectly bolsters the function of the immune system.

As has been noted, numerous studies have documented that stress hormones can destroy vital disease-fighting cells in the immune system, leaving us vulnerable to disease. In fact, many researchers have come to the conclusion that the decline in the ratio between DHEA and corticosteroids may be the primary reason that the immune system is thrown out of whack in the first place. This makes perfect sense. When we are young, our high levels of DHEA help keep stress hormones under control, giving them enough slack to do their job but reining them in before they can inflict damage. As we age, our levels of DHEA decline, allowing our stress hormones to run amuck, slowly and insidiously damaging important organ systems. By restoring our levels of DHEA to their youthful peak, it is possible to prevent this damage from occurring. By maintaining a strong and youthful immune system, it is possible to stave off the diseases of aging and doing so, maintain our youthful health and vigor.

Several studies—those of Dr. Kalimi and myself—demonstrate that DHEA has a protective effect against potentially lethal stress hormones, and I would like to turn to them now. As you will see, restoring DHEA to youthful levels may indeed serve as a buffer against these stress hormones, which is one reason it is such a potent anti-aging weapon.

Taming Killer Stress

One of the areas that I personally have devoted much study to is the effect of stress hormones on immunity and, in particular, how DHEA protects the body against the ravages of out-of-control stress hormones.

Given the responses of those people taking DHEA, it really should come as no surprise that our studies are proving DHEA has a demonstrable effect on stress hormones. People who take DHEA often talk about feeling better able to handle stress, feeling calmer, and, in sum, having a better outlook on life. What they are really experiencing is DHEA's unique ability to tame the hormones that are produced when their bodies are under stress.

When we are under stress, our adrenal glands produce corticosteroids, chemicals that pump the body up for action. Corticosteroids raise blood sugar levels and speed up the heart to get the blood pumping, giving the body a burst of energy to cope with a physical challenge. Under ideal conditions the surge of corticosteroids is quickly used up during a burst of physical activity. Most of us, however, do not live under ideal conditions. In many cases we internalize stress, and the destructive stress hormones linger in our bloodstream. Illness places a tremendous amount of stress on the body, and often when we are sick, our corticosteroid levels are very high. Although elevated levels of stress hormones may provide a short-term burst of energy to the body, they can have a dampening effect on the immune system. In fact, studies have shown that after periods of extreme stress, our T "helper" cells, which protect us from infection, do not work efficiently and are unable to protect us against disease. That is why it is not uncommon for college students to come down with bad colds or flu after completing their final exams. The same hormones that give them the energy to cram all night and take tests all day leave them vulnerable to infection.

Extreme stress, which often accompanies or can even induce depression, can also make us particularly vulnerable to viral disease. Several years ago a fascinating study was done at a military base in Maryland that clearly documented the potentially lethal effect which stress hormones can have on immunity. At the time of the study, Asiatic flu was rampant throughout Europe and was expected to reach the United States within a short time. Before the flu epidemic reached our shores, all military personnel on the Maryland base were psychologically evaluated, to determine their mental state. Of those who later came down with the flu, researchers found that 90 percent of them had been classified earlier as either being depressed or stressed out. Interestingly, it took three weeks for the soldiers who had been classified as depressed or stressed out to recover from the flu. In contrast, it took only five days for the soldiers who were not depressed or under stress to recover fully from their illness. This study clearly demonstrates to me the lethal effects of stress.

As the years pass, the corticosteroids we produce under stress remain in our bloodstream for longer periods of time. In other words, as our bodies age, we become less efficient in coping with these hormones, giving them more opportunity to inflict their damage on the immune system. (The immune system is not the only system in the body that is affected by elevated levels of stress hormones. There is good evidence that stress hormones can have disastrous effects on the heart and brain, points I will turn to later.) Our inability to cope with stress hormones as we age is a prime example of how we lose our resiliency through the years. In chapter 1, I noted that when we are young, we are better equipped to bounce back from life's stressors, and by "stressors" I meant any of the literally thousands of challenges in which our bodies are forced to respond. As we age, we are less able to meet these challenges successfully and to move on to the next. The change in the way our bodies handle stress hormones clearly demonstrates this critical point.

From the first moment I heard about DHEA, I was struck by the fact that as levels of DHEA decline in our bodies, we begin to suffer the damaging effects of stress hormones. I knew from existing research that DHEA had an inverse relationship with stress hormones —meaning that as levels of stress hormones rise, levels of DHEA drop. But then I connected this fact to another puzzling phenomenon: When younger people are under extreme or chronic stress, their DHEA levels tend to plummet to levels much like those of older people! My experience as a physician and a medical researcher taught me that this could not be a coincidence. Over the years I have learned that there are always interconnections among such biological events even though they may not be readily apparent.

To test my emerging hypothesis about the role of DHEA in the immune system, back in the early 1980s we devised an experiment to test whether DHEA could actually "rescue" the immune system from the damaging effects of stress hormones. My close friend Dr. Vernon Riley was a pioneer in the field of neuroimmunomodulation, the study of the relationship between the endocrine system (which produces hormones) and the immune system (which protects us against disease) and the brain (which regulates them both). The work of Riley and other innovative thinkers, including Dr. Walter Pierpaoli, my coauthor on *The Melatonin Miracle,* provided the foundation for what we now call "mind/body medicine." Thanks to them, we now know that our emotional state can profoundly affect the state of our overall health and, in particular, the condition of our immune system.

I had an idea, and I turned to Dr. Riley for help in implementing it. In past experiments Dr. Riley had shown that extreme stress could produce some very real and tangible physical effects in animals and that in some cases it could actually kill them. Dr. Riley discovered that when he placed a mouse in a stressful situation for a long period of time—for example, when he put the animal on a rotating platform, tied it up and placed it in a refrigerator, or dunked it in icy water—its immune system would undergo some peculiar changes. Its thymus gland (located under the breastbone), where the all-important T cells are stored, would cease functioning, shrivel up, and die. Dr. Riley also found that giving the mice an injection of stress hormones produced the same disastrous effect on the thymus. Interestingly, in older animals, including humans, the thymus gland becomes shriveled—or, as we scientists say, involuted—as we age. But Dr. Riley was able to cause thymus involution in young animals by subjecting them to stress or injecting them with stress hormones! In other words, stress literally *aged* a young immune system.

Knowing that stress hormones could produce thymus shrinkage and that DHEA appeared somehow to modulate the levels of stress hormones, I suggested the following experiment to Dr. Riley: Give the mice a shot of DHEA, subject them to stress by placing them on a constantly rotating turntable, and see what, if anything, happened to their thymus glands. He performed this experiment on dozens of young adult mice, and the results were quite remarkable. When the mice were given DHEA, they did not show signs of damage to the thymus. Their thymus glands remained in their strong, youthful state and did not exhibit any of the telltale signs of stress. In other words, DHEA had served as a buffer against the potentially damaging stress hormones.

Dr. Riley and I tried another variation on the same experiment, and the results are important to our understanding of how to use superhormones effectively. Instead of trying to prevent thymus damage, this time we tried to rejuvenate the thymus after the damage had already been done. We gave older animals DHEA and put them through the same ordeal. Nothing happened. This time the thymus gland remained shrunken and "sick." Although DHEA was a powerful protector against stress-induced thymus damage, it could not reverse the damage. I mention this because there is another superhormone that has been shown to rejuvenate the thymus gland, and that hormone is melatonin, which was the subject of my last book. This is a prime example of how one superhormone can pick up where another has left off, and it is why the hormone "cocktail" promises to be more effective than taking a single hormone.

Perhaps the most compelling experiment documenting DHEA's positive effect on stress hormones—and one that most clearly highlights DHEA's power as a superhormone—was one performed with my esteemed colleague Mohammed Kalimi, Ph.D., at Virginia Commonwealth University. In our study we gave rats a hefty dose of dexamethasone, a hormone that mimics the release of stress hormones and sends blood pressure levels soaring to deadly heights. Shortly after they received a shot of dexamethasone, the animals typically died of heart failure or stroke. We found, however, that if the animals were given an injection of DHEA before the injection of the lethal drug, they not only survived, but their blood pressure was normalized. This demonstrated that DHEA offers powerful protection against stress-induced disease.

More recently, DHEA's effect on stress and immunity was tested by a group headed by Dr. Ben Nathan in Israel. In their study they subjected mice to viruses that under normal conditions are benign and can easily be resisted by the animals. When the animals were then exposed to extreme cold, however, which is highly stressful, they succumbed to the viral infections and died. When the animals were given DHEA before being exposed to the cold, they all survived. DHEA provided the animals with 100 percent protection against the potentially lethal effect of stress on their immune systems.

Why is the fact that DHEA can protect against stress so important? Since many of the most common diseases that afflict us today, from heart disease to arthritis, are believed to be at least partly the result of stress, and since nearly all illnesses are aggravated by stress, any substance that can soften the blow inflicted by chronic stress is truly valuable.

By now I think you are beginning to see why I called DHEA the ultimate anti-aging superhormone, why I feel so strongly about this superhormone, why I take it myself and give it to members of my family, and why I have devoted twenty years of my life to studying it. DHEA not only makes people feel strong and vigorous, but it has a markedly positive effect on the immune system, which is one way it helps to keep the diseases of aging at bay. But I want to stress that its effect on the immune system is not the only way that DHEA fights against disease. What is truly extraordinary about this superhormone is that it attacks disease on many different fronts. It bolsters our body's ability to resist disease and has some unique disease-fighting properties in its own right. There is some incredible work currently being done, for example, on DHEA's role in the prevention and treatment of specific diseases, and some of the most fascinating research is in the area of cancer, to which we will now turn.

Cancer Fighter

Chemotherapy was killing me. . . . DHEA saved my life.

—ALEX T., 84, cancer patient

Cancer is very much a disease of aging. It is no coincidence that cancer tends to strike us when we are older, when our immune systems begin to "retire." A sixty-five-year-old is fifty times more likely to get cancer than is a twenty-five-year-old. Studies show that even when exposed to the identical cancer-causing agent, a young animal will be able to resist cancer, but an old animal will succumb to it. That is why much of the research on aging has centered on cancer prevention strategies.

When I first began studying DHEA, it was with the modest hope that DHEA might one day prove to be a useful tool in the treatment of cancer. Now, nearly two decades later, I firmly believe that DHEA has proven to be far more than just another chemotherapeutic agent. Please don't think that I regard chemotherapy drugs as unimportant; indeed, I regard them as critically important, and they have been the prime focus of my cancer research. But these drugs are useful only after cancer has taken hold. What other scientists and I find so exciting about DHEA is that it appears to be an entirely different type of anti-cancer drug—perhaps the ultimate cancer fighter—that is, a true *anticarcinogen* in that it can actually *prevent* the onset of this deadly disease.

This hope is shared by Dr. Arthur G. Schwartz of Temple University, one of the world's leading DHEA researchers and the scientist who, as mentioned earlier, first introduced me to DHEA. As far back as 1974, long before I or most other members of the scientific community had ever heard of it, Dr. Schwartz was testing DHEA's anti-cancer properties. Dr. Schwartz and his colleagues have documented DHEA's cancer-fighting power in hundreds of other studies, using both test tube and animal models. DHEA appears to protect against a wide range of carcinogens and many different forms of cancer. For example, DHEA supplementation in their food prevented breast cancer in a strain of female mice that are prone to die of it. In other animal studies, DHEA inhibited the growth of chemically induced tumors of the skin, colon, and lungs.

These and other experiments demonstrate that DHEA offers protection against cancer, but they did not explain how DHEA performed this feat. Indeed, it has taken Dr. Schwartz and his colleagues more than twenty years to begin to unravel this mystery, and although they have developed some answers, there is still much to learn.

Here is what we know so far. When you think of cancer, you probably think of a cell that somehow turns "bad," replicates rapidly, and produces more "bad" cells that devour the body by sapping it of its nourishment. That is basically correct, but the process is far more complicated and involves many different levels. In order to understand how DHEA works, you need to think of cancer as a process involving not just one chemical or cell but a whole cascade of events. The process begins with the introduction of a carcinogen, or initiator, a substance which initiates the early changes in the cell that can result in the growth of cancer down the road. The list of probable initiators includes ultraviolet light, tobacco, heavy metals, fats, alcohol, and radiation. A damaged cell can remain dormant for decades until it is "awakened" by a tumor promoter, a substance that encourages these cells to start dividing.

DHEA appears to thwart the cancer process in its earliest stages by foiling the action of these tumor promoters. DHEA does this by inhibiting the action of an enzyme (a chemical in the body) called glucose-6-phosphate dehydrogenase, or G6PDH for short. When left to its own devices, G6PDH stimulates another chemical, NADPH, causing a chemical reaction that converts dormant carcinogens into very active ones. Inactive or sedentary carcinogens are not much of a problem because they are not activated and leave the other cells alone. But when carcinogens are awakened by G6PDH and NADPH, they become active, and the more active a carcinogen, the more mischief it can inflict on other cells. DHEA prevents cancer by intercepting these cellular wake-up calls.

THE ULTIMATE ANTIOXIDANT

But DHEA may play an even more important role in helping to prevent cancer as well as other diseases. Here's why: NADPH, the enzyme that turns on or awakens carcinogens, is also a key player among a group of enzymes that generate oxygen-activated free radicals. Oxygen is involved in metabolism, the process by which cells make energy. Obviously, oxygen is essential for life, and we cannot live very long without it. In terms of biochemistry, however, oxygen is a double-edged sword. When we produce energy, we also produce free radicals, very unstable atoms whose sole purpose is to bond with other atoms. In the process of uniting with other atoms, these free radicals emit very high quantities of energy that can destroy or damage the cells of the body. Free radicals can damage sensitive cell membranes that protect the cells and then can infiltrate the cell nucleus and damage DNA, our precious genetic material. When DNA is damaged, it can cause the kinds of mutations that trigger irregular cell growth, which in turn can lead to cancer.

You have undoubtedly heard of antioxidants, and some of you are probably already taking antioxidant vitamins and other supplements, such as vitamins C and E and beta-carotene. Melatonin and estrogen, two superhormones that will be discussed later in this book, are also powerful antioxidants. Antioxidants are substances that protect against damage inflicted by free radicals. Free radicals are implicated not only in cancer but in many other diseases as well, including atherosclerosis (hardening of the arteries), inflammation, and autoimmune diseases such as lupus and rheumatoid arthritis. Increasing numbers of researchers are touting free radical damage to key organs as the primary reason we age. I personally don't agree that free radical damage is the sole cause of aging—and believe there are other factors at play—but I do agree that free radicals are a major culprit in the aging process. Antioxidants such as vitamins C and E are free radical scavengers because they mop up free radicals after they are formed and disarm them. There is good reason to believe that DHEA is the ultimate antioxidant because it appears to prevent the formation of free radicals in the first place by, in effect, disarming NADPH before it can generate free radicals. This theory makes a good deal of sense because the body often has backup systems to compensate when one system fails. It seems unlikely that a job as important as fighting free radicals would be relegated to a small group of free radical scavengers that mop up after the fact; the body is too smart for that. There must also be some mechanism to prevent the formation of free radicals early on, and evidence points to DHEA as the chief of the body's "free radical police."

DHEA TO THE TEST

I have been an oncologist for forty years, and during that time we have made tremendous strides in the treatment of certain types of cancers. When I began practicing medicine, leukemia was a fatal diagnosis for children, the odds were heavily against women with breast cancer, and most young men with testicular cancer or people with Hodgkin's disease did not live to see their fortieth birthdays. Thanks to traditional medicine and the research of many dedicated scientists, childhood leukemia is often curable, women who are diagnosed with early breast cancer stand a 90 percent or better chance of survival, and testicular cancer and Hodgkin's disease can now be cured. When it comes to the treatment of cancer, I have been accused of being somewhat of a conservative. I am the last person to recommend experimenting with untried and unproven cancer treatments, and it infuriates me when I hear of patients seeking "alternative" treatments for cancers that I know can be successfully treated with conventional therapy. I think that this is irresponsible and can lead to tragic consequences. Yet I also know from firsthand experience the limitations of modern medicine. Although we have come a long way in treating cancer, much about this disease still eludes us and remains a mystery. We still do not know precisely what causes cancer, and in some cases our standard treatments are harsh, have serious side effects, and fail to work. Regrettably, our track record for treating certain cancers is abysmal. Although I believe we need to do more research on DHEA before we can routinely include it in our arsenal of chemotherapy agents and we need to conduct clinical trials of DHEA against many different forms of cancer to see where it might prove most effective, I see great promise in DHEA for cancer treatment. One of the primary reasons I am writing this book is to spark public and professional interest in this research. Given what we already know about DHEA, however, I feel that physicians should consider it as a cancer treatment especially for people who have not been responsive to conventional chemotherapy.

I myself have tested DHEA as a cancer treatment on both humans and animals with some success. I first used DHEA to treat an intractable tumor on Kitty, our beloved tortoiseshell family cat. Kitty had developed a mast cell sarcoma, a bulging tumor on the orbit of her eye. Although this particular type of cancer does not strike humans, it is the most common cancer among dogs and cats, and is not unlike a human cancer in terms of how it develops and grows. In Kitty's case the tumor was growing rapidly and had spread to the point that her eye was literally being pushed out of its socket. Our veterinarian felt that nothing could be done for Kitty, and he recommended that we put her to sleep. I decided to treat the cat with high doses of DHEA. Within three months the cancer had literally melted away, and the cat was in remarkably good health. Although Kitty died three months later, it was apparent to me that the DHEA treatment had extended her life by close to six months and had improved her overall health.

Encouraged by DHEA's effect on Kitty's cancer, I decided to see what effect, if any, it would have on other veterinarian tumors; this was done in collaboration with Greg MacEwen, D.V.M., now a professor of veterinary medicine at the University of Wisconsin. Similar to what I had seen in Kitty, we observed a significant regression in other mast cell tumors in dogs and cats after they had been put on DHEA. Although we gave the animals very high doses of DHEA, there were no untoward side effects.

Based on the fact that the animals had tolerated such high doses of DHEA, I felt confident that it was safe to use on humans. I decided to test DHEA, in what is called a phase I study, on my advanced patients who had been diagnosed with terminal cancer. The purpose of my study was to determine the optimum dose for humans as well as overall tolerance to the drug. Over the course of two and one-half years I gave nineteen patients extremely high doses of DHEA—up to 40 mg. per kilogram of weight daily in a divided dose. Considering that the average patient weighed between 70 and 80 kg., this was an astonishingly high dose, between 2800 and 3200 mg. daily. In nearly all cases the DHEA was well tolerated, which to me further attested to the safety of this superhormone. Nearly all the patients said they felt better and reported a reduction in fatigue. What was particularly interesting was that the patients with the poorest prognosis—two patients with advanced renal (kidney) cancer, a particularly lethal malignancy—seemed to fare the best. Although these terminal patients had limited life expectancy, DHEA arrested the growth of their cancers. One survived for another two and one-half years; the other lived for another two years without regression but without further growth. The true leavening grace in this is that my patients were in stable condition and out of pain for most of their "borrowed time." Thus, although DHEA may not have "cured" the cancer, it improved the overall physical condition of these patients and greatly enhanced the quality of life they had left.

I am not the only physician who has had some success in treating advanced cancer with DHEA after other conventional treatments have failed. For example, one physician I know has been using DHEA in his practice for several years and recently decided to try it on terminal patients. One such patient, Alex, was an eighty-four-year-old man who had been recently diagnosed with advanced lymphoma. After two treatments of chemotherapy, the cancer had not shown any signs of regression, but the side effects of the chemo were harrowing. Alex had lost feeling in his arm and had developed deafness in one ear. His mouth was so swollen he couldn't eat. He was in pain and was so weak that he could barely move. All this was a tremendous blow to the once vigorous, active man. "The chemo therapy," Alex recalls, "nearly killed me. I said, 'Enough.' " That was when he went to see a physician who was traditionally trained but practices a combination of conventional and alternative medicine. Alex remembers that at their first meeting he told his new doctor, "I have lumps all over my body. They've given up on me. I think I'm dying."

The new physician prescribed DHEA along with antioxidants. The results have been impressive. Today Alex says, "I'm more energetic. I'm no longer in pain. Although I can't go running anymore, I can still walk. I can shovel snow, and I can cut wood. I'm not quite my old self—now I have to use an electric saw—but I'm feeling much better."

Granted, these are anecdotal reports, and the effectiveness of DHEA as a cancer treatment has not yet been evaluated in rigorous clinical studies. Nevertheless, I believe there is a large and credible body of evidence that suggests DHEA may be a useful cancer treatment in combination with traditional chemotherapy. I hope by writing this book to succeed in fueling interest in this type of research and to get DHEA and other potential lifesaving treatments into clinical trials where they can be properly investigated.

DHEA: The Heart-Healthy Hormone

At the turn of the century the average life span was 49 and the most common cause of death was from infection. Thanks to the discovery of antibiotics and vaccines, death by infection is now rare. The average life span has increased by more than thirty years, which is certainly something to cheer about. Yet it is important to note that despite these advances, few of us reach our maximum potential life span of 120 years, because most of us are struck down earlier by one or another of the illnesses of aging.

More often than not, the disease that stops us in our tracks is heart disease. More than any other disease, heart disease can cut life short and is the number one killer of both men and women. In fact, according to the American Heart Association, if heart disease was eliminated, total life expectancy would rise by nearly ten years! Not only that, heart disease can rob us of the kind of quality of life that makes our extended life span worth living. The good news—and there is good news—is that I believe it is possible to remain free of heart disease. In order to achieve this goal, however, we are going to have to radically change our approach to treating heart disease. Instead of waiting for the disease to strike and treating the symptoms, as we do now, we must focus instead on what is happening within our bodies that creates the environment in which this disease is allowed to take hold in the first place.

I am convinced that the decline in DHEA and other superhormones is a key factor in the progression of heart disease. Within the past decade there has been some compelling evidence, albeit circumstantial, that DHEA—or, more precisely, a lack of it—is a major factor in the onset of atherosclerosis. I do not mean to suggest that DHEA is a cure for heart disease, but what many other researchers and I now believe is that the age-related decline in DHEA levels creates an environment in which heart disease is permitted to take hold. This is yet another example of how DHEA functions as a buffer hormone, helping our bodies to maintain normalcy, and demonstrating how, when our DHEA levels decline, "abnormal" events that trigger the disease process begin to occur.

To prevent yourself from becoming a victim of heart disease, you need to know something about how a healthy heart becomes a diseased heart. When we use the term "heart disease," we are actually referring to atherosclerotic disease, or atherosclerosis, a disease in which the arteries delivering blood to the heart become narrowed or blocked entirely. (Atherosclerosis is sometimes referred to as coronary artery disease, or CAD.) The flow of blood is blocked by deposits of plaque, a thick, yellowish, waxy substance that consists of a variety of cells that includes cholesterol, which is a type of fat produced by the liver and can produce blood clots. If the heart is deprived of blood, heart muscle will die, resulting in a heart attack.

What makes atherosclerosis such a deadly threat is that despite decades of research, we still do not fully understand what causes it, and we do not have any "magic bullets" to treat it. Most researchers believe that atherosclerosis is caused by a combination of factors, including diet, a genetic predisposition to develop the disease, and lifestyle. For example, we know that people who smoke are more likely to develop atherosclerosis and that obesity and diabetes substantially increase the odds that someone will die from a heart attack.

We also know that atherosclerosis is very much a disease of aging. With each decade of life past fifty, the odds of developing it increase exponentially. In fact, one out of two Americans will die from heart disease. This is true for both men and women. Although men typically suffer heart attacks earlier than women, once women hit menopause, they quickly catch up to men, and heart disease becomes the leading cause of death for both sexes.

Why does the risk of heart disease increase so dramatically with age? What role does DHEA play in protecting us against heart disease? The relationship between falling DHEA levels and heart disease has been debated for more than forty years. As far back as the 1950s a lone researcher reported a puzzling finding: People with heart disease had lower levels of DHEA. Several studies have shown that levels of DHEA are indeed lower in people with heart disease, and the connection between low DHEA and heart disease is a particularly strong one for men.

What is especially interesting about the way DHEA functions vis-à-vis the heart is that it does not protect us in one specific way but rather appears to shield us in many different ways, each of which I will explain in some detail.

The insulin connection One of the main points of this book is that superhormones such as DHEA do not operate in a vacuum; they interact with or regulate one another and also other hormones. As levels of superhormones drop, the role and influence of these other hormones may change, often with detrimental effects on our health. The critical relationship between DHEA and insulin is a prime example of this process, because it demonstrates how a decline in DHEA allows a life-sustaining hormone, insulin, to become a potentially lethal one, especially for our hearts.

Insulin is a hormone that is secreted in the pancreas (a gland below and in back of the stomach and the liver) by special cells called the islets of Langerhans. Insulin is essential for regulating the body's metabolism of sugars and starches. It breaks down sugar or glucose so it can be utilized by the body's cells. The inability to produce enough insulin can lead to diabetes, a disease characterized by excess sugar in the blood or the urine.

There are two types of diabetes. *Type I Diabetes* (also called *juve-*

nile diabetes) typically occurs during childhood. Type I diabetes is caused by a failure of the pancreas to produce enough insulin, and people with this disease must take supplemental insulin by injection. *Type II Diabetes* (also called *adult-onset diabetes*) is the most common form of this disease. It is not caused by a lack of insulin; paradoxically, there is more than enough insulin to go around. The problem is that the insulin works less efficiently and does not break down sugar as fast as it should. As a result, blood sugar levels rise as they would in Type I diabetes. Because the body has become resistant to the action of insulin, Type II diabetes is sometimes referred to as *insulin resistance*. Type II diabetes can often be treated through weight loss and diet. Patients are typically put on low-fat, high-carbohydrate diets. Sometimes Type II patients are given oral medication or insulin to control blood sugar surges.

Some 14 million Americans have some clear-cut form of diabetes, and 85 percent of all cases occur in people who are thirty-five or older. The older we are, the greater are our odds of getting Type II diabetes. Although Type II diabetes is not life-threatening per se, it is a major risk factor for atherosclerosis and high blood pressure, two potential killers, and should not be taken lightly. High blood levels of insulin pose a particular risk for children and young adults. According to the famous Bogalusa Heart Study, a twenty-two-year examination of heart and blood vessel disease risk factors, chronically elevated insulin levels (a sign of insulin resistance) from childhood through adulthood greatly increased the risk of developing heart disease, high blood pressure, high cholesterol, kidney damage, obesity, and other serious health problems. In fact, the Bogalusa researchers say that a diagnosis of high insulin, standing alone with no other risk factors, is reason enough to begin medical treatment for diabetes early in life.

Although we do not fully understand why insulin resistance is a risk factor for heart disease, we do know that the condition itself can have devastating effects on blood vessels. For example, under normal conditions insulin helps dilate or relax blood vessels, improving the flow of blood through the body. When people are insulin-resistant, however, their blood vessels are more prone to spasm; that is, they may suddenly constrict, inhibiting blood flow and increasing the risk of heart attack or ischemic injury to lower extremities. Interestingly, women are twice as likely to develop diabetes as men and are also more prone to suffer from arterial spasms.

There also appears to be a direct relationship between insulin resistance and blood vessel obstruction due to plaque formation, and this, too, may be due to insulin's effect on blood vessels. A blood vessel is much more than a hose through which blood flows passively; it is also a pump that must actively push the blood through the body. Thus, it needs to be elastic enough to have some flexibility. Insulin resistance appears to stiffen blood vessels. This not only interferes with the blood vessels' ability to pump blood but can actually injure the vessels. Such injury to blood vessel linings may be the first step in the very complicated and lethal process by which artery-clogging plaque and blood clots are formed.

Insulin resistance does even more damage to tiny blood vessels, called capillaries, which deliver blood to the peripheral (outer) tissues of the body. Insulin resistance appears to inhibit the growth of capillaries, reducing the blood supply and resulting in serious conditions such as peripheral neuropathy, or nerve damage, to the extremities (legs, hands, and feet).

Clearly, insulin resistance is a potentially serious problem that under certain circumstances can be disastrous. In fact, if we could prevent insulin resistance, it would probably result in a significant decline in deaths from heart disease. We know that maintaining youthful weight and avoiding obesity helps control insulin resistance. There is also compelling evidence that DHEA plays a role in controlling the ill effects of insulin. My colleague Dr. John Nestler at the Medical College of Virginia has reported that the levels of DHEA and insulin are inversely related; that is, as one goes up, the other goes down. As we age, our levels of DHEA naturally decline and our levels of insulin rise. Dr. Nestler has proposed an intriguing theory. He suggests that the age-related rise in insulin actually causes the decline in DHEA. Thus, if we can treat insulin resistance at its earliest stages, we may be able to restore DHEA to youthful levels.

Furthermore, Dr. Nestler suggests that DHEA may be the "missing link" between insulin resistance and atherosclerosis. He believes that the decline in DHEA may precipitate the damage to the cardiovascular system that leads to heart disease. In clinical studies Dr. Nestler gave insulin-resistant men medication to normalize their insulin and lower blood sugar. After taking the drug, the men experienced a marked increase in DHEA levels, confirming that there is an inverse relationship between these two hormones.

I find Dr. Nestler's work fascinating, and I would take his findings one step further. It seems logical to me that DHEA must somehow buffer or shield us from the harmful effects of insulin, and as we age and our DHEA levels drop, the balance between these two hormones is upset, and insulin is allowed to do its damage, thereby increasing our vulnerability to Type II diabetes.

This is not just speculation on my part. There is strong evidence that DHEA plays a protective role against diabetes, which is a primary risk factor for heart disease. For example, as far back as 1983, Les Coleman, Ph.D., of the Jackson Laboratories in Bar Harbor, Maine, at my urging, tested DHEA on mice that were specially bred to develop diabetes. Despite a strong genetic predisposition to develop both diabetes and obesity, these mice remained free of diabetes and maintained their normal weight. This and other experiments like it tell us that DHEA could be a potent tool in the prevention of diabetes. (In the bibliography on DHEA, I include several studies that further document DHEA's potential as a treatment or preventive agent against diabetes.)

As you will see, a number of other researchers have shown that DHEA has a beneficial effect on many different aspects of the cardiovascular system and appears to correct the types of problems that may be caused by insulin resistance and injury to blood vessels. There are also other factors at play that can injure blood vessels, as I will address next.

PREVENTS "STICKY BLOOD"

Platelets are the particles in blood responsible for the formation of blood clots. Platelets are Mother Nature's version of the Band-Aid. When we are injured, platelets rush to the site of injury and clump together to form a protective covering to stop the bleeding. Platelets perform an important job. If we did not have functioning platelets, we would bleed to death. Overzealous platelets, however, can also cause real problems. In fact, some people have "sticky" blood, which tends to form excess clots that can lodge in arteries, blocking the flow of blood through the body. Many of these people must take blood thinners such as Coumadin or aspirin.

Out-of-control platelets may also be a primary cause of the formation of plaque deposits. As mentioned earlier, no one knows precisely what causes plaque deposits to form, but there are some likely explanations. Many scientists believe in the injury response theory, that is, that plaque begins to grow when injury occurs in the inner layers of an arterial wall. If you sliced open an artery, you would see layers of concentric circles, similar to those of an onion. The inner core of the artery through which the blood flows is called the lumen. The lumen is surrounded by the endothelium, a thin lining of protective cells. According to the injury response theory, atherosclerosis begins when an injury occurs to the precious endothelium. In this context, injury is defined rather liberally to mean any "insult" that could affect cell function. For example, as mentioned earlier, an excess amount of oxidized fat in the bloodstream could "injure" the cell by upsetting the normal chemical balance in the body. As explained earlier, many researchers also believe that high insulin levels somehow "injure" the artery wall. Usually, the endothelium (cell lining) is able to heal itself, but if the injury is severe, other cells from the area race in to fill the damaged site. Sometimes a cellular riot ensues, with cells pouring madly onto the scene. Platelets are quickly dispersed to the area and release a substance that causes them to stick together and form a blood clot. Other factors, including cholesterol, smooth muscle cells, and foam cells, join the commotion and become part of what grows into a thickened plaque deposit. If a piece of plaque breaks off, it can lodge in an artery leading to the heart, causing a heart attack, or in an artery leading to the brain, causing a stroke.

Both test tube and human studies have shown that DHEA can prevent the formation of such life-threatening blood clots. In one study, at my medical school, the Medical College of Virginia, platelets derived from human blood were put into a test tube, and a substance that promotes platelets to stick together was added. Under normal conditions the platelets would form a clot, but when DHEA was added to the test tube, the platelets proved much less likely to clump together. In a second study, patients who suffered from clotting problems were given DHEA. When researchers then examined the patients' blood, they found a significant decline in their propensity to form blood clots. By preventing excess blood clot formation, DHEA may protect against both heart disease and stroke.

Lowers Cholesterol

Cholesterol is a type of fat produced in the liver and found in certain foods, primarily animal products. Our bodies can convert fat, particularly saturated animal fat, into cholesterol. Cholesterol is not all

bad; in fact, it is from cholesterol that all our superhormones, including DHEA, are made. Nor is all cholesterol the same. There are two
types of cholesterol: LDL (low density lipoproteins) and HDL (high
density lipoproteins). LDL is the body's major carrier of cholesterol
in the bloodstream. Excess blood levels of LDL are believed to be a
major factor in the formation of plaque. HDL is known as the good
cholesterol because it transports excess cholesterol from the blood to
the liver and intestines where it can be excreted from the body.

Although cholesterol is essential for the normal functioning of our
bodies, high levels of cholesterol can be dangerous. Several studies
have shown a direct connection between elevated cholesterol levels
and heart disease. Organizations such as the American Heart Association therefore recommend that we try to maintain cholesterol levels
of 200 milligrams per deciliter and lower. As your doctor has probably told you, it is also important to try to maintain a good ratio
between total cholesterol and HDL. For example, if total cholesterol
is 240, HDL should be 40 or more.

Lowering elevated cholesterol levels is not so easy. Reducing your
intake of saturated fat and cholesterol-rich foods can help, but very
often medication or other supplements (such as niacin or newer cholesterol-lowering drugs like lovastatin) may be required, particularly
if there are other factors involved that increase the risk of developing
heart disease. Since many of the medications used to lower cholesterol have potentially serious side effects, the discovery of a substance
that can safely and effectively reduce cholesterol is an important one.
DHEA is such a substance. In the 1980s I was medical advisor to a
study in which DHEA was administered to postmenopausal women
to determine its effect on blood cholesterol levels. After menopause,
women's cholesterol levels tend to rise, and so does their risk of
having a heart attack. (In fact, by the time a woman is sixty-five, she
is at equal risk with men for having a heart attack!) After three
months of taking DHEA, the women in our study showed an 8 to 10
percent decline in total cholesterol levels, which is quite significant
given the fact that for every 1 percent drop in cholesterol, there is a
2 percent drop in the risk of developing heart disease. Other studies
have since confirmed our findings.

Why does DHEA lower cholesterol? One likely reason is that
DHEA enhances the ability of the liver to utilize or dispose of lipids,
which means that less cholesterol is released throughout the body.
Another reason could be that DHEA is an antioxidant, as explained
below.

ANTIOXIDANT ACTION

Previously, when DHEA's role as the ultimate anticarcinogen was discussed, I explained how DHEA helps protect cells against damage inflicted by free radicals, those highly unstable oxygen molecules that destroy cell membranes and damage DNA. Free radicals are not only implicated in cancer but also appear to play a significant role in heart disease. Here's how: Free radicals are believed to damage LDL, the so-called bad cholesterol. Such "injured" LDL attracts other cells, known as scavenger cells, which gobble it up and form what we call foam cells, and these begin the formation of plaque in the artery. DHEA appears to stop this insidious process in its earliest stages by blocking the enzyme sequence that triggers the formation of these troublesome free radicals. Once again, this is a prime example of a superhormone preventing the onset of disease by intercepting it at its earliest stage, long before the disease can take hold.

There is yet another important way that DHEA can save us from heart disease, and this is by controlling obesity, a major risk factor for both heart disease and stroke.

Fighting Fat

Our goal is to help people enjoy a bowl of low-fat salad with the same gusto as a heaping plate of high-fat french fries.

—DR. FRANK SVEC, Louisiana State University

Weight "creep" is one of the biggest problems of middle age and beyond. Each year most of us gain girth, and as the years go by, it becomes increasingly difficult to take off the excess baggage. Our metabolism slows down, and as a result we don't require as much food as we did when we were young, yet few of us actually cut back. Whether we like it or not, the pounds begin to accumulate. The result is that the flabby, out-of-condition, out-of-shape body is what has become the norm for aging. I can't help but think that this is very sad. Our physical appearance goes to the very core of our self-esteem, and it is extremely difficult to feel good about yourself if you do not look good. And this is true for both men and women.

Many of us spend the second half of our lives trying to recapture our sleek physiques. Many of us even manage to shed a few pounds from time to time. No matter what method we use to take the weight off, however, the risks of gaining it back are high. As many as 90 percent of all dieters regain the lost weight within a year. Clearly, losing weight and keeping it off is a complicated process, about which there is still much to learn. One of the most intriguing and promising areas of research deals with the effect of hormones, especially DHEA, on appetite and weight loss. Combined with other medications and weight loss strategies, DHEA appears to be a formidable weapon in the ongoing battle of the bulge.

In 1977 DHEA's role as a "fat fighter" made headlines when a pharmaceutical company researcher discovered that DHEA could literally melt fat off obese mice. What was particularly interesting about this study was that it showed DHEA could produce weight loss even if the mice did not reduce their food intake. In other words, DHEA appeared to have an effect on metabolism, the process by which the body converts food into energy. The prospect of a pill that could "up regulate" or turn up metabolism was so tantalizing that it attracted the attention of other scientists, including Dr. Greg Mac-Ewen at the University of Wisconsin. Dr. MacEwen knew that humans were not the only species that had difficulty maintaining their weight; obesity is also a big problem for dogs that can cause serious health problems. Like humans, many dogs simply do not know when to stop eating and will gobble up whatever food their owners give them—and more if they can get it. Also, like humans, for many overweight dogs, losing weight can be a slow and difficult process, especially as they get older. Dr. MacEwen decided to test the effect of DHEA on obese dogs. In the first experiment he gave a group of obese dogs a very high dose of DHEA supplement and allowed them to eat their usual diet. At the end of three months, two-thirds of the dogs showed significant weight loss (in addition to a reduction in their cholesterol levels). One-third of the dogs showed no change at all. In a second study, Dr. MacEwen put two groups of obese dogs on a reduced-calorie diet. One group was given a DHEA supplement, and the other group was given a placebo. At the end of three months he found the dogs that were given the DHEA lost 10.7 percent of their excess weight per month. The dogs that were given the placebo lost only 5.5 percent of their excess weight per month. In other words, the dogs on DHEA had double the weight loss of the untreated dogs, indicating that diet alone was not solely responsible for the weight loss.

Curiously, Dr. MacEwen found that a small group of dogs, about

10 percent of the total, did not respond to the DHEA/diet regimen. No matter what they ate or did, their weight remained stable. Notably, all of these unresponsive dogs were considered "morbidly obese." Obesity is said to begin at 20 percent above ideal body weight; these dogs exceeded their ideal body weight by more than 40 percent. The fact that these dogs were unresponsive to DHEA could indicate that the factors at play in cases of morbid obesity are different from those in "normal" obesity and that significant alterations in hormonal interactions either contribute to the onset of morbid obesity or just make it more difficult to treat. This finding also strongly suggests that obesity—in either dogs or humans—may not be one disease but may be the result of many different biochemical abnormalities. Perhaps that is why one treatment approach does not work for everybody.

Despite the failure of DHEA to help that small group of morbidly obese dogs, the majority did lose significant amounts of weight. How does DHEA stimulate weight loss? It appears to have several effects on metabolism that could explain how it enhances the body's ability to shed pounds and, more important, keep them off.

DHEA Turns Up the Heat

From many different studies we know that DHEA can trigger weight loss even if diet remains the same, although weight loss is most dramatic if DHEA is used in conjunction with a low-calorie diet. Still, the fact that weight loss was achieved even when diet was not changed clearly demonstrates that food intake alone does not determine DHEA's effectiveness as a weight reduction tool. Many scientists have come to believe that DHEA has an enhancing effect on the way the body breaks down and utilizes food. Although it may strike you as counterintuitive, DHEA may actually make the body less efficient in energy conservation, and here's why, in this particular case, less is better. When it comes to weight loss, we humans are often working at odds with nature. From nature's point of view, survival often depends on an animal's ability to endure periods of famine. We convert food into energy, and we measure in terms of calories the energy we derive from food. Food is not always plentiful for many species (and, sadly, even for some humans); thus nature has designed us to run on as little energy (or few calories) as possible. We humans, however, typically eat much more food than necessary to keep our bodies running. The excess caloric intake is converted into stored fat, and fat is what puts on extra pounds. In order not to gain weight, we must burn up those extra calories before our body turns them into fat. That is why very active people can eat vast quantities of food and stay slim, and why sedentary people need to watch every calorie.

When we metabolize, or break down, food, our body burns energy in the process—it is the fuel that helps keep the body running. From nature's perspective it is beneficial to metabolize food as efficiently as possible. This means that nature wants us to utilize as little energy or fuel as possible so that we store the excess energy (calories) as fat in preparation for the next period of famine. DHEA appears to alter this equation; it makes the body burn more energy to do the same work, thus metabolizing or utilizing the food that would be converted into fat and result in a weight gain. In other words, in order to perform a given task, the body needs to burn up many more calories. Clearly, this is a less efficient way to operate, but it is a wonderful way to get rid of excess calories.

BLOCKS FAT FORMATION

Other scientists explain DHEA's effect on weight loss in a completely different way. They believe DHEA may actually block the formation of fatty acids that are stored as fat in our bodies. The process by which the body makes fat is a complicated cascade of biochemical events that involves many different enzymatic reactions. Somewhere along this complex trail, DHEA may block the action of a particular enzyme, inhibiting the synthesis of fat. DHEA's blocking the production of fat could explain why animals were able to lose weight even though they were eating the same amount of food.

EATING LESS AND LIKING IT

Perhaps the most interesting effect of DHEA on weight loss is its effect on appetite. DHEA appears to be a natural appetite suppressant. It does this by altering the brain's hunger signaling system (the brain's satiety center) so that an animal reaches its satiation point after eating less food. Not only that, DHEA seems to lessen an animal's desire to eat one particular type of calorie-laden food—fat. Since fat has more than double the calories per gram than protein or carbohydrates (fat has 9 calories per gram versus 4 calories per gram for protein or carbohydrate), a lower fat diet would naturally result in a loss of weight.

Some of the most interesting studies on DHEA, fat intake, and weight control are being performed in the laboratory of researchers Frank Svec and John Porter at Louisiana State University. Drs. Svec and Porter devised an experiment to test the effect of DHEA on food selection of the Zucker rat, a breed that if left to its own devices would eat a diet that was 50 percent fat or more. Drs. Svec and Porter developed three different rat chows with varying amounts of fat, protein, and carbohydrate. One chow contained 90 percent fat, 5 percent carbohydrate, and 5 percent protein. The second chow contained 90 percent protein, 5 percent fat, and 5 percent carbohydrate. The third, of course, contained 90 percent carbohydrate, 5 percent fat, and 5 percent protein. A group of Zucker rats was given the option to feed from any of the three chows. Under normal circumstances the Zucker rats would opt for the chow with the highest fat content. When given DHEA, however, the rats not only ate less food in general but showed a marked preference for the lower-calorie, carbohydrate-rich chow. In other words, even though they could eat whatever they wanted, the rats had actually developed a preference for less food and less fat!

Can DHEA do the same for humans? The high-fat diet typical of many Americans has been implicated as a risk factor for many serious diseases, including heart disease, diabetes, and cancer. Getting Americans to reduce their fat intake even slightly could have a profound impact on their overall health. In this regard, the results of laboratory studies with DHEA and weight loss are very promising. What makes DHEA so unique as a "fat fighter" is that unlike so-called diet pills that offer at best a temporary solution to weight loss by dampening appetite but not changing eating habits, DHEA has the potential to offer a long-term solution to obesity in that it not only quells appetite but appears actually to change food preferences. DHEA could be the tool that helps overweight people take off the weight and keep it off permanently.

The only stumbling block to using DHEA as a weight control agent is that the dose required to achieve weight loss in animals was extremely high, and we prefer to use lower doses of DHEA in people, more in keeping with our natural DHEA levels. But that problem is not insurmountable, and I believe it may soon be overcome. For DHEA to be used as a human weight reduction tool, it would have to be effective in lower doses, and that could be achieved by combining it with another drug that would synergize or enhance its action. That is precisely the approach that Drs. Svec and Porter are taking in their latest studies. They have tested DHEA in conjunction with a clinically available antidepressant (fenfluramine) that has also been used with some success as a weight reduction aid. Similar to a better known drug, Prozac, fenfluramine is a serotonin re-uptake inhibitor, a class of drugs which has a distinct effect on the brain centers that control appetite and satiety. Fenfluramine has been shown not only to reduce food intake but to actually reduce the desire for carbohydrates.

The problem with fenfluramine is that although it initially causes weight loss, patients quickly develop a tolerance for it, rendering the drug ineffective. In addition, fenfluramine may be habit forming, and the FDA does not allow it to be prescribed long-term. (The FDA prohibition may soon end, however. There will soon be available a new and more biologically active form of fenfluramine called deoxy-fenfluramine that is believed to be both safe and effective.)

Drs. Svec and Porter wondered whether DHEA and fenfluramine could pick up where the other had left off; that is, they wondered whether DHEA could enhance the action of fenfluramine, extending the period that it is effective, and whether fenfluramine could enhance the activity of DHEA so that it would be effective in lower doses. They repeated their initial study with obese Zucker rats, allowing the rats to choose freely among the high-fat, high-protein, and high-carbohydrate foods. This time, however, one group of rats was given a combination of a low dose of DHEA and fenfluramine. Another group of rats (the control group) was given no drugs and was also allowed to eat freely from any of the three bowls. The results were remarkable. The control rats gained 30 percent more body weight during the study, but the rats on the drugs dropped 20 percent of their body weight. The animals on DHEA and fenfluramine did not develop a tolerance to their weight loss cocktail and continued to lose weight for the entire twenty-eight days of the study. "As long as we gave them the drugs, the animals had dramatic weight loss," reported Dr. Svec, who added that although the rats had stopped eating, sometimes for days, they appeared to be healthy and energetic.

Having documented the dramatic effect of DHEA and fenfluramine, Drs. Svec and Porter said that their next task is to identify the precise mechanism which makes the combination work. They will be looking at how DHEA and fenfluramine affect the neurotransmitters in the hypothalamus, the brain center that controls appetite. The answer may pave the way to a similar treatment for humans. "Our interest is finding out what goes on in the brain that makes it change its food selection and food amount," said Dr. Svec.

What is particularly interesting about this approach is that it targets a major and seemingly intractable problem confronting most dieters. Even though they may lose weight while they are adhering to a strict calorie-controlled diet, restricted diets cause boredom and the temptation to revert to old eating habits. Thus, it is almost a foregone conclusion that a dieter will eventually regain lost weight. "The trouble with the standard diet and exercise approach," noted Dr. Svec, "is that although it does help to keep weight down, people still want to eat. There is something pleasurable about eating. The combination of DHEA and fenfluramine worked for the Zucker rat. They could eat all the fat they wanted, but they didn't want to. We can't answer all the questions at once, but if the DHEA and fenfluramine combination does influence food intake and if we can find a way of amplifying and zeroing in on excessive food intake, we would really have something unique and exciting."

How exciting? "Our hope is that one day if you take DHEA and fenfluramine, you might be able to go over to the salad bar and actually like the salad and not even want the rich dressing on top!"

Of Special Interest to Women

SUPERHORMONE THERAPY FOR MENOPAUSE

Menopause is a time when women often feel that they are mere bystanders as their hormones rage out of control, wreaking havoc on their bodies. Many women feel as if they are hapless victims of a biological event that is completely out of their hands. That is why there is no better time in a woman's life for her to take command of the situation.

It is imperative for every woman to understand what menopause is about, and its potential impact on her health and emotional well-being. From this knowledge she and her doctor can design a super-hormone program tailored to her individual needs. Taking a proactive stance can make a real difference between feeling hopeless and helpless, or feeling hopeful and very much in control, not just of menopause but of the entire aging process. The subject of menopause will be covered in greater detail in the chapters on estrogen and progesterone. Here, however, I want to tell you about an exciting new breakthrough in the use of DHEA for postmenopausal women that warrants discussion.

Among the questions I am most frequently asked is whether postmenopausal women can turn to DHEA instead of the typical estrogen/progesterone combination now used. More specifically, women want to know:

- Does DHEA offer the same benefits as estrogen, without some of the negative side effects?
- Can DHEA prevent osteoporosis, a serious disease in which bone becomes brittle and thin, leaving it vulnerable to fracture? (Osteoporosis tends to strike after menopause and is believed to be caused by the loss of female hormones.)
- Can DHEA protect women against heart disease?
- Will DHEA help relieve some of the unpleasant symptoms of menopause, such as hot flashes and vaginal atrophy, which can be very painful?

For several decades DHEA, marketed under the name of prasterone, has been used in Europe to treat menopause-related depression. In Italy a combination of estrogen and DHEA, known as astenile, is being used to treat hot flashes and other forms of menopausal discomfort. To those of us who have been studying DHEA's properties, it makes perfect sense that DHEA would be a useful treatment for menopause because DHEA is an estrogen precursor. This means that DHEA is converted to estrogen in the body. After menopause, when the ovaries stop making estrogen, small amounts of estrogen continue to be manufactured in the adrenal glands from hormones, including DHEA. Supplementing DHEA in postmenopausal women therefore appears to be a way of increasing estrogen levels naturally. Not only that, DHEA has some unique properties of its own that make it a boon for postmenopausal women.

My wife, Sylvia, who began taking DHEA several years before menopause and who has been taking it for sixteen years, chose not to use estrogen replacement therapy after she became menopausal. She never needed to. Sylvia has never had a hot flash, nor has she experienced any of the normal discomfort associated with the loss of estrogen. Although osteoporosis runs in her family, she stands straight and tall, and does not suffer from this disease. Sylvia credits

DHEA with helping her make menopause what she coolly refers to as a "nonevent" in her life.

Several clinical studies of DHEA's potential as a substitute for estrogen replacement therapy are now under way, and several that have been completed have produced positive results. Preliminary findings indicate that DHEA offers many of the same benefits of estrogen without many of the potentially harmful side effects. Although DHEA may not do everything that estrogen does, it does do a lot in terms of relieving menopausal symptoms and protecting against disease, and it may even offer a few benefits that estrogen does not.

At a recent meeting on DHEA in Quebec City, Canada, Dr. Pierre Diamond reported on a study he conducted at Le Centre Hospitalier de l'Université Laval. In his study, Dr. Diamond gave DHEA replacement therapy to twenty postmenopausal women, aged sixty to seventy, for a year. None of these women was taking estrogen. DHEA was administered in the form of a cream that the women applied daily. The women's blood levels were measured periodically to ensure that DHEA had been restored to twenty-year-old levels. After a year on DHEA, the women, without their knowledge, were switched to a placebo.

According to Dr. Diamond, during the period that the women were taking DHEA, they showed significant improvement in several key areas. Nearly all the women reported an increase in energy and an improvement in general well-being. Dr. Diamond also detected some important physical changes during the period of time the women were on DHEA, including the following:

1. He observed a reduction in both blood insulin and glucose (sugar) levels, reinforcing our belief that DHEA has a positive effect on insulin resistance. Since insulin resistance is a risk factor for heart disease, this suggests that DHEA shields postmenopausal women from heart disease, the number one killer of postmenopausal women.
2. Although the women's weight remained the same, they did show a change in "body mass index," the ratio of fat to muscle. Their levels of fat decreased, and their levels of muscle increased.
3. Typically, during the decade after menopause, women begin to lose roughly 2 to 4 percent of their bone mass each year. As a result of this bone loss, many women suffer from hip and spinal

fractures. The good news is that while the women were taking DHEA, they showed a marked increase in bone density. In fact, after a year on DHEA, the average bone mass density of the women was increased at the hip and spine, two sites that are particularly vulnerable to osteoporosis.

4. DHEA produced a modest drop in blood cholesterol of 3 to 10 percent in the women. In this context, modest does not mean insignificant: Even a modest drop in cholesterol can offer a significant reduction in heart disease.

5. At least half the women in the study had suffered from vaginal atrophy, that is, a thinning of the vaginal wall (the endothelium), which occurs commonly after menopause, and a reduction in the production of vaginal secretions that lubricate the vagina. These changes not only produce discomfort but they also promote vaginal infections and can make intercourse painful. Estrogen taken orally, or an estrogen cream applied directly to the vagina, can help relieve this problem, and it appears that DHEA may also be a good remedy. Eight of the women with vaginal atrophy showed a marked improvement after taking DHEA, and, indeed, DHEA did appear to stimulate growth of the vaginal endothelium and increase vaginal secretions, thus restoring the vagina to its youthful condition.

As an oncologist, what I find even more interesting was what DHEA *did not* do: Although DHEA did stimulate growth of the vaginal lining, it did not stimulate the growth of the uterine lining. In this regard, DHEA offers a distinct advantage over estrogen replacement therapy. Remember, estrogen is the hormone that stimulates the monthly buildup of tissue on the lining of the uterus to ready it to receive a fertilized egg in the event of pregnancy. When a woman is still menstruating, the hormone progesterone triggers the sloughing off of this tissue, which is expelled during menstruation. When a woman is postmenopausal, however, and no longer has a monthly progesterone surge, this excess tissue builds up on the uterine lining and can turn cancerous. That is why postmenopausal women on estrogen who have not had hysterectomies are usually also given synthetic progesterone (progestin), the hormone that stimulates the monthly menstrual flow. As a result, these women experience regular monthly bleeding, much the same as they do during the menstrual cycle. In fact, many women stop taking hormones because they do not want to have monthly cycles. Other women find that the progestin makes them moody and produces many of the symptoms associated with premenstrual syndrome (PMS) such as bloating and irritability. Researchers at major pharmaceutical companies are racing to find a safe form of estrogen that offers all its positive effects without stimulating the growth of uterine tissue, thus eliminating the need for progestin. If such an estrogen were developed, many more women would undoubtedly be eager to try it. (I discuss this in more detail in the section of the book entitled "The New Estrogens" in chapter 5.) Interestingly, DHEA appears to offer many of the benefits of estrogen, but without producing the unwanted effect on the uterus. In fact, the only negative side effect recorded by Dr. Diamond was that a few patients had some very mild facial blemishes which were treated successfully with a topical cream.

I am particularly intrigued by Dr. Diamond's findings on bone, which clearly demonstrate that DHEA can help preserve bone mass. Dr. Diamond's study is the first to test and establish this effect on postmenopausal women, and his results are consistent with the findings of other researchers. For example, Dr. Raymond Daynes (whose work is described in the section of this chapter on DHEA and the immune system) demonstrated that DHEA reduces the levels of IL 6, a hormone believed to stimulate the activity of osteoclasts, special cells that cause the breakdown of bone. When we are young, we produce new bone faster than our old bone is broken down. Thus, our bones remain strong. As we age, however, bone is broken down faster than we can replace it, and our bones grow weaker. By inhibiting IL 6, DHEA may be blocking this destructive process.

Other fascinating DHEA/osteoporosis studies are currently under way that may help us to better understand the complex relationship between hormones and bone. One of the most innovative is being performed at Brigham and Women's Hospital at Harvard Medical School by Dr. Julie Golwacki. Dr. Golwacki explains that all women experience a decline in estrogen as they age, and yet all women do not get osteoporosis. Dr. Golwacki believes that the decline in estrogen is not the sole reason women get osteoporosis but that other factors are at work. She hypothesizes that there may be a difference in the hormone content of the bone marrow of women who are prone to develop osteoporosis and women who don't. Here is why: When you think of estrogen, you probably think of the hormone produced by the ovaries in women, but, in fact, estrogen can be produced in other sites of the body outside of the reproductive system called the peripheral tissue. Some researchers believe that estrogen produced by peripheral tissue is actually safer than estrogen produced by the reproductive organs because it does not enter the bloodstream and circulate throughout the body. Rather, it stays locally in the tissue in which it is produced. The bone marrow may be a site where estrogen is produced, at least in some women and perhaps even in some men.

In her study, Dr. Golwacki is taking bone marrow samples from women who are undergoing orthopedic surgery for noninflammatory conditions, that is, for breaks and fractures typical of osteoporosis. She is testing the marrow for, among other things, levels of key hormones, including DHEA (which, as we have seen, is converted to estrogen in women). Her purpose is to determine if women with osteoporosis have lower than normal hormone levels in their marrow. If DHEA proves to be a factor in the production of estrogen in the bone marrow, then DHEA may actually turn out to be as effective as estrogen in the treatment of osteoporosis and perhaps be even better, because it may trigger the production of estrogen at precisely the site where it is needed.

DRY SKIN

There are certain age-related changes in our bodies that, though not life threatening, can seriously interfere with the quality of our lives. One of these problems is dry skin. As we age, our skin becomes dry, itchy, and flaky. Dry skin can afflict men and women, but it is particularly common among women past menopause. Scores of creams on the market that are designed to ameliorate the annoying symptoms of dry skin, but none gets to the cause of the problem. Dry skin is actually a result of a drop in the production of sebum, an oily substance produced by special glands in the skin known as the sebaceous glands. Sebum lubricates the skin. Renowned dermatologist and researcher Dr. Norman Orentreich has shown that the function of sebaceous glands is directly linked to DHEA levels. Our sebaceous glands produce huge quantities of sebum when our DHEA levels rise during puberty. (As a matter of fact, excess sebum can result in acne, a problem typical of adolescence.) Then, as our DHEA levels drop, sebum production falls off, and our skin gets dryer.

Dr. Orentreich has also shown that replenishing DHEA levels (via oral supplements or a skin cream) can restore oil gland activity, returning sebum production to more youthful levels. The effect is to "plump up" the skin, giving it a more youthful appearance. One of the most frequent (and delighted) comments I have heard from people taking DHEA is that their skin looks and feels better. I know what they mean. My face is virtually wrinkle free, which is quite remarkable considering that I am seventy-one. I was tickled to discover in an article that appeared in *The Sciences,* a popular magazine published by the New York Academy of Sciences, a reporter's description of me as someone who "looks twenty years younger than his age." Fancy that!

Dry Eye

Dry eye, characterized by irritated, red, and itchy eyes, is another troublesome condition that becomes more common as we reach middle age. Although men are also affected, it primarily strikes women, usually starting during perimenopause, the years leading up to menopause when estrogen levels begin to decline sharply. This condition is particularly problematic for women who wear contact lenses, and, in fact, many women with dry eye must stop wearing contacts. Several over-the-counter and prescription eyedrops are designed to lubricate eyes, but none of these products truly solves the problem. The problem with these artificial drops, according to Dr. Michael Zeligs, a physician studying aging intervention in Boulder, Colorado, who has done extensive research on dry eye syndrome, is that they are missing some important substances found in real teardrops. Although most people think of teardrops as little pools of water, they actually contain a highly complex combination of lipids, or fats. Without these lipids, the teardrop would not be able to stretch over or cover the eye but would evaporate rapidly when exposed to air. Although artificial tear products contain lubricants, these lubricants are not nearly as good as those that are produced naturally by the eye. The lipids found in tears are produced by special glands called the meibomian glands, which are actually highly specialized, sebum-producing sebaceous glands.

Aware of Dr. Orentreich's work showing that DHEA stimulates the sebaceous glands to produce sebum, Dr. Zeligs wondered whether it would have the same effect on the meibomiam glands, the glands that produce the lipids for the eyes. Dr. Zeligs developed an eyedrop containing DHEA and first checked his theory on Pekingese dogs, a breed that frequently suffers from dry eye. The eyes of dogs given the DHEA eyedrops showed dramatic improvement. Not only were they less irritated, but the function of their natural tears improved. Dr.

Zeligs then gave the DHEA eyedrops to women in their forties who, plagued by dry eye, had given up wearing contact lenses. After taking the DHEA drops, these women experienced less eye irritation, and their natural tear production was improved. Many of the women were able to resume wearing their contact lenses comfortably. (For information on how to obtain these DHEA eyedrops, see chapter 10, How to Take Superhormones.)

On the Horizon

As I have mentioned, one of my primary goals in writing this book is to alert the public to important research that is being done on superhormones such as DHEA. In the following section I will review some of the newer groundbreaking research that is under way on DHEA that has the potential to both extend life and improve the quality of life for countless numbers of people.

NEW HOPE FOR LUPUS SUFFERERS

Some of the most exciting work being done with DHEA is in clinical studies involving one of the most common and most difficult to treat of the autoimmune diseases: systemic lupus erythematosus, more commonly known as lupus, or SLE. In clinical trials, DHEA has been shown to be effective in treating the autoimmune disease we call lupus.

Auto- (for "self") immune diseases are those that occur when the cells of our immune system, for no apparent reason, attack our own bodily tissue. When our immune system is in its youthful prime and working well, it dispatches special cells—appropriately named "suppressor" cells—that prevent the immune system from engaging in so-called "friendly fire," on its own tissues and organs. As we age, these suppressor cells become less effective and have more difficulty distinguishing friend from foe. As a result, our immune system runs amuck, and the army of disease-fighting cells that is supposed to protect us turns on us. Autoimmune diseases are more common among older people as the immune system begins to run down and become less efficient. That is why the risk of getting a disease such as rheumatoid arthritis or Hashimoto's disease (a thyroid disorder) increases with age. Some autoimmune diseases, however, are also common in younger people, especially women. We do not know what causes the autoimmune response to occur in these people; we think it may be triggered by an undetected viral infection, a genetic defect, a defect in the production or metabolism of sex hormones, or a combination of all these factors.

Lupus is a chronic inflammatory disease that can affect virtually any part of the body. It is characterized by a hyperactive immune system that produces *auto*antibodies. These are antibodies that attack the body's own tissues. Lupus cases can be mild or severe. In a severe case these autoantibodies can wreak havoc on the body, attacking many different sites including bone marrow (resulting in severe anemia), connective tissue (causing joint pain, arthritis, and inflammation of muscle), and organs such as the kidneys, heart, and brain.

About half a million Americans have lupus, and 90 percent of them are women. Although lupus can develop during childhood, it most often strikes women of childbearing age, that is, between fifteen and forty. The symptoms of lupus vary widely from patient to patient; the most common complaints include excessive fatigue, joint pain, skin rashes, chest pain (caused by inflammation of the lining of the heart and lungs), headaches, dry eyes and dry mouth, cold hands and feet, and difficulty concentrating. Lupus can be very mild at times and go into remission for months or even years. Then lupus patients may experience a period of severe symptoms, called a "flare."

Although, as I have noted, the precise cause of lupus is not known, scientists have identified certain changes in the immune system that are characteristic of the disease. Medical researchers now believe that the glitch in the immune system, which triggers the production of autoantibodies, may be caused by a communication gap within the cells of the immune system. The immune system must maintain a delicate balance between aggression and inactivity. White blood cells called lymphocytes are key players in the production of antibodies. The B lymphocytes produce antibodies as the body needs them, and they are regulated by T cells. One group of T cells, which we call helper cells, encourage the B lymphocytes to produce more antibodies, shoring up the body's defenses. Another group of T cells, which we call suppressor cells, tell our B cells when it is time to retreat. Lupus appears to occur when the suppressor cells are not communicating properly with the B cells, and the command to cease production of antibodies goes unheard or unheeded. As a result, the B cells run amuck, producing antibodies against the very tissue that the immune system is supposed to protect.

There is no cure for lupus, but there are some effective treatments, each of which has its drawbacks. In mild cases, for example, any number of several nonsteroidal anti-inflammatory medications (NSAIDs) may be prescribed. Although these medications may offer some relief, their effectiveness often declines after a year or so, and the medication must be changed. NSAIDs can also produce some undesirable side effects, ranging from mild stomach upset to gastro-intestinal bleeding, fluid retention, liver problems, and abnormalities in kidney function. Antimalarial drugs are also effective against lupus; however, they, too, can cause potentially dangerous side effects, including damage to the eye, mild hair loss, and peripheral neuropathy (nerve damage).

Patients who do not respond well to NSAIDs or antimalarials may be given corticosteroids, which, as we have seen, are hormones that the body produces during time of stress. These work very well—patients feel better almost overnight—but corticosteroids can produce serious side effects, including weight gain, diabetes, high blood pressure, a rise in cholesterol, premature osteoporosis, and increased susceptibility to infection. (By suppressing our immune function, corticosteroids reduce not only our production of autoantibodies but also our production of disease-fighting antibodies.)

Still stronger immunosuppressive drugs, the kind that are used to treat cancer, may be given to lupus patients. These drugs, such as methotrexate or Cytoxan, target rapidly dividing cells, and while they "turn down" immune function, they can have some devastating long-term side effects, including liver damage, hair loss, infertility, and an increased risk of cancer. These drugs are therefore prescribed only when absolutely necessary to treat the most severe lupus cases.

As you can surmise, the challenge of treating patients with lupus is to find a therapy that relieves the symptoms—and controls the overactive immune system—without inflicting further harm on the patient. Two small but successful studies conducted at Stanford University Medical Center have shown DHEA to be an effective treatment for lupus. A group headed by Ronald F. van Vollenhoven tested the effect of DHEA on women patients with mild to moderate lupus. In the first study, the researchers gave 200 mg. of DHEA orally to ten patients for three to six months. During the DHEA treatments, eight out of ten patients reported that they were not only feeling and doing better (an impression shared by their physicians) but they showed actual improvement in their immune function. There was significantly less autoimmune activity, and other markers of the disease, such as abnormal kidney function and red blood count, were also significantly improved. What is especially encouraging about this study is that patients were able to reduce their dose of prednisone, a corticosteroid used to control lupus symptoms.

These results were so encouraging that the researchers decided to do a more ambitious study. They undertook a double-blind study involving another twenty-eight women who suffered from mild to moderate lupus. For three months one group of the women with lupus (the control group) received a placebo, while another group received DHEA. Neither group's members knew whether they were taking the DHEA or the placebo, nor did the researchers who were conducting the study. After three months, two-thirds of the women on DHEA showed a marked improvement, and they were able to reduce their dose of prednisone. The women who received the placebo showed virtually no improvement. The only negative side effect from DHEA was an outbreak of blemishes in eight of the women, and that was treated successfully with topical creams.

Dr. van Vollenhoven says that he cannot yet explain why one-third of the women did not appear to be helped by DHEA, but he remains heartened by the fact that a majority of the women did experience great improvement. As Dr. van Vollenhoven explained, "Scientifically, you go for averages, and what I did not write in the study, but to me was the biggest sign of hope and was especially encouraging, was the sizable number of patients who told us things such as: 'You know, this has really turned things around for me. For years I've had lupus and I've had flares on and off, but I never felt really healthy, I've never felt really well. But it seems with DHEA I'm back to normal.' "

Dr. van Vollenhoven also thinks it is noteworthy that the majority of patients said they had more energy. "Fatigue is always a big factor in lupus. It has been clearly documented that the vast majority of patients with lupus have fatigue even if their disease has been otherwise treated and under control. Fatigue gets dramatically better in the majority of patients on DHEA. For example, some patients who had never been able to go Christmas shopping told me that after being in the study, they were able to go shopping for the first time in years. To us this was most exciting."

Dr. van Vollenhoven says that the effect of DHEA on lupus is not fully understood, but he theorizes that it works by correcting certain abnormalities in the immune system. For example, there is a hormone produced by our immune cells called cytokine IL 6. IL 6 levels are increased in patients suffering from lupus and other inflammatory diseases. DHEA appears to restore IL 6 levels to normal. Similarly, levels of cytokine IL 2 (which is believed to control the production of suppressor cells) are abnormally low in lupus patients. Once again, DHEA appears to normalize IL 2 levels. "DHEA appears to correct an imbalance that is expressed in lupus patients," observed Dr. van Vollenhoven.

As a lupus treatment, DHEA offers significant benefits over other drugs, particularly corticosteroids. One of the problems with long-term use of corticosteroids is that it causes the bones to thin, promoting premature osteoporosis, a condition in which the bones are prone to breaks and fractures; in severe cases it can lead to bone necrosis, or bone death. Preliminary studies suggest that DHEA may actually have a bone-sparing effect, providing many of the benefits of corticosteroids without the damage.

Dr. van Vollenhoven says that although the results of the Stanford study are very promising, the treatment group was small, and it is necessary to verify the results in a larger population. Currently, a large clinical trial involving twenty-five universities and more than two hundred patients is in progress. Dr. van Vollenhoven's group is also investigating whether DHEA would be a useful adjuvant therapy in patients with severe lupus and whether DHEA would help to control mental function in lupus patients who often have difficulty with mental tasks such as memory and concentration.

Dr. van Vollenhoven thinks that, ideally, it is better for lupus patients to wait for the results of the larger clinical trials before starting on DHEA, but he receives queries from rheumatologists who are interested in using DHEA to treat their lupus patients. Dr. van Vollenhoven stresses that any lupus patient who is interested in taking DHEA should do so only under the care of a rheumatologist or trained physician, and the patient must be closely monitored. (I am in complete agreement with this.) In the bibliography of this book is a list of articles on the use of DHEA in lupus cases. If you are a lupus patient and your rheumatologist or physician is interested in learning more about DHEA, please refer him to that list.

Given the fact that DHEA has worked so well for lupus and appears to be both a safe and effective treatment with virtually no side effects, I feel it is imperative that more research be done on DHEA's potential as a treatment for other autoimmune diseases. It makes sense that if DHEA can enhance the quality of life and reduce the level of disease in women with lupus, it may work just as well as a treatment for similar conditions.

HEALING BURNS

The immune system is not just involved in fighting disease. It is also a key player in recovery from injury. In fact, some of the most interesting work being done in Dr. Daynes's lab deals with DHEA's effect on burns and wound healing. In recent years researchers have discovered that a serious burn is not just skin deep; it can have a profound and negative impact on immune function. We know, for example, that people who are seriously burned are particularly vulnerable to infection, not only because the loss of skin provides a convenient way for bacteria and viruses to enter their bodies but perhaps because their levels of stress hormones are so high, which dampens their immune function. The same is true for animals. If an animal (after being anesthetized) is given a small scald on its back, its immune system will be depressed for weeks following that injury. Dr. Daynes found, however, that if the animal is given just one injection of DHEA sulfate within 3 days after receiving the burn, its immune function will bounce back to normal. Moreover, if the DHEA is administered within three or four hours after the burn, the burn heals faster.

To understand why DHEA promotes healing, you need to know a bit about the anatomy of a burn. A burn is rarely even or uniform throughout. When you get a serious burn, you may have areas that are not quite as deep or as acute as others; in other words, you can have a second-degree area and a third-degree area in the same burn. Burn care specialists know that a serious burn often gets worse before it gets better, simply because the injury will progress to its maximum depth around the burn during the first two to three days. That is because immediately following the burn, platelets clump together at the site of the injury and block the blood supply to the entire area, depriving it of oxygen. In the absence of oxygen, certain enzymatic changes occur in the tissue that in the presence of oxygen would cause damage. When the platelet plug dissipates and the blood flow is restored, a sudden "blast" of oxygen can promote the formation of free radicals, which in turn can cause further injury to the surrounding tissue. Dr. Daynes suspects that DHEA actually helps prevent this sort of propagated injury, which is why the animals treated with DHEA heal faster. DHEA has worked to promote wound healing in mice, rats, and pigs, and although it has not yet been clinically tested in humans, Dr. Daynes suspects it will do the same thing.

Here is a prime example of why more studies are needed on DHEA and why this important research must continue.

WILL DHEA HELP YOU LIVE LONGER?

When we wrote *The Melatonin Miracle,* we reported that there were only two proven ways to extend the life span of an animal. The first method was to put an animal on a severely restricted diet. We said this because a number of studies have documented that when mice or rats are given just enough food for survival, they live considerably longer than those that are allowed to eat at will. The second method —and one we and undoubtedly the animals found much more palatable—is to take a melatonin supplement. Indeed, when melatonin was added to the nighttime drinking water of many different strains of mice, the animals lived up to 40 percent longer, and not only that, they stayed healthy and vigorous. The good news is that some exciting research being done at the University of Wisconsin in Madison suggests that DHEA may also help extend life.

Richard Weindruch, an associate professor of the department of medicine, is conducting a carefully designed laboratory study to test the effect of DHEA on the life span of mice. In his study Dr. Weindruch is tracking the progress of four different groups of mice; there are seventy-five mice in each group, all of which begin their treatment at age one. Mice in the first group (the control) are being fed a normal diet. Mice in the second group are being fed a normal diet with DHEA sulfate added to their drinking water. Mice in the third group are being fed a calorie-restricted diet. Mice in the fourth group are being fed a calorie-restricted diet with DHEA sulfate added to their drinking water. If DHEA can indeed increase the life span, the animals taking DHEA should fare better than the animals that are not. By adding a food-restricted group to the study, Dr. Weindruch can compare the effect of DHEA to that of a low-calorie diet. As the study progresses and each animal dies, it is autopsied to determine the cause of death. The results of the study will not be known for at least another year, and Dr. Weindruch, who is a careful scientist, is reluctant to release any information prematurely. He does admit, however, that based on preliminary data, half of the control mice are still alive, but the DHEA mice are doing better. We have heard from colleagues of Dr. Weindruch's that the DHEA mice are actually doing much better than the control mice, and they are very optimistic that DHEA will prove to be a tool which will extend life.

I agree. Given everything that we know about this extraordinary superhormone, and the vast and truly astonishing scope of health benefits already documented, it would not surprise me at all if future research reveals that DHEA is the second superhormone to be credited not only with the power to rejuvenate, but also with the power to actually extend life.

CHAPTER 2

Pregnenolone

THE SUPERHORMONE FOR YOUR BRAIN

Potent memory enhancer
Improves concentration
Fights mental fatigue
Relieves arthritis

MY FORTY YEARS as a physician and medical researcher have taught me that nothing which happens in the body occurs in an isolated vacuum. One event leads to a cascade of events that can eventually be felt in every cell of every organ system throughout the entire body. This is precisely what happens when the aging clock runs down and our levels of superhormones decline. We do not merely experience a shift in our hormone levels, we experience profound changes that affect every aspect of our physical and mental well-being.

These changes are reflected not only in our behavior but in our outlook on life itself. We lose our joie de vivre. We lose our psychic energy. We lose the mental vitality that keeps us excited and part of the world in which we live. We lose our desire to learn and to try new things. One of the expressions we often hear used to describe an older person is that he is "set in his ways." I believe that it is the loss of psychic energy, which is responsible for the fear of trying something new. As we age, we feel overwhelmed by new experiences, and we respond by trying to avoid them. This can be deadly. To me it's even worse than deadly. It is monotonous. It saps our joy and enthusiasm for life. *It should not and need not be this way!*

We have always assumed that the changes in mental function that occur among older people are perfectly normal and are merely an inevitable part of the aging process. Just as we believed it was normal for older people to experience a physical downward spiral, we expected that their brains would deteriorate as well. I am hoping through this book to put this sort of nonsense to rest once and for all. There is absolutely no reason that men and women should sit back and allow their brain function to decline, any more than they should sit back and allow the diseases of aging to take hold of their bodies. With superhormones at our disposal, we need not allow our brains to "rust," nor should we experience a diminished capacity in either memory or alertness. With superhormones we can stay smart and sharp for our entire lives. The promise of superhormones is that we will have the mental wherewithal to welcome new experiences, and the physical stamina to enjoy them.

Pregnenolone is a superhormone that is key to keeping our brains functioning at peak capacity. Some scientists believe it is the most potent memory enhancer of all time. Perhaps what is even more amazing are the studies that demonstrate pregnenolone enhances our ability to perform on the job while heightening feelings of well-being. In other words, this superhormone appears to make us not only smarter but happier. It improves memory and mental function, and I believe it can restore the psychic energy, which I feel is absolutely critical to our capacity to enjoy a full and happy life at any age.

Most of you probably have never heard of pregnenolone, so let me tell you what it is, where it comes from, and the role this superhormone plays in your body.

Like the other steroid superhormones (DHEA, testosterone, and estrogen) pregnenolone is synthesized from cholesterol. As you know, cholesterol is a kind of fat (or "lipid") found in certain foods (primarily meat and dairy products) and is also produced in our bodies. In recent years cholesterol has gained a reputation as being unhealthy and something to avoid, because people with high levels of blood cholesterol are at higher risk of developing heart disease. As a result, we go to great lengths to cut our intake of cholesterol-rich foods, and some of us take cholesterol-reducing drugs if our levels are too high. Cholesterol, however, has gotten a bad rap. Having too much cholesterol can increase the risk of heart disease, but it is also dangerous to have too little cholesterol. Let me put it this way: Without cholesterol, you could not live. Cholesterol is essential for many bodily processes; it is needed to produce vitamin D, which is necessary for the absorption of calcium and for the production of bile, used to absorb fat from the intestines. It is needed to make myelin, the fatty coating that surrounds nerves, including the nerves in the spinal cord and brain. Studies have shown that people with very low cholesterol levels are more likely to develop cancer or to suffer from mental illness.

Cholesterol is also a critical component in the production of steroid hormones. In a complex series of steps, cholesterol is broken down into different steroid hormones as the body needs them. It is first synthesized into pregnenolone and used by the body in that form. What is not utilized undergoes a chemical change that "repackages" it into DHEA. DHEA, in turn, is used by the body as DHEA and is also broken down into estrogen and testosterone. This chain of hormones is known as the "steroid pathway." Because pregnenolone gives birth to the other hormones, it is sometimes referred to as the "parent hormone," which is probably the origin of its odd-sounding name.

Pregnenolone is produced both in the brain and in the adrenal cortex, the glands that sit above the kidneys. Like the other superhormones, pregnenolone production declines with age. By the time we are seventy-five, we are making 60 percent less pregnenolone than we did in our thirties.

As our pregnenolone production drops, so does production of the other hormones in the steroid pathway. Since pregnenolone is the parent hormone from which other hormones are made, this makes perfect sense. Pregnenolone provides the raw material for these other hormones, and as levels of pregnenolone decline, so will the levels of the other hormones that are made from it.

For the first time pregnenolone, like DHEA, is now being sold over the counter and is available in natural food stores and pharmacies. Pregnenolone is also available by prescription from compounding pharmacies. I have no doubt that, given pregnenolone's ready availability and great potential, it will soon be eagerly embraced by a generation of men and women who are unwilling to allow their bodies and minds to deteriorate with age, and who want to grow older and wiser but with a brain and a body that still enjoys the "youthful advantage" in terms of mental acuity and physical function.

Pregnenolone and Your Memory

Although few people may have heard of pregnenolone before, ironically, this superhormone was one of the first to be studied and the first to be proven both safe and effective. In fact, in the mid-1940s, a group of industrial psychologists tested pregnenolone on students and workers, and discovered that it markedly improved their ability to learn and remember difficult tasks. And as mentioned earlier, pregnenolone has recently been rediscovered as a potent memory-enhancing agent.

To understand why the latest findings on pregnenolone and memory are so exciting, you need to know a bit about memory drugs in general. There are numerous substances that can improve memory, but they are far from perfect. The problem is that many of them work within a very limited dose range, and if the optimum dose is exceeded, the drugs can be rendered ineffective or, even worse, can cause amnesia. As you can well imagine, it is imperative to use precisely the right dose for each patient, and figuring out the right dose can be very tricky. If a researcher were to design an ideal memory-enhancing agent, it would be one that is so powerful only the tiniest amount would be required to produce the desired result. It would be one that works in a number of different dose ranges so that there is little or no risk of over- or underdosing a patient.

Recent studies in both animals and humans indicate that pregnenolone may be this ideal memory-enhancing drug and also that it is the most potent memory-enhancing substance known. This exciting research on pregnenolone and memory is being conducted jointly at two distinguished institutions, the Beekman Research Institute at the City of Hope Hospital under the direction of Eugene Roberts, Ph.D., a brilliant researcher and long-distance friend whose work I have followed for more than two decades, and at St. Louis University School of Medicine by two noted researchers and physicians in the field of gerontology, John E. Morley, M.D., and James F. Flood, M.D. In one of their studies, hormones, including pregnenolone, were given to mice who were being taught to run through a maze. The purpose of the study was to see whether any of these hormones had an effect on memory and learning. Mice, like humans, are either right-handed or left-handed. Consequently, if they are placed in a maze, they will automatically run to one side or the other, depending on which side they favor. In the study, the researchers tried to retrain the mice to go in a direction other than the one they naturally preferred. Every time the mice tried to go in the "wrong" direction, they were given a tiny electric shock. After a few false starts, the mice typically learned to navigate the maze correctly. Once the mice learned their way around the maze, they were divided into two groups. One group of mice received a hormone injection directly into the brain center that is believed to control memory. The injections contained either DHEA, testosterone, or pregnenolone. The other group received no injections. A week later the mice were again placed in the same maze and retested to see if they remembered the correct way out. The mice that received each of the hormone injections remembered their lesson well; they quickly made their way through the maze. It emerged that the important difference was in the dose required to produce the memory-enhancing result. Only a minuscule amount of pregnenolone—just 15 to 145 molecules—was required, whereas much higher doses of testosterone and DHEA were needed to gain the same effect. This experiment dramatically showed how potent a memory enhancer pregnenolone is.

As Dr. Morley explained, "Pregnenolone makes sense potentially. It is clearly by far the most potent of the neurosteroids for improving memory by light-years, and it has a much broader memory response than any of the other neurosteroids. This makes it almost an ideal agent for looking at memory and the consequences of the age-related deterioration of memory."

We've seen that pregnenolone works for mice, but will it work as well for people? Happily, the answer is a resounding yes. As mentioned before, more than fifty years ago researchers showed that pregnenolone had a remarkable effect on memory and mental function. Back in the 1940s, researchers at the University of Massachusetts devised a study to test the effect of pregnenolone on psychomotor performance, including hand-to-eye coordination, learning, memory, and stamina. In their study the researchers trained fourteen subjects to operate an airplane flight simulator machine. This contraption looked and worked oddly like the joystick-controlled video games that our children and grandchildren play. The idea was to "fly" the "plane" correctly, avoiding obstacles and crashes. If you're having trouble picturing this experiment, go watch the kids play their video games for five minutes, and you'll see just how difficult and harrowing this task can be—at least for adults. In any case, seven of the subjects were airplane pilots, whereas the other subjects had no previous flight experience. Before each of the "test runs," the subjects took either 50-mg. capsules of pregnenolone or a placebo. Tests conducted over a period of several weeks showed that the ability of all the subjects to "fly" the imaginary airplane improved significantly after they took pregnenolone. The improvement was especially profound after the subjects had been on pregnenolone for at least two weeks, suggesting that pregnenolone's effect on mental function may be cumulative. What was even more interesting was the report by the professional pilots that while they were participating in the study, they found they performed better in their real flying jobs and that they fatigued less easily.

The same research group tested pregnenolone supplements on factory workers to see if it could affect their productivity on the job. Interestingly, the effect on productivity was most noticeable in those who worked in stressful situations, such as those who were paid by the piece and therefore had to produce a certain number of items in a given amount of time in order to make a living. These workers showed more improvement on pregnenolone than those who were working for a fixed hourly wage. Pregnenolone not only improved productivity, but many of the workers reported that it enhanced their mood. They said that they felt happier and better able to cope with the pressures of the job when they were taking pregnenolone.

Now, some fifty years later, pregnenolone is once again the subject of intense medical interest. At St. Louis University School of Medicine, researcher Rahmawhati Sih, Ph.D., has conducted several studies to test the effect of pregnenolone on mental function. Although the results are very preliminary, Dr. Sih was kind enough to share them with us. In one of her studies, Dr. Sih administered a 500-mg. capsule of pregnenolone or a placebo to a small group of older men and women. Three hours later the men and women were asked to perform a variety of standard memory tests, including paragraph recall, block design, and tests of concentration. The men and women who were given pregnenolone showed an improvement in memory, but the nature of the improvement varied by sex. Men tended to improve in visual spatial tasks; that is, they performed better at block building, trail making (connecting the lines), and other jobs that required three-dimensional thinking. Women, on the other hand, showed an improvement in verbal recall. For example, if they were read a list of words and later asked to recall the words on the list, they were able to remember more of those words after taking pregnenolone. In other studies, when older men were given testosterone, they also showed an improvement in visual spatial tasks, and when older women were given estrogen, they scored better on verbal recall tests. We will again encounter this issue of gender differences in the chapters on estrogen and testosterone. Dr. Sih's study not only shows that pregnenolone helps restore flagging mental function but also points to something even more intriguing. Her results suggest that pregnenolone is being broken down differently by men and women; that is, it appears to have a testosteronelike effect in men and an estrogeniclike effect in women. This makes sense because, as explained earlier, pregnenolone is the precursor hormone from which some of the other superhormones—DHEA, estrogen, testosterone, and progesterone—are made.

This, in turn, leads to a very intriguing question: If as we age we restore our pregnenolone levels to their youthful values, will we also be able to replenish levels of all the other hormones that are made from pregnenolone? In other words, by simply taking pregnenolone will we be able to reverse the decline in all of the superhormones? This is an intriguing question, and no one knows the answer as yet. Some researchers who have pondered this question do not believe that pregnenolone supplementation alone will be enough to correct the age-related decline in other superhormones but that a combination of DHEA and pregnenolone will do the trick. This also makes a lot of sense to me. Many of us who have studied both hormones believe that the two appear to work in harmony. Well, you may be thinking, if pregnenolone breaks down into the other superhormones, won't it also increase the level of DHEA on its own? Why bother to take extra DHEA? The answer is really quite simple. As you now know, as we age, our production of DHEA declines. Why? The decline in DHEA is due to a drop in production of an enzyme that is necessary to break pregnenolone down into DHEA. Therefore, if we take pregnenolone supplements, we still may not be able to produce enough DHEA because we will still be lacking this essential enzyme. As a result, pregnenolone may bypass the DHEA stage and instead be broken down directly into the sex steroids or to other hormones in the pathway.

By the way, there is another reason to add DHEA to the pregnenolone cocktail. If pregnenolone does indeed prime the pump that produces other hormones, there is a chance that it may also turn up the production of corticosteroids, or stress hormones, at least in some people. Since we know that DHEA dampens the effect of corticosteroids and is a potent stress reliever, this is all the more reason to include DHEA in the pregnenolone cocktail even if pregnenolone turns out to be all that these researchers believe it to be. For me, this just confirms my assertion that the "cocktail" approach is the right one and that our superhormones work best when they work in tandem.

Pregnenolone and Depression

As discussed earlier, as the levels of superhormones decline, we run out of psychic energy, the fuel that keeps us interested and connected to the world. When we run out of psychic energy and we lose our connection with the world, it is not uncommon for us to become isolated and withdrawn. This, in turn, sets the stage for depression.

In recent years we have learned that many cases of depression are actually caused by an imbalance of substances called neurotransmitters, chemicals in the brain that are intricately involved in how we think and feel. For example, Prozac, probably the best known of the antidepressants, works by restoring the normal balance of a neurotransmitter known as serotonin. In addition to performing the routine functions of regular hormones, we now know that superhormones are also similar to neurotransmitters; they are located in the brain and have a profound impact on mental function. That is why I believe that many cases of depression in older people are actually caused by the decline in superhormones and, in particular, pregnenolone and/or DHEA. I believe that restoring the superhormones such as pregnenolone to their youthful levels will prevent many of the cases of depression that occur among older people and that are all too frequently written off as part of the "normal" aging process.

My belief has been confirmed by a recent study conducted by the National Institutes of Mental Health; it showed that people with clinical depression have lower than normal levels of pregnenolone in their cerebral spinal fluid (the fluid that bathes the brain). Although this study did not look specifically at older people, this finding is relevant to anyone who is producing lower than normal levels of pregnenolone, and that is precisely what happens in aging. What is the connection between pregnenolone and depression? Let me explain the theory. The nerve cells in our brains are constantly being bombarded with stimuli and receiving and transmitting information. Our brains contain a neurotransmitter called GABA, which literally cools the brain and protects our nerve cells from burning out in the course of all this activity. GABA performs an important function, but too much GABA may make the brain too sluggish and produce a dampening effect that depresses brain function. It appears that pregnenolone mitigates the effect of GABA and restores balance to the brain. You may remember that in the earlier studies performed on pregnenolone in the 1940s, the researchers noted that the participants reported an enhanced sense of well-being and an improvement in mood. This could also be due to pregnenolone's effect on GABA.

Although there have been no official studies done on the treatment of depression with pregnenolone, based on all we know about this superhormone, I believe that in cases of mild depression pregnenolone should be very helpful and certainly should be tried before bringing on the "heavier guns," stronger medication that can cause substantial side effects. We know that pregnenolone is safe, well tolerated, and causes no known side effects, so it just makes good sense to try it first.

A Treatment for Arthritis?

In the 1940s, pregnenolone was used quite successfully as a treatment for rheumatoid arthritis, the disease that causes severe joint pain and fatigue, and that continues to plague millions of sufferers. As you may remember from the chapter on DHEA, rheumatoid arthritis is an autoimmune disease that is more likely to strike as we get older. There is as yet no cure for rheumatoid arthritis, and the symptoms are usually treated with anti-inflammatory medication. Nearly a half-century ago, rheumatoid arthritis patients who took pregnenolone reported that they felt less pain and were less tired, and much stronger.

Despite the fact that pregnenolone showed promise as a treatment for rheumatoid arthritis, all research on pregnenolone as an arthritis treatment ended abruptly in the 1950s. One reason the medical community lost interest was that, like the other superhormones, pregnenolone was a natural substance produced by the body and therefore could not be patented. As a result, no drug company was interested in investing the time or money to bring pregnenolone to market. As previously mentioned, it is a sad fact of life that in the United States, no matter how effective a substance may be in treating illness or extending and improving the quality of life, if it is not patentable, it stands a good chance of falling by the wayside. Again, that was a primary reason for writing The Melatonin Miracle and for writing this book. I hope to awaken public interest in these extraordinary natural substances; they are doomed to oblivion unless someone steps forward (I feel it must be the government) to fund these important studies.

There was another reason that pregnenolone was forgotten: It was completely overshadowed by the discovery of an exciting new drug, synthetic cortisone, in the late 1940s; it was thought to be the cure for arthritis. When cortisone was first introduced, it received as much hoopla as did penicillin when it launched the antibiotic revolution a decade earlier. Unlike pregnenolone, the effects of which were cumulative and felt over a period of weeks, cortisone also produced almost overnight relief from arthritis symptoms. From the point of view of pharmaceutical companies, which could make real money selling cortisone, and of patients who understandably wanted fast, fast, fast relief, cortisone was a dream come true. The problem is that by the time we woke from the dream and realized that cortisone and its related compounds have some pretty nightmarish side effects—such as a dampening effect on the immune system that makes patients susceptible to infection, and a destructive effect on bone mass, leaving patients vulnerable to osteoporosis—we had forgotten that once upon a time there was a substance called pregnenolone, which produced relief from arthritis symptoms much more safely, albeit more gradually.

I hope *The Superhormone Promise* ensures that pregnenolone does not stay forgotten. I want to spread the word that pregnenolone has a vast therapeutic potential, which deserves further investigation. This superhormone is not only a kinder and gentler treatment for arthritis, but it is a proven strategy for enhancing memory and brain function and elevating mood. I suspect that it may one day be proven useful for combatting symptoms of Alzheimer's disease. These are just some of the things that we know pregnenolone can do, and there are probably many as yet undiscovered uses for this superhormone.

There is even evidence that pregnenolone may be the long-sought-after drug that can reverse paralysis in victims of spinal cord injuries.

On the Horizon: Pregnenolone and Spinal Cord Injuries

One of the most exciting reports I've seen in years deals with the use of pregnenolone in combination with other drugs as a treatment for spinal cord injuries. As you may know, when the brain and spinal cord are injured, they are unable to repair themselves. The central nervous system, of which the brain and spinal cord are parts, regulates the peripheral nervous system, that is, the nerves in the arms and legs. Moreover, when the spinal cord is injured, the body tends to aggravate the injury by producing swelling and inflammation, which can do further damage and also can interfere with healing. That is why if the spinal cord is severely injured, partial or total paralysis can result. To date there are no drugs or effective treatments for spinal cord injuries.

Every year some two hundred thousand people suffer spinal cord injuries. After a tragic riding accident that resulted in such an injury, actor Christopher Reeve called attention to the plight of spinal cord injury victims and pleaded for more funding of research to find effective treatments. A promising study performed by Drs. Lloyd Goth and Ziyin Zhang at the College of William and Mary in Williamsburg, Virginia, with Eugene Roberts at the City of Hope Hospital, suggests that pregnenolone may play an important role in treating at least some types of spinal injuries. In this study the researchers anesthetized rats and then inflicted compressive injuries on their spinal cords. (A compressive injury is a very common spinal cord injury and is caused by a sudden blow to the back or head, or a crushing injury to the spine. A typical compressive injury might occur, for instance, when someone hits his head very hard on the roof of a car during an automobile accident.) Afterward, the rats were divided up into several different treatment groups. One group received no drugs. A second group was given a combination of three drugs including an anti-inflammatory substance (indomethacin), a drug that stimulates immune function, and pregnenolone. The third group was divided into subgroups that were treated with either one or two of the various drugs used in the three-drug cocktail. According to the researchers, the drug cocktail that included pregnenolone not only reduced the amount of swelling and inflammation but resulted in a dramatic improvement for most of the rats. In fact, eleven of the sixteen animals were able to stand and walk within twenty-one days after injury, and four of them regained almost normal function. The other combinations of drugs provided only modest improvement, and the rats that received no treatment did not improve at all.

Does this mean that this combination of drugs, or some other combination utilizing pregnenolone, could work as well on people? We'll never know unless this important research is continued, and with that in mind, I would like to close this chapter with an appeal for more clinical studies on the long-term effects of pregnenolone, similar to those done on DHEA that I reported on earlier. Since pregnenolone research is not likely to get major funding from a drug company, the only way that research is going to be done is if we, the tax-paying public, pressure the government to fund it.

Whether or not pregnenolone gets the attention it deserves or once again becomes the memory drug that is forgotten depends on educating the public. Pregnenolone may offer far greater benefits than we ever imagined, but we'll never know unless the right studies are done. The promise of pregnenolone is simply too great to let another fifty years go by before its potential is explored.

PART II

The Superhormone for Sex and Strength

Introduction: Testosterone

TESTOSTERONE IS A male hormone, or what scientists call an androgen, but women, too, produce testosterone—although in much smaller amounts than men do. In men, testosterone is produced primarily in the testes (or testicles), but a small amount is also manufactured in the adrenal glands. In women, testosterone is produced in the adrenal glands and—what may surprise you—the ovaries.

Although testosterone was discovered more than sixty years ago, only very recently have we begun to fully understand and appreciate the power of testosterone—and, now, the role it will also play in the superhormone revolution. It is, as you will see, one of the most potent weapons in our arsenal of anti-aging superhormones.

Testosterone behaves differently in the bodies of men and women, but what may be less obvious is that it plays a very important role in the overall health and well-being of both sexes. We will examine the many roles testosterone plays in a man's body and what happens when testosterone levels decline with age, and then we will take a thorough look at testosterone and women.

Now hold on! Before you begin turning pages to get to the section that applies to you, I want to urge all women readers to read chapter 3, Testosterone: For Men, and I also want to urge all male readers to read chapter 4, Testosterone: For Women. If you take my advice, you will acquire not only an understanding of this fascinating hormone and the role it plays in your life but a better understanding of the role it plays in your lives together.

CHAPTER 3

Testosterone

FOR MEN

Enhances sex drive
Builds muscle
Elevates mood
Prevents osteoporosis
Improves memory
Lowers cholesterol
Protects against heart disease

I have a number of patients whom I've been treating with testoster-
one for the past five years, and most of them would not come off it
even if you offered them a small piece of the Federal Reserve.

—DR. FRAN KAISER,
Medical Researcher
St. Louis University School of
Medicine

I take testosterone because I want to feel the same way I did when I
was in my prime. I want to have the same sexuality that I did when
I was young. I want to maintain my muscle strength. I want to feel
vital. Testosterone makes it all possible.

—DR. NORMAN ORENTREICH, 73
New York City physician and
medical research scientist

SEX.
   Strength.
   These are the words that men most frequently invoke when describing the effects of testosterone. They consistently report that they
feel sexier, stronger, and healthier. They say that testosterone makes

them feel as they did when they were—as the saying goes—"in their prime."

This is, after all, what superhormones are all about. It is about restoring your superhormones to their youthful levels so that you feel as you did when you were at the peak of your physical and mental prowess. *The Superhormone Promise* is about not having to regret your "lost youth," because you will stop feeling as though you ever lost it. Nor will you wish that you could "look that way again," because you will still look good. *The Superhormone Promise* is about living life with passion and gusto . . . and staying in the game.

Testosterone can stop and reverse the physical decline that otherwise robs men of their energy, their strength, and their libido. Testosterone can restore muscle tone and improve stamina. And for men who have lost interest in sex—and perhaps in life itself—testosterone can restore healthy sexual excitement and desire.

I've observed that once a man starts taking testosterone, he is very quickly aware of its benefits. Most men enjoy a palpable improvement in mood, libido, and strength. That men on testosterone feel stronger and sexier is not surprising. In a very real sense, testosterone is the ultimate aphrodisiac. Testosterone is responsible for the sex drive of both men and women; it is the hormone that stimulates our desire for sexual activity and orgasm. But as you will see later, testosterone is not the only hormone that affects our sexual functioning and health. For example, the superhormone melatonin influences the functioning of the pituitary gland and our ability to perform and respond sexually in a number of ways. Testosterone is, however, the hormone that makes us desire sex in the first place, and this is so for women as well as men.

As testosterone levels decline through the years, many men feel the loss acutely, and a common symptom of low testosterone is a lack of sexual desire. Many men who experience this loss of desire assume that they are impotent. Let me reassure you that for most men this is not the case. The fact that a man is low in testosterone does not mean that he is physically unable to maintain an erection and enjoy sex. The problem is that a man low in testosterone may simply not care enough to pursue it. He may feel impotent even though he is technically not.

Happily, restoring testosterone to youthful levels can turn this situation around, practically overnight. Once testosterone levels are replenished, a man will find that he has recaptured a healthy interest in sex—as well as the capacity to enjoy it. That was the experience of Jerry K., a fifty-nine-year-old divorced businessman from California who began taking testosterone when he realized that his lack of sexual interest and energy was having a chilling effect on a new and important relationship. "The woman that I loved felt I was losing interest in her, and this simply wasn't true. The real problem was, even though I cared about her, I just couldn't become sexually aroused. I didn't think there was anything I could do about this, but when I mentioned it to my doctor, he decided to check my testosterone level. When he saw that it was low, he put me on testosterone. The difference in how I feel now is incredible. Within ten days I went from zero libido to a vigorous sex life."

This is the kind of testimonial about superhormones that I find particularly heartening because it underscores an important point: There is no reason that the ability to enjoy a good sex life should be solely the perogative of youth. All too often men and women automatically assume that, as they age, their sexual capacity will steadily diminish until sex is no longer a part of their lives, merely a part of their pasts. They are willing to settle for less than what they really want or deserve. Just as I believe that there is no need to accept disease and debility as a normal part of aging, I do not believe that we are forced to accept the loss of our sexuality. Sex is the kind of life-affirming activity that should be cherished throughout our lives. For both men and women, superhormones such as testosterone, DHEA, estrogen, and melatonin can play a critical role in helping to preserve and even restore sexual desire and function so that we can live out our extended life span with the same excitement and enthusiasm we enjoyed in our youth.

The number of men, midlife and older, who are using testosterone has grown exponentially over the past few years, and many distinguished institutions, including the National Institute on Aging, are exploring the benefits of boosting testosterone to youthful levels. Although no one knows precisely how many men are currently taking testosterone, experts predict that within the next five years there will be as many men taking testosterone as there are postmenopausal women taking estrogen, and I predict this will soon be viewed as a vital component of our superhormone profile.

The explosion of interest in testosterone is the result of the growing realization that our testosterone levels decline with age, and that, as they fall, many of us suffer serious palpable consequences in terms of our physical and mental health. It is becoming apparent that many of the symptoms we men have come to accept as a normal part of the aging process are actually due to low testosterone levels and are easily correctable. This realization has sparked a tremendous interest in testosterone among men who see no reason to surrender to the physical and mental deterioration some call "aging" when they now have a choice and simply don't have to.

The desire to look and feel strong is one of the primary reasons that New York physician Norman Orentreich, who is seventy-three, has used a topical form of testosterone (which his pharmacist compounds) for more than fifteen years, and why he prescribes it to his patients who need it. Dr. Orentreich achieved fame as the inventor of the hair transplant, but he is also a major figure in the field of aging research. As explained earlier, Dr. Orentreich was among the first researchers to document the decline in DHEA that occurs as we age and to show that our DHEA levels are themselves a measure of how and how well we are aging. Dr. Orentreich heads a thriving medical practice in New York, serving as guide and mentor to his son and daughter, who are also dermatologists. He also serves as director of a major research center in upstate New York. The waiting room of his Fifth Avenue office is a study in diversity and a measure of his breadth of expertise. His services are sought by victims of burns and troublesome skin conditions as well as by the world's "beautiful people," models, actors, and major political figures whose success depends on maintaining their youthful good looks. Dr. Orentreich works long hours and clearly loves his busy, active life. He looks and moves like a man who is ready to take on the world, not like a man well beyond conventional retirement age.

"I can assure you that if I were not on testosterone, I would not be what I am now," says Dr. Orentreich. A handsome man, he has remarkably smooth skin; a full head of thick, white hair; a trim, youthful body; and powerful biceps that he is willing to flex in order to make an important point. "I was a great athlete as a kid, but now most of the day I'm forced to be sedentary. I take testosterone to maintain my muscle strength, which is something I could not do at my age through exercise alone. My energy level is up, my musculature is up, and my fat is down because of testosterone. I feel the same way sexually as I did in my forties. Maybe I should accept the fact that at seventy-three things change and I should just let it happen, but I don't want to, and with testosterone, I don't have to."

To me, Dr. Orentreich presents the model of the man in the forefront of the Superhormone Revolution. He is a man active in mind and body who refuses to accept physical and mental decline as inevitable components of aging. Moreover, he is *living proof that the decline need not occur.*

The superhormone revolution will undoubtedly increase interest in testosterone as a potent anti-aging tool. As more and more men become aware of the fact that there is no reason to accept less from life with each passing year, they will want to have their testosterone levels checked and will want to add testosterone to their superhormone cocktail if necessary.

Interest in testosterone will also be fueled by the recent FDA approval of a new testosterone patch that, like the better known estrogen patch, can be worn on any part of the body; it makes using this superhormone easier than ever. Formerly, testosterone was available in the United States only by injection, which made it somewhat difficult to use, or via a patch that had to be worn on the scrotum, which presented other difficulties. Testosterone pills are available in Europe but have not yet been approved for use in the United States, and most researchers believe that the shot and patch are the most effective and safest delivery methods.

Until recently, testosterone was used primarily as a treatment for young men suffering from severely low testosterone levels, a rare condition that can cause serious health problems. The realization that older men might need testosterone to stave off some of the most troublesome symptoms of aging is a recent phenomenon and, in fact, may come as a surprise to many men and their doctors. When they think of hormone replacement, many men—and, I might add, physicians—immediately think of women and hot flashes. This may have been appropriate at one time, before we understood the power of superhormones, but today this view is not only decidedly archaic, it is decidedly unfair to men! Superhormones are for everyone—male or female—who wants to stay healthy and vital. As you will see, men need superhormones for many of the same kinds of reasons that postmenopausal women need estrogen.

In the introduction to this book, I told you about an aging clock, a point in the brain that controls how and when we age. By around age forty-five, the aging clock signals throughout the body that it is time for testosterone levels to begin to decline, and from that point on, testosterone production drops slowly but steadily with each passing year. In women the midlife decline in female hormones is called menopause, but there is no corresponding word in our lexicon that describes the hormonal decline experienced by men. In recent years the decline has been called many names, including "male menopause," "andropause," "viropause," and "age-related testosterone decline." The last is the term favored by researchers, but none has been officially or uniformly adopted.

But whatever you call it, the decline in testosterone is very real, although it may affect individuals differently. Interestingly, some men do not experience any untoward symptoms of testosterone loss, whereas others feel the loss acutely. One reason for this difference is that testosterone levels vary widely among men, even when at their highest points. So, if a man starts out with a "high normal" level of testosterone he may in his later years, even after the decline has occurred, still have more testosterone than a man who started out with a "low normal" level. Indeed, the man who starts out with the "high normal" level may never experience the same kind or degree of symptoms as those experienced by a man who started out in the "low normal" range. It is the man who starts out with lower (but still in the normal range) levels who may run into problems later, since the natural decline may bring his level down too low for proper function.

Nevertheless, at least 30 percent of us will eventually confront lower than normal levels of testosterone, a condition called hypogonadism, and with this deficiency of testosterone comes a host of significant emotional and physical problems. These may include loss of libido, depression, fatigue, irritability, muscle weakness, and a thinning of bones that could lead to osteoporosis—which, popular belief to the contrary, is not just a problem of small-boned women.

Not all men are going to suffer all these symptoms, nor will they experience them to the same degree, but many men will reach a point when they become aware of the fact that something is not quite right. As one sixty-one-year-old man recalls, "Before I began on testosterone, I didn't feel like myself. I can't say that I felt sick, but I tired easily, I looked old, and what was worse, I *felt* old."

Now that he is on testosterone, however, he feels, in his own words, "recharged": "I'm stronger, I'm happier, and what I notice most is that I feel like my old self. I have gotten back my drive and ambition, and it feels wonderful."

The majority of doctors are still only prescribing testosterone to men whose testosterone levels are extremely low, that is, who are hypogonadal. For these men the benefits of testosterone are well documented. But physicians and researchers are now beginning to ask whether all men past fifty who have experienced declining levels, though technically within the "normal" range would nonetheless benefit if testosterone levels were restored to their youthful levels. I believe that for many midlife men whose testosterone levels are normal, albeit lower than they were during youth, testosterone is not necessary if they are already taking DHEA. I say this because DHEA is converted into a small amount of testosterone in the body, and this, I believe, will provide enough of a testosterone boost to counteract the decline. I also believe that because DHEA is what we call a testosterone precursor, it may at least postpone the need for testosterone. Thus, a man in his forties or fifties may do well on DHEA alone until he reaches his sixties or seventies, at which point he may require testosterone. At that time, he and his physician may decide to include testosterone in his personalized superhormone ℞.

These recommendations are in keeping with my philosophy that your personal ℞ for superhormones is not carved in stone and that, in fact, it is likely to evolve with you as your needs change over the years. This is also why I believe it is critical for patients to understand that my program of restoring superhormones to their youthful levels is not about simply checking your blood levels and filling a doctor's prescription. Paying attention to how you *feel* is also relevant in determining what superhormones you should be taking and in what dosages. If a man is in the low end of the normal range for testosterone but is exhibiting the symptoms of testosterone deficiency, I feel that it is reasonable for him to add testosterone to his superhormone regimen.

Testosterone: A Measure of a Man's Health

Although low testosterone levels are not unusual among older men, they are rare among younger men, and when they do occur, they are usually the result of a chronic illness or glandular malfunction. Yet younger men who have abnormally low testosterone levels experience many of the same symptoms that older men who are low on testosterone suffer. They are weak, uninterested in sex, and give the appearance of having aged prematurely. If this makes you think that the effects of low testosterone in the young are strikingly similar to the physical and mental deterioration that we sometimes refer to as "the ravages of age," you are not alone.

This striking parallel has not gone unnoticed by Dr. Fran Kaiser, a pioneer researcher in the field of testosterone who also runs a sexual dysfunction clinic at the St. Louis University School of Medicine. Dr. Kaiser and her colleagues have conducted the longest clinical trial to date involving older men on testosterone. In her medical practice Dr.

Kaiser has also prescribed testosterone for many of the men who have come to the school's sexual dysfunction clinic for help. Years of treating men with low testosterone levels have brought Dr. Kaiser to the realization that low testosterone in men is a paradigm for the aging process. She explains: "Low testosterone levels at any age are associated with many of the same symptoms that we have come to associate with aging, including loss of muscle mass, loss of mobility, loss of bone, anemia, loss of sense of well-being, alteration in sexual function, and diminished libido. There are really many commonalities." In other words, a man with insufficient testosterone will not feel well, look well, or function well, regardless of his age; indeed, testosterone insufficiency accelerates the aging process.

To me Dr. Kaiser's astute observation highlights yet another important point, which, I might add, is one of the central themes of *The Superhormone Promise.* I cannot fathom why the symptoms of testosterone deficiency in the young are immediately recognized as abnormal and a "disease state," and yet, when precisely the same symptoms occur in older men, we are quick to accept them as the symptoms of "normal" aging. This is a prime example of ageism at its very worst. There is absolutely nothing normal about being tired, being sick, being weak, or being depressed at any age! There is nothing normal about being frail or being disinterested in sex, whether you are in your twenties, forties, or eighties. These conditions should not go untreated in either the young or the old. To me they are clear and obvious symptoms of a superhormone deficiency, and there is now a remedy.

If testosterone deficiency accelerates the aging process, the good news is—and I cannot stress this enough—that this decline is neither irreparable nor irreversible. Replacing testosterone to youthful levels can stop and even reverse the downward spiral caused by low testosterone. As I will explain, all the symptoms caused by low testosterone can be easily corrected by simply restoring testosterone to youthful levels. First, I want to tell you a few things about testosterone itself.

It is not surprising that the drop in testosterone levels can create so many problems for men or that restoring testosterone to youthful levels should have such a salutary effect. Testosterone is the primary male hormone, the one that is responsible for how men look and feel and think. Although there are other important hormones in a man's body, testosterone is the dominant one.

Just as estrogen controls the traits that are defined as "typically female," testosterone is the defining hormone for all that is typically "male." Even before birth, testosterone endows the male body with qualities that are masculine. The sex of a child is determined at conception. If a sperm carrying an X chromosome unites with an egg, a female child is produced. If a sperm carrying a Y chromosome unites with the egg, the child is male. All fetuses, however, start out female. Sex is not finally determined until the development of the testes in males, which begin to pump testosterone, stimulating the development of male genitals. If testosterone is missing from the womb, the male fetus cannot develop normally.

Throughout a man's life, testosterone travels through the blood-stream and binds to target tissues via special receptors on cell membranes. Once bound to these receptors, testosterone triggers a reaction within the cells, helping to control the various organ systems that run the body. There are testosterone receptors throughout the body, including key areas of the brain.

Puberty is a time when the effects of testosterone are felt most acutely. Testosterone is the stuff that turns a boy into a man. During puberty, rising testosterone levels cause the voice to deepen, the penis and testicles to grow and mature, hair to sprout on the face and body, and muscles and bone to develop, giving the body a male "definition." As it courses through the bloodstream, testosterone turns on libido, or sexual desire. Testosterone is instrumental in the production of sperm and the ability to maintain an erection. It is also associated with assertive behavior and feelings of well-being in both sexes. In sum, it is a superhormone that has become synonymous with robustness, vigor, and vitality of youth.

A Brief History

Testosterone is a superhormone that has a mystique all its own. From the earliest days of recorded history, healers and shamans have intuitively sensed that there was a vital substance in men's bodies that governed their strength and sexuality. Throughout history, glands and sexual organs from male animals have been used to create medicines designed to restore potency and revitalize men. Although these ancient healers did not know it at the time, these glands and organs undoubtedly contained small amounts of animal testosterone. Ancient Greek physicians believed that there was a life-giving substance in men that was somehow connected to the function of the sexual glands and was essential for good health. Nearly two thousand years later, in 1889, French physiologist Charles-Edouard Brown-Séquard wrote of experiments in which he injected himself with the fluid he extracted from the testicles of animals. The results, he reported, were nothing short of miraculous. "The question," he wrote in his journal, "is certainly not whether the injections . . . rejuvenate. . . . To me that appears certain."

In the first few decades of the twentieth century, treating sexual problems with various potions made from the testicles of animals became quite a fad, and although doctors and their patients were convinced they had found a "cure" to male potency problems, more serious researchers recognized that there was too little residual testosterone in animal testicles to have long-term impact on the men who ingested or injected them. These more serious scientists understood that if men were responding to these treatments, it was purely a placebo effect. They understood that if testosterone were to be used as a medical treatment, it would have to be available in a synthetic form. The problem, though, was that no one knew how to synthesize testosterone in the laboratory. Then, in 1934, two Eastern European chemists discovered the chemical formula for testosterone and were actually able to synthesize it from cholesterol. They were awarded a Nobel Prize for their work. More important, once the chemical structure for testosterone was available, pharmaceutical companies were able to develop the synthetic versions of the hormone that are used in testosterone treatment today.

Since the discovery of testosterone, there has been a great deal of controversy over what role, if any, it plays in the aging process. For most of this century, endocrinologists insisted that there is no age-related decline in testosterone, and only within the past decade has the fact that testosterone levels actually decline as we age been proven conclusively. Moreover, science has only recently come to understand that testosterone is not merely a male hormone but a superhormone that plays a profound role in our ability to maintain a strong body and a well functioning mind—in essence, in when and how well we age.

Why the Lag?

Considering the fact that menopausal women have been restoring estrogen to more youthful levels for more than forty years, why did it take so much longer for scientists to figure out that older men would benefit by replenishing their flagging testosterone levels? Scientists who are involved in this field often say that testosterone research today is roughly where estrogen research was fifteen years ago. In other words, research on the role of testosterone and aging has lagged far behind that of estrogen. I believe that this information lag is due primarily to three obstacles: ignorance, denial, and the simple fact that researchers had no idea what they were looking for.

Let's begin with ignorance. In recent years, women have complained that medicine has been dominated by a male model; that is, the male body has been the one most studied, and the lessons learned by studying men have been applied to women without regard to the fact that the physiology of women is completely different. What they say is largely true. Men *have* been the favored subjects in many areas of medicine—with one exception. Ironically, when it comes to men and their male hormones, quite the opposite is true. Science has devoted inestimably more time to women and their age-related decline than it has to men.

One reason may be that at midlife women experience a more dramatic shift in hormone levels, resulting in menopause. Once past menopause, women lose their reproductive ability; they are no longer able to conceive or carry children. Men do not experience a parallel event. They do not stop producing sperm, nor do they become infertile. Men do experience changes, however, in sexual desire and function—a subject to which I will return—but these changes tend to be subtle and occur gradually over time. So if you're not looking for them or don't know what to look for, these changes can be easy to miss—at least until they reach a critical mass, at which point they are too easily attributed to and dismissed as old age. In other words, because there is no single dramatic event signaling a hormonal decline in men, most researchers simply assumed that no such decline occurred.

But I think there is another reason that science has taken so long to recognize that men undergo a midlife change similar to that experienced by women. Frankly, by and large, male researchers and physicians were not overly interested or eager to discover the truth. I believe that testosterone is so intertwined with the male ego that it was virtually impossible for men to accept that their testosterone levels might actually go down. What I find even more interesting is that even though there is solid, indisputable evidence today, which proves unequivocally that men do indeed experience a midlife decline, there are still some men, including some wonderful scientists, who will argue until they are blue in the face that no decline exists. Why are they so blind to the facts? The answer is: denial.

"In many cases, men were totally incapable of studying themselves and didn't want to look at themselves because they couldn't believe that men could be anything but wonderful macho men," observed Dr. John E. Morley, who has conducted many groundbreaking studies on testosterone and other hormones. Dr. Morley, who is chairman of the Department of Geriatric Medicine at St. Louis University School of Medicine, adds, "Men don't like to admit that they may actually decline; it's not a sort of 'male' thing to do. It's not by coincidence that a large number of people pursuing this area of study today are women."

Even in these "enlightened" times, when many older men complain to their physicians of classic low testosterone symptoms—reduced sex drive, muscle weakness, even depression—the proper diagnosis isn't made. These men get shuffled from doctor to doctor until, if they are fortunate, one of the doctors decides to "look under the hood" and check their testosterone levels. Clearly, prejudice and denial have thwarted the progress of testosterone research and contributed to the resistance of otherwise able physicians and scientists to realize that we men experience a midlife decline in male hormones. I must add, though, in fairness to my colleagues, that until very recently it was difficult to document the decline. The studies were often contradictory and confusing, some clearly showing a drop in testosterone and some showing no drop at all. One reason it is so difficult to get an accurate reading of testosterone is that there is a diurnal rhythm to the release of testosterone. At least in younger men, testosterone levels may vary throughout the day (with higher levels in the morning) and even from season to season (with one study finding that levels peak in December). As noted earlier, there is also a wide variation in levels among individual men. As a result, if a researcher did a cross-sectional study by comparing, for example, the testosterone levels of a group of men aged forty to fifty with a group of men aged fifty to sixty, a clear pattern of decline might not emerge. On the other hand, a researcher who tracked the same group of men over a period of a decade or longer, in what we call a longitudinal study, would see an obvious and striking decline in each man over the course of time. That is one of the reasons that some test data from different studies seem to conflict, some showing a decline and others not.

Perhaps the biggest problem in documenting the decline in testosterone is that for years researchers were looking at the wrong numbers. Most of them were measuring the amount of total testosterone in the bloodstream, but that measurement can be quite deceptive. Much of the testosterone in the body is tightly bound to a protein called sex hormone binding globulin, or SHBG. The testosterone that is bound to SHBG is not readily available for use by the body; in order for testosterone to be available to body tissues it must be in the form of unbound or free testosterone, also called bioavailable testosterone. Only a small amount of testosterone, about 4 percent, is actually free or unbound. As we age, the amount of testosterone that is bound to SHBG actually increases, leaving less testosterone free for the body to use. Therefore, it is possible to have a normal testosterone reading but still be low in bioavailable testosterone. Savvy researchers and physicians now know that in order to get an accurate testosterone level, they must measure the amount of free or bioavailable testosterone. Once researchers began looking at the levels of free testosterone, the decline in testosterone in older patients became immediately more apparent.

We now know that there is not only a decline in testosterone in men as they age but that there is a reduction in the number of special Leydig cells in the testes that produce testosterone. In fact, the reduction in Leydig cells is one reason that the level of testosterone declines. There are also subtle changes in interaction among hormones that result in lower testosterone levels. The secretion of testosterone is actually regulated by the brain through the pituitary gland. When the body needs testosterone, the pituitary gland prompts the release of LH-RH (luteinizing hormone-releasing hormone), a hormone that, in turn, stimulates the testes to pump out testosterone. As men age they appear to grow less sensitive to the signals sent by the pituitary—giving rise to a condition called secondary hypogonadism. It is yet another possible cause of declining testosterone levels.

Revving Up Your Sex Drive

Libido, or sex drive, is the term used to describe our ability to become sexually aroused. Libido is strongest in adolescent boys and young men, and typically subsides with age. Nearly all studies of men have documented a decline in sexual desire and function beginning at around midlife.

For most men, some decline in sexual activity is not necessarily a problem; and as young men learn (and wise men know), the quantity of sexual encounters is not nearly as important as the quality. Many men and women feel that sex actually improves through the years, particularly as they gain an increased understanding of their own needs and the needs of their partners. If you are feeling content and fulfilled, if you and your partner are happy, that is all that matters.

But for men with low testosterone levels, it is a completely different story. These men often experience this sexual decline keenly and severely. A severely diminished sex drive can cause real and profound problems, especially when it interferes with the ability to sustain a relationship and enjoy life. It can make men feel old before their time, isolated, and very unhappy. These men are not dealing with an occasional sexual setback; for them, gratifying sexual activity has become a fond memory. "Their interest in sex isn't the way it used to be. Their ability to have sex isn't the way it used to be. They can't get an erection anymore, or when they do get an erection, they lose it quickly. If they do manage to have sex, they don't ejaculate any fluid. These are all things related to sexual function that can be associated with low testosterone," explains Johns Hopkins Medical School researcher Dr. Adrian Dobs, who is conducting studies on testosterone.

Before moving on to the specific benefits that result from boosting the levels of testosterone to youthful values, I want to say I am not suggesting that taking testosterone is going to cure all sexual problems or turn all men into sexual supermen. Not at all. Sexuality is too complex a human activity to be reduced to a few micrograms of any chemical. Our ability to become aroused, and to function accordingly, involves a wide range of factors—some physical and some emotional, which I will discuss later. Yet the role that testosterone can play in helping men in their later years regain the sexual vigor and endurance they enjoyed in youth should not be understated. Especially for men whose testosterone levels have dropped, restoring testosterone to youthful levels can have a profoundly leavening effect on their sex lives and hence their overall quality of life.

Many men who experience signs of sexual malaise suffer in silence and do not seek help unless they are forced to, usually by a disappointed and hurt sexual partner. The situation is particularly problematic when one partner in a relationship has a drop in libido while the other partner is still going strong. A case in point is that of someone we'll call Sam J., who at age seventy, after a decade-long

struggle with impotency, finally sought help from the sexual dysfunction clinic at St. Louis University School of Medicine. Sam's inability
to have an erection was putting a serious strain on his marriage. He
was caught in a vicious cycle. Fearful that he could not perform
sexually, Sam would pull away when his wife Susan would make
romantic overtures. Unaware of Sam's problem, Susan assumed that
Sam had simply lost interest in her. She felt rejected. Sam turned to
the sexual dysfunction clinic to find out what, if anything, could be
done to help restore potency—and, he hoped, their once satisfying
relationship. At the clinic Sam's hormone levels were checked as part
of his routine physical. The test results were clear: Sam had very low
levels of testosterone. Sam's doctor recommended that he try boosting his testosterone levels, which entailed receiving an injection of
testosterone every three weeks. Almost immediately following his
first treatment, Sam reported that his impotency problem was over.
For the first time in years Sam found that he was not only interested
in sex but was able to sustain an erection long enough to have
satisfying intercourse with his wife. "I feel alive again," Sam said. "I
feel more content, more relaxed, and generally healthier. My muscles
are stronger, I can perform better sexually, and I can do a lot more
things than I could before." Sam's marriage is also stronger than ever,
and, Sam says, "I plan on taking testosterone forever."

Dr. Fran Kaiser, Sam's physician, is quick to point out that Sam's
problem, which included the loss of sexual interest, was a clear-cut
one of testosterone deficiency. She cautions that not all cases of impotency can be traced to testosterone deficiency and, therefore, won't
be resolved by taking testosterone. In some cases, she notes, there
can be an underlying organic problem, such as atherosclerosis or
diabetes—two conditions which may impair blood flow to the penis
—that can prevent a man from having an erection. Other treatments,
either in conjunction with or instead of testosterone, may be warranted.

A man's inability to achieve an erection may instead be due to a
lack of interest in sex. In other words, his problem is not mechanical
dysfunction—he has the tools but lacks the motivation or inspiration
to use them. In such a case, testosterone restores the man's ability to
become aroused and with it his ability to function. But some studies
show a link between testosterone levels and performance in men
whose levels are so low that they simply cannot maintain an erection.
For these men, testosterone may enhance their sexual performance.
Researchers suspect that testosterone may stimulate the nerves and

skeletal muscles responsible for erection, but the precise mechanism is not yet fully understood. "We know more about sending a rocket to the moon than we actually understand about the physiology of erections," observes Dr. Kaiser. "It appears as if testosterone is a major regulator, probably via a whole slew of other neurotransmitters, most of which we haven't yet identified."

Easing Depression

We know that testosterone restores libido and revitalizes the sex lives of men, but testosterone's effect on libido is not solely through its effect on the reproductive system. Testosterone is also a superhormone that enhances the feeling of well-being, and when we are in a good mood, we are more inclined to sexual arousal and enjoyment. Men who take testosterone typically report that they feel happier, more energetic, and more full of life. I personally believe that the fact they are feeling more sexual may very well be as much a result of these good feelings as it is of any direct effect that testosterone has on libido per se. I say this because when it comes to something as complex as sexuality, it is very difficult to separate the physical and emotional. Nowhere is the mind-body connection more conspicuously at work than it is here. Sexual arousal begins above the neck, in the brain, which, by releasing hormones, instructs the other parts of the body to respond to sexual stimulation.

Skeptics have suggested that at least some of the men who are taking testosterone are merely experiencing a placebo effect. It has been well documented that the power of suggestion can indeed be very strong, and if a patient believes he is receiving a medication that is going to make him better, he may improve even if the medication is worthless. But this does not appear to be the case with testosterone. Consider the findings of a study involving thirteen older men with low testosterone levels conducted at Emory University in Atlanta, Georgia, by Dr. Joyce S. Tenover, a well-known researcher in the field of testosterone. For three months the men were given testosterone, and for another three months they were given a placebo. Since it was a double-blind study, neither the men nor the researchers knew when the testosterone or the placebo was being given. At the end of the study, the researchers noted that the effect of testosterone was so pronounced that twelve of the thirteen men were able to correctly distinguish between the months they were on testosterone and the months they were on the placebo. How did they know? According to Dr. Tenover, they were able to tell the difference based on their own sense of heightened libido, their aggressiveness in business transactions, and their generally elevated sense of well-being. What is so striking here is the ability of nearly all the men to sense such a palpable difference in their mood and behavior after taking testosterone.

More than a decade ago, while American researchers were still debating whether or not men experienced a meaningful decline in testosterone levels, British physicians had already begun to use hormones to treat men who showed signs of testosterone deficiency. John Moran, M.D., of the Hormonal Health Care Center in London, one the earliest proponents of the so-called "male menopause" theory, observed that men experience many of the same emotional upheavals during their midlife testosterone decline as do women during menopause. "Men will often experience a mild depression that is quite similar to the type of depression we see in women. On testosterone, that depression will lift. They will become less irritable, happier, and more content."

The role that testosterone plays in elevating mood and combating depression has been well documented in England where testosterone is routinely used to treat mood disorders attributed to midlife depression in men. Dr. Moran's typical patients are often men in their early fifties who are undergoing a period of extreme stress and are also suffering from an underlying hormonal deficiency. At Dr. Moran's clinic the men receive a careful physical and psychological examination. Their levels of key superhormones, including DHEA, testosterone, and thyroid, are checked. If any levels are low, they are restored to their youthful levels. Even if a man is at the low end of normal for testosterone, Dr. Moran prescribes a short-term course of testosterone accompanied by psychological counseling. "I find that testosterone definitely helps men who are under intense stress, and when the stress levels are reduced, they may not need testosterone anymore. It is not necessarily a permanent therapy for every man. Some may need it for a short time, others may need it for a longer period."

In some cases Dr. Moran takes patients off testosterone after a year if the depression lifts and switches them to DHEA. As noted earlier, a small amount of DHEA is converted into testosterone, which may provide enough of a testosterone boost. (As we know,

DHEA also has a powerful effect in its own right on mood and behavior, and can also help to ward off depression. See the chapter on DHEA for a full discussion of this topic.)

Energy Booster

We consistently hear from men taking testosterone that it restores energy, which helps explain its libido-enhancing and depression-easing effects. Testosterone has other effects on other systems of the body that may explain why the men who take testosterone often talk about experiencing a surge of energy such as they have not felt since they were young. One is testosterone's effect on red blood cells. Men experience a decline in the production of red blood cells as they age. This decline is especially marked in men who are in their seventies and eighties. Red blood cells are important because they transport oxygen throughout the bloodstream. Oxygen is essential for the normal metabolic processes in every cell. Deprived of oxygen, our cells would starve and die. Indeed, if our brains are denied oxygen for more than a few minutes, every organ system in our body shuts down, and we soon die. When men take testosterone, their red blood cell count rises, which means they are getting more oxygen throughout their bodies. Dr. Kaiser explains: "For example, if somebody who is a runner has blood removed before he goes on a race, and then suddenly gets infused with blood right before the race, his oxygen-carrying capacity is increased. There are more red blood cells to carry oxygen, and his endurance improves and his energy improves. That may be part of the mechanism that makes men on testosterone feel better."

The increase in red blood cells results in an increase in energy, which is good. As a rule men who take testosterone feel reinvigorated and have more physical stamina. Dr. Kaiser cautions, however, that it is important not to let the rise in red blood cells climb too high because that can cause a condition called thrombocytosis, which can increase the risk of blood clots. This situation can be avoided, however, which is why men on testosterone should be monitored by their physicians and should have their red blood cell levels checked routinely. (In addition, before starting testosterone, all men should have a thorough physical examination that includes a PSA (prostate specific antigen) test, which can help to detect any latent prostate tumors. Although testosterone is not carcinogenic, it can stimulate the growth of existing prostate cancer, so men need to be certain they are cancer free. I believe that all men over fifty should be doing this anyway. Just as all women over fifty should have mammograms each year whether or not they are taking estrogen, all men over fifty should have their prostates checked each year whether or not they are taking testosterone. (For more information on other things that need to be monitored while you are taking testosterone, see chapter 10, How to Take Superhormones.)

Strong Body, Strong Bones

Throughout this book I have proclaimed my belief that it is possible to live out our lives in strong, healthy bodies that remain in the "youthful state." By that I mean that we need not suffer the ravages of age and can maintain in our upper decades the same vigor and vitality that we had in our youth. Yet I am not oblivious to the fact that as we age, most of us find it is tougher to maintain strength and stamina, and we often need to work harder to stay in shape. Working out becomes more of a chore, and once we reach our middle years, it can be a very real challenge to keep our weight down and our muscle strength up.

Until recently it was widely believed that there was little a man could do to overcome this physical decline and that becoming fat and flabby was an inevitable part of the normal aging process. It was widely believed that beyond a certain age, all you could hope for was to keep whatever muscles you still had from sagging and that it was nearly impossible to make new muscle. I am happy to report that we now know these beliefs were completely off base. Physical deterioration is not—I repeat, *not*—a normal part of aging. It is becoming apparent that the decline in superhormones is a key factor in accelerating the physical downward spiral that affects so many men. In fact, there is good evidence that the midlife change in body composition—from muscle to fat—is directly related to the decline in testosterone and that by restoring testosterone to youthful levels, this "meltdown" can be slowed and even reversed.

Researchers around the country have begun to investigate testosterone's role in helping men preserve muscle and prevent weight gain. These researchers are confirming the fact that testosterone is *the* superhormone when it comes to helping a man keep fit and trim while maintaining strong muscles. Consider the following:

Testosterone pumps muscle   In a groundbreaking study just published in the prestigious *New England Journal of Medicine* (July 1996), researchers made the stunning announcement that testosterone can significantly enhance muscle size *even in men who do not exercise*. In their study, which involved male weight lifters, the researchers gave one group of men weekly testosterone injections and another group of men a placebo. Of the men receiving testosterone, one group was put on an exercise regimen, while the other group did not exercise. The men on the placebo were also put on an exercise program. At the end of ten weeks, the men who took the testosterone had more muscle to show for it; in fact, they had much more muscle whether or not they exercised. All the men taking testosterone—including the nonexercisers—had significantly bigger triceps and quadriceps than the men in the placebo group.

Testosterone's effect on muscle is not just for weight lifters. In an article published in the *American Journal of Physiology,* six men (average age sixty-seven) were given testosterone injections for four weeks. The men showed increased strength in their leg muscles as well as an increase in the production of muscle protein, clearly demonstrating testosterone's ability to *restore aging muscle*.

Testosterone trims the fat   Here is more good news about this superhormone! At a study at the University of Washington in Seattle, men aged sixty-plus with low testosterone levels who received weekly testosterone injections for three months showed a significant increase in "lean body mass." That is, the men lost fat and gained muscle without going on a diet!

Before continuing, I want to make one thing clear: I am not suggesting that testosterone or any of the other superhormones alone are going to turn all men into muscle-bound hunks, regardless of their health habits. As stated at the beginning of the book, if you smoke, abuse alcohol, take drugs, or are careless about your diet, your body will suffer, notwithstanding anything else you do. If, however, you safeguard your health—if you exercise and eat wisely—you will enhance the effect of your superhormone program, and you will look as good as you feel.

Why does the decline in superhormones have such a profoundly disabling effect on our ability to maintain muscular strength? Obviously, as the studies cited earlier have shown, testosterone itself has an effect on creating and preserving muscle. I also believe, however, that there is another, equally important—if less "scientific"—reason that declining superhormone levels make us weak. When our levels of superhormones decline, we lose our vitality; when we lose our vitality, we become tired; and when we become tired, we don't exercise. Without exercise, our muscles cannot stay as strong, and we simply don't feel as well.

The decline in superhormones begins during the middle years when most of us are consumed by work and family responsibilities. At precisely the time when we most need to take care of ourselves, we find it very difficult to do so. A jog in the park or a trip to the gym becomes a luxury. When we become sedentary, we lose our muscle strength. The flab/fatigue cycle feeds on itself, and unless we actively intervene to stop it, it can accelerate through the years.

This is true for all men, but it is particularly true for men with low testosterone levels. Testosterone is not only vital to staying strong and energetic but, as studies have shown, it is also a key factor in the maintenance of muscle. Therefore, if you are low in testosterone, you not only lack the get-up-and-go to get to the gym or the jogging track, but your muscles will deteriorate more rapidly.

Older men who are taking testosterone say, to a man, that they feel not only more energetic but stronger and more vigorous. They have not only more stamina and endurance but actually feel a palpable difference in muscle strength.

A case in point is John T., seventy-four years old, who began taking testosterone two years ago because he felt exhausted and worn-out. "I was weak and flabby, and I knew that I should be doing more exercise. But I didn't have the energy to make it to the gym, let alone get through a workout," he recalled.

Within two months after starting on superhormones, he felt markedly better and began a regular exercise program. Today he gets to the gym at least three times a week to work out with a trainer, and his body shows it: He is strong and sleek, and looks and acts like a much younger man. Needless to say, John is delighted with the change. "I'm more muscular, my workouts are getting better, and I feel twenty years younger."

Clearly, testosterone has a positive impact on the maintenance of muscle and can help to keep our bodies strong and looking good. In John's case, the effect of testosterone was twofold: First, it gave him a much needed energy boost so that he had the stamina to work out.

Second, the testosterone enhanced the effect of his exercise regimen, and I do not believe he could have achieved the same effect without it.

Wanting to be able to flex your muscles at the gym or in the bedroom may be a compelling enough reason for most men to take steps to maintain muscle strength, but it is certainly not the only reason or perhaps the best reason. Preserving muscle will also help prevent another serious problem that affects older men (and one that younger men rarely think about): osteoporosis, or the thinning or wearing away of bone. Muscles support bone, and as we age, our bones need all the help they can get. We tend to think of osteoporosis as a disease that afflicts only women, but this is not the case. Men are also vulnerable to osteoporosis, and the longer we live, the more vulnerable we are.

When we are young, old bone is constantly being broken down and new bone is constantly being produced in a process called remodeling. By our thirties, however, we begin to lose bone faster than we can replace it. Although the loss of bone progresses faster in women, men (who are fortunate in that they start out with more bone to begin with) do lose significant amounts of bone.

I am telling you this not to scare you but to give you ample warning. The less bone you lose, the better off you will be in your later years, and the time to build up your bone reserves is *now*. Exercise, vitamin D, and calcium-rich foods will help you maintain bone, but it will not prevent bone loss. It so happens that one of the major reasons women take estrogen is that it slows the rate of bone loss, which accelerates in women after menopause. There is tantalizing new evidence that testosterone may have the same bone-protecting effect in men.

Although no long-term studies have been completed, preliminary studies of older men suggest that testosterone has such a bone-sparing effect. In these studies, researchers have measured blood levels of substances such as hydroxyproline, a compound that is key to the formation of collagen and bone. As we age, our hydroxyproline levels decline. In one study performed at the University of Washington, the amount of hydroxyproline excreted in the urine was reduced in men taking testosterone, suggesting that more of this compound was being retained by the body to create bone. In another study done at St. Louis University School of Medicine, researchers found that testosterone injections raised the levels of osteocalcin in the blood. Osteocalcin is a protein associated with the maintenance of bone, and a rise in this protein could mean that less bone was being lost during remodeling. Studies have also shown that in men with abnormally low testosterone levels, restoring testosterone to youthful levels can actually increase bone density.

Alzheimer's Disease

We all want to remain steady, smart, and sharp throughout our lives. In other words, we want to keep our brains functioning at full capacity regardless of our age. Restoring testosterone to youthful levels can play a major role in helping us do just that. In fact, there is a growing body of scientific evidence that like the other superhormones, DHEA, estrogen, and pregnenolone, testosterone also plays a protective role in Alzheimer's disease (AD). To understand how, you need some understanding of what we know about the disease itself. In AD, key portions of the brain are destroyed by an overgrowth of beta amyloid, a protein found in the brain and other parts of the body. In normal amounts, beta amyloid is harmless, but in AD the protein literally overtakes the brain, resulting in the characteristic plaques or tangles that lead to the memory loss, irrationality, inability to communicate, and loss of ability to function that are characteristic of this devastating condition. AD is perhaps the most dreaded of all the diseases of aging because it renders its victims completely helpless and dependent on others. Science has yet to identify the precise cause or a cure for AD. What is becoming increasingly evident, however, is that the decline in superhormones that we experience as we age may somehow trigger its onset.

Women who take the superhormone estrogen have a substantially lower risk of developing AD than do women who are not taking estrogen. As explained in chapter 5, estrogen is the "oil" that keeps the brain from getting rusty. Estrogen improves memory and overall mental function, and many women say they take estrogen for the simple reason that they can "think better" when they are on it. Testosterone plays a similar role in men.

In order to understand about the brains of men, I shall tell you about the brains of some special mice, specifically the SAMP8 breed. What makes these mice so unique? The SAMP8 mouse was bred to grow old quickly and die young. For this reason, the SAMP8 mouse provides an excellent model for researchers who study the aging process. What is also particularly interesting about the SAMP8 mouse is that at an early age its brain begins to develop the same brain abnormalities that are characteristic of AD in humans. You begin to see why scientists regard the SAMP8 mouse as a wonderful, living, breathing laboratory for the study of AD.

At around eight months of age, a point when other mice can learn simple tasks such as navigating their way through a maze with relative ease, the SAMP8 mouse already exhibits signs of senility and slowing down. Compared to normal mice of the same age, the SAMP8 mouse has much more difficulty learning tasks. That old saying about old dogs applies to SAMP8 mice: They can't be taught new tricks.

You may have already anticipated that the testosterone levels of SAMP8 mice drop rapidly and dramatically early in their life cycle. That's exactly right. Between the ages of four to twelve months, the testosterone levels of male SAMP8 mice decline by 71 percent. This represents a huge dip compared to the 26 percent decline experienced during the same time period by normal mice. This difference in testosterone levels was so significant that researchers began to wonder whether the drop in testosterone was the reason SAMP8 mice grow old and senile prematurely. A group of scientists at St. Louis University sought to answer this question. They implanted testosterone pellets in a group of twelve-month-old SAMP8 mice and then tested them for any improvement in their ability to learn and retain new information. The tests measured how fast the mice could be taught to find their way through a maze, and how well they could "memorize" the road map. Normally, by twelve months, these mice would have been extremely slow learners and quick forgetters. After receiving the testosterone implants, however, they behaved like veritable whiz kids. They were able to learn and memorize the way out of the maze as well as four-month-old SAMP8 mice whose brain is far less damaged. Although this study does not prove that testosterone can "cure" AD in men, it does strongly suggest that this superhormone has a positive impact on both learning and memory, and it offers some protection from the destructive changes typical of AD. Many scientists believe that testosterone helps modulate the production of beta amyloid, the protein responsible for forming the destructive tangles and plaques in the brain. This should come as no surprise. We know that there are testosterone receptors in the brain, and we also know that testosterone can profoundly affect mood and libido. We also know that testosterone has a direct effect on our ability to perform certain tasks, such as those involving visual spatial acuity. I am talking here about the effects of testosterone on separate functions controlled by different regions of the brain, and yet I believe this is a case in which the whole really is larger than the sum of the parts. There is no doubt that testosterone plays a major role enhancing our mood, our spatial visual acuity, and our ability to learn and retain information. These are among the core functions that AD steals from us when it robs us of our personalities and our "personhoods." This is why I believe that testosterone offers protection against the ravages of Alzheimer's disease, similar to the other superhormones.

Testosterone and Your Brain

The more we learn about superhormones, the more we come to appreciate the profound effect they have on brain function and, in particular, on the aging brain. Superhormones influence the way we learn and the way we think, and each hormone appears to have its own unique effect.

Research on superhormones is even shedding some interesting light on the ongoing gender debates in science. Those who maintain that there are gender-based differences in mental function will find support in some recent findings. Well-known researchers Doreen Kimura and Diane Lunn of the University of Western Ontario have found that from early childhood through adulthood males are better than females at what are called visual spatial tasks; for example, men tend to be better at dart throwing, skeet shooting, and map reading. What is so interesting about the work of Drs. Kimura and Lunn is that it clearly shows that these sexual differences in mental acuity are not due to environment or conditioning but are present in children as early as age three. Researchers Kimberly Kerns and Sheri A. Berenbaum at the University of Chicago have shown that even at very young ages boys are also better at three-dimensional thinking than are girls and that this difference begins in infancy and continues throughout adulthood. If a man and woman are shown a picture of a geometric figure, instructed to mentally rotate that figure by, say, 45 degrees, and then draw a picture of what that figure would look like from that new view, the man will usually perform this task better. Many scientists believe that testosterone, which is present in the brain, plays a role in these differences.

• • •

Interestingly, older men perform less well than younger men on these visual spatial tasks. Scientists now speculate that the decline in testosterone in men as they age accounts for their diminished capacity to perform these tasks. In a study conducted at Oregon Health Sciences University, for example, a group of older men with testosterone levels that were "low normal" for their age wore testosterone patches for three months. The actual purpose of the study was to investigate whether testosterone had any affect on bone loss, but the researchers also took this opportunity to test the subjects' mental function. At the beginning of the study, the men were given patches that, unbeknownst to them, were placebos—that is, they did not contain testosterone. During the week that they were wearing the placebo patches, the men were given a battery of tests to assess cognitive function. In a test designed to test visual spatial acuity, the men were asked to build a figure with colored blocks by following a two-dimensional drawing. A week later half the men were given real testosterone patches, while the other half continued to wear a placebo patch. Three months later all the men were then retested. The men using testosterone did not show any improvement in mental function over the placebo group—except in one area: the building block test. Here they showed what the researchers called a modest improvement, and yet the researchers were very excited by this result.

Why? To the casual observer the fact that older men do better with building blocks when they take testosterone may not seem to be big news, but, in fact, the implications of this finding are profound. Many researchers believe that visual spatial ability is a key factor in helping us perform a critical task: maintaining our balance. As we age and our visual spatial ability declines, we suffer a marked increase in injuries due to falling. Unsteadiness is not so much a problem for men in their middle years; it is more likely to strike during later decades. Older men—in their eighties and beyond—often complain of feeling off balance and out of control. Researchers suspect the area in the brain that is used to build blocks—that enables us to think in a three-dimensional way—is the same area that helps us maintain our balance when we are walking down the street or getting out of an easy chair in our living rooms. It does this by helping our muscles interpret our surroundings in a three-dimensional framework. Think about it. When you take a step, your muscles need to know when to shift weight and in which direction to move, and all this activity must be synchronized by your brain—or you will fall flat on your face. Without this brain/body connection, it is impossible to be steady on your feet. Although testosterone produced a modest improvement in visual spatial function, even a small but subtle change in mental function can be very significant in terms of someone's ability to perform a particular task. By replenishing the testosterone, I believe it will be possible to prevent the loss of visual spatial acuity in the first place, which will enable men to remain both strong and steady on their feet.

The Hearts of Men

Heart attack is the number one killer of men in their middle years and beyond. If you are a man under the age of forty-five, your risk of dying from heart disease is extremely slim, but as we age, that risk rises dramatically and continues to do so with each passing year. According to the American Heart Association, every year some ninety thousand men between the ages of forty-five and sixty-four will die from a heart attack or a related ailment. These are sobering statistics, and every man should be aware of them because, in my opinion, heart disease is a very preventable disease. I am convinced that the decline in superhormones that we all experience—and, in particular, the decline in testosterone—is what sets the stage for heart disease. It creates an environment that is hospitable to heart disease and permits it to take hold.

In Europe testosterone has been used for more than fifty years to treat a wide range of circulatory problems, from clogged arteries to gangrene to diabetes. European medical journals are full of articles reporting about testosterone's beneficial effect on the heart. We in the United States tend to ignore these reports. Why? The answer, I think, is that at some point during the 1960s our cardiologists decided the treatment of choice for coronary artery disease would be by the surgeon's knife; they decided the trauma of open heart surgery was preferable to the exploration of other options. I do not dispute that bypass surgery has saved and improved lives, but it is not the panacea that we doctors had hoped for. Very often the surgery needs to be redone after a few years, and the risk of disability and death rises with each successive surgery. Surgery not only exacts a steep toll on the patient but is also the most expensive of all medical options, running into the tens of thousands of dollars for every procedure. As a result of our disappointment with the surgical approach, medical professionals have started to rethink the issue and propose alternative treatments. Some physicians advocate the use of supplements, such as antioxidants, and changes in diet. Others, feeling that the control of stress through meditation and other lifestyle changes is key, dispatch patients to spas and yoga retreats. I do not reject these approaches. Lifestyle changes—giving up smoking, exercise, eating properly—can all help to reduce the risk of heart disease. So can the use of antioxidants. But these measures alone are not enough. I believe that *we cannot prevent heart disease unless we alter the inner environment in the body that allows it to take hold*. I also believe that the judicious use of superhormones will do just this and thereby significantly reduce the risk of heart disease in men.

As pointed out earlier, the incidence of heart disease and heart attack in men rises sharply when they reach their mid-forties. Among women of that age, heart disease is rare, and it does not become the leading cause of death in women until they reach their sixties. Why the difference? Why does heart disease strike men earlier and harder than it strikes women? Researchers have suspected for years that, since the risk of heart disease rises so significantly after menopause in women, estrogen must somehow protect them. Indeed, there is compelling evidence that taking estrogen after menopause greatly reduces the risk of heart disease in women. Not only that, some studies also suggest that women with abnormally high testosterone levels are more prone to heart disease. From these findings researchers concluded—not completely illogically—that: (a) estrogen must protect against heart disease, and (b) testosterone must increase the risk of developing heart disease. In other words, they concluded that estrogen is good for the heart, and testosterone is bad for the heart. If you are thinking, "Hey, wait a minute. Aren't you guys forgetting something?" You are in very distinguished company, including that of Dr. Gerald B. Phillips, Professor of Medicine at Columbia University's College of Physicians and Surgeons, working out of St. Lukes–Roosevelt Hospital Center in New York. "When I went to medical school," he explained, "it was assumed that hormones acted the same way in men and women. I was told that it was the robust man who was most prone to get a heart attack, the most 'masculine' man, whatever that meant, the man who had the highest levels of testosterone."

If medical schools are no longer teaching this faulty logic, it is in large part due to the work of Dr. Phillips, who investigated the relationship between hormones and heart disease in men. In the 1970s, Dr. Phillips began research to determine what other factors, if any, might increase the risk of heart disease in men. At that time Dr. Phillips was studying the role of cholesterol and other lipids (fatlike substances) in causing heart disease, but early on in his research Dr. Phillips decided that there was more to this story than simply elevated cholesterol levels and that there must be other factors that make some people more prone to heart disease. Dr. Phillips then decided to study young men who had heart attacks, and soon thereafter focused his work on hormonal abnormalities. Much to Dr. Phillips's surprise, he discovered a distinct pattern among young men who had heart disease, but it was not the one he had been taught to expect. What he found was that young men who suffered heart attacks had significantly higher than normal levels of *estrogen*!

Dr. Phillips then confirmed his findings by checking the hormone levels of blood samples of men who participated in the world-famous, long-term Framingham Study of heart disease conducted by the National Heart, Lung and Blood Institute. Dr. Phillips learned that those who had had heart attacks had higher than normal estrogen levels.

Dr. Phillips's research suggested that estrogen does not offer men the protection against heart disease that it offers women and that it might even promote it. More generally, but no less important, his studies also indicated that hormones work differently in men and women. The next obvious question to consider was whether testosterone influenced a man's risk of developing heart disease.

Dr. Phillips made several observations that helped answer these questions. He noticed that a particular group of risk factors for heart disease tended to occur together. In other words, if a man had one of these risk factors, he very likely had the others. These risk factors included an abnormal glucose tolerance test with high insulin values (a sign of insulin resistance), high blood cholesterol levels, and high blood pressure. Further studies also revealed that in men there is an inverse correlation between heart disease risk factors and testosterone levels. In other words, the higher a man's testosterone level, the less likely he is to have heart disease risk factors.

Here was evidence that the hormone once believed to cause heart attacks more likely prevented it. But the most compelling evidence on testosterone's role as a heart protector was still to come.

Dr. Phillips and his colleagues recently studied the testosterone levels of fifty-five men undergoing coronary angiography, an X-ray examination of blood vessels. The X-ray images showed the degree of atherosclerosis, or hardening of the arteries, in each vessel and how much the vessel had narrowed due to deposits of plaque. The narrower the vessel, the less able it is to carry blood to the heart, and the greater the risk of a heart attack. Dr. Phillips found that the men with the lowest levels of free testosterone had the most serious cases of atherosclerosis. He also found that the men with the highest levels of free testosterone had the highest levels of the so-called good cholesterol, HDL. In both men and women, high levels of HDL are associated with a lower risk of heart disease.

Dr. Phillips concludes: "In men, the higher the testosterone, the less coronary artery disease. In other words, it appears as if *testosterone is good for men.*"

I think you can now see why I consider testosterone to be such a critical superhormone. Although all the superhormones are important in their own way, for a man, testosterone is the most critical in terms of its profound effect on his body and mind. Low testosterone levels can age men long before their time, accelerating their descent into old age. It is heartening to me that testosterone is fast becoming an option for men who need it. For these men, boosting testosterone to youthful levels can make the difference between leading a life of sickness, depression, and inactivity, and leading a full, vigorous, lusty, and healthy life.

Testosterone is of no less importance to women, as you will see in Testosterone: For Women.

CHAPTER 4

Testosterone

FOR WOMEN

Enhances sex drive
Helps relieve menopausal symptoms
Restores energy
Strengthens bone
Relieves depression

Testosterone is also a female *sex hormone.*

—SUSAN RAKO, M.D., AUTHOR OF
The Hormone of Desire

FULFILLING THE SUPERHORMONE promise means restoring the natural balance of hormones that we enjoyed when we were at our physical and mental peaks. It means following the entire blueprint that nature wrote for us, not just a fragment of it. Let me explain what I mean and why this concept is so very important.

If you are a woman, at twenty years old your body produces peak levels of estrogen, progesterone, and testosterone. At fifty your body produces far less of each. If you receive standard treatment, however, chances are you will take estrogen and perhaps progesterone. As a result, like many women who take only estrogen or estrogen with progesterone, you may find yourself thinking, "I don't feel like myself." And you may not feel like yourself for a good reason: You're not yourself. The reason is that by ignoring the superhormone testosterone, doctors who prescribe conventional estrogen replacement therapy are heeding only part of nature's superhormone command, only part of the superhormone promise. In other words, for many women who feel they are not quite themselves, the ingredient missing from the blueprint is testosterone.

Although testosterone is widely known as the male hormone, it is less well known that it is also a critically important hormone for women. There is a great deal of misunderstanding and confusion about the role that testosterone plays in the physical and emotional health of women. As a result there is also great confusion as to whether testosterone should be routinely included with the estrogen/progesterone given to menopausal women. Today, fewer than 5 percent of menopausal women who are using estrogen are taking testosterone along with other hormones. This omission is due, I believe, to the fact that there is a definite (and I believe irrational) resistance to giving women what is mistakenly regarded as a purely male hormone. This resistance is based on groundless fears that testosterone will somehow masculinize women, causing them to grow facial hair, become overly aggressive, and, in sum, look and behave too much like the stereotypical male. As one of my male colleagues admitted to me rather sheepishly, "I know that I'm not being fair, but I don't like the idea of giving male hormones to women." If, as suggested earlier, male researchers had difficulty accepting the reality that men experience a decline in testosterone as they age, a similar resistance seems to be in force when it comes to acknowledging that women produce testosterone in the first place!

Candidly, I think this resistance is not rooted merely in the perceived close association between testosterone and male development and behavior. I think this resistance also has to do with the fact that testosterone is so closely identified with sexuality and lust. Well, it's true. The ebb and flow of testosterone does control sex drive for both men and women. It may be hard to believe, but many physicians still sincerely feel that it is unseemly to give women (especially menopausal women) anything that will enhance their libido.

It is time to shatter the myth that testosterone is exclusively a male hormone. It is not. Testosterone is produced in both the ovaries and adrenal glands of women, just as a small amount of estrogen, the so-called female hormone, is produced in men. Although women make only about one-tenth of the testosterone that men do, it is nevertheless an important hormone for normal female sexual development. In fact, puberty and the onset of menstruation in girls is triggered by the revving up of the production of testosterone and DHEA by the adrenal glands. This process is known as adrenarche. In women, testosterone levels fluctuate throughout the menstrual cycle, rising just before ovulation, creating a surge in libido. Mother Nature knew what she was doing! That is the point in the cycle when a woman is most fertile and most likely to conceive!

As women age, there is a dramatic drop in the production of testosterone. By age forty, a woman has half the amount of testosterone that she had at age twenty. One factor contributing to this decline is that at this age a woman's adrenal glands are pumping out less DHEA. DHEA is broken down into a small amount of testosterone when it is metabolized, and for women this is a main source of testosterone. By the time they reach menopause, many women are testosterone deficient.

In women, as in men, the extent of the drop in testosterone varies from individual to individual, and while some women may not experience adverse symptoms from the decline in testosterone, others will feel the loss more acutely. In most cases if a woman feels that she needs testosterone after menopause, she will have to raise the subject with her doctor.

I want to assure you that there is nothing unseemly, unnatural, or otherwise unsound about giving women testosterone if they need it. Just as boosting testosterone levels can reinvigorate men, it can be a boon to women, provided it is given to the right women in the right fashion. Restoring testosterone to youthful levels may not be appropriate for every woman, but it is certainly the right treatment for women who are testosterone deficient and who are suffering the effects of this deficiency.

Who Needs Testosterone?

What happens when a woman does not produce enough testosterone? The most striking effect is her loss of libido, a symptom that is far too common in menopausal women. In her groundbreaking book, *The Hormone of Desire: The Truth About Sexuality, Menopause and Testosterone*, Dr. Susan Rako, a psychiatrist, described the feelings of utter despair she experienced after menopause. She wrote that she had lost not only her interest in sex but her interest in life. After her physician placed her on estrogen and progesterone, she actually felt worse. She said that she felt "flatter and flatter" and that she started "seeking out alternative methods to try to pick up my energies and revitalize my turned-off body." Unable to find the appropriate treatment from a physician, Dr. Rako devoted the next five years to doing research on women, hormones, and menopause. She ultimately learned that what she really needed to do was add another hormone to her hormone cocktail, and that hormone was testosterone. She began using a topical testosterone preparation, and, she explained, within two months she felt like herself again.

There are a handful of researchers who have investigated the role of testosterone in postmenopausal women. Dr. Barbara Sherwin, a professor of psychology at McGill University in Montreal, is one of them. She began research on testosterone in women more than a decade ago and is the undisputed leader in the field. In one innovative study, Dr. Sherwin investigated the effect of using either estrogen alone or small amounts of testosterone in combination with estrogen in young women who had undergone hysterectomies and as a result suffered premature menopause. Since one-third of the testosterone produced by women is made in the ovaries, these women experienced a dramatic decline in testosterone when their ovaries were removed. Dr. Sherwin's study showed clearly that the women taking testosterone and estrogen were more interested in sex, enjoyed intercourse more, and even had more orgasms.

"There was a dramatic effect on libido," says Dr. Sherwin, who feels that testosterone can be beneficial for many women who experience a decrease in sexual desire around menopause. According to Dr. Sherwin, the length of time needed to be on testosterone varies from woman to woman. "Each woman is different. Some may need to stay on testosterone for a long time, while others may only need it for short-term therapy."

What about the fears that testosterone will masculinize women by, for example, encouraging the growth of excess body hair? If correct doses of testosterone are given, there will be no such negative side effects. As long as the dose is the lowest possible, there should be no problems.

Questions have been raised about whether testosterone might actually increase the risk of heart disease in women or at least negate the positive effects of estrogen. Oral testosterone does appear, however, to lower levels of cholesterol and LDL, the so-called bad cholesterol, which is good. But oral testosterone also appears to lower levels of HDL as well, the so-called good cholesterol. This is bad because low HDL is a major risk factor for heart disease in women. The effect of testosterone on cholesterol depends, however, on the way the hormone is administered. The good news is that if it is given by injection instead of orally, testosterone does not appear to lower HDL or cause any negative effects. A recent study conducted at the Bowman-Gray School of Medicine at Wake Forest University suggests that women have little to fear. In this study, researchers performed hysterectomies on female macaque monkeys, which made them menopausal. Macaques are a good model from which to study humans because, similar to humans, they can develop heart disease. The postmenopausal macaques were then given estrogen alone, estrogen/testosterone together, or no treatment at all. The researchers found that the monkeys receiving either form of hormonal therapy had significantly lower levels of LDL (the "bad cholesterol") than did monkeys in the control group. What was most striking to the researchers was that there was no difference in cholesterol levels that could be attributed to using estrogen alone or in combination with testosterone.

Despite these positive findings, I still believe that any woman who is taking testosterone should have her cholesterol levels checked every six months, just to make sure that she is not losing too much HDL. If a woman is at particular risk of developing heart disease (if she has high blood pressure, diabetes, atherosclerosis, or a parent who died from a heart attack at a young age), I would think twice about putting her on testosterone unless she absolutely needed it. I would then recommend monitoring her cholesterol even more closely, but I would not altogether rule out using testosterone. A woman's emotional well-being—feeling good about herself and, more important, feeling "like herself"—is critical for good mental and physical health. If a woman finds that a lack of libido due to low testosterone is ruining her sex life, adding testosterone to her superhormone cocktail for even a short period may make a real difference in helping to restore her interest in sex and her ability to enjoy it. (For more information on other things that need to be monitored when you are taking testosterone, see chapter 10, How to Take Superhormones.)

Testosterone Builds Bone

Throughout this book I have shown how one superhormone complements the action of another, and how the cocktail approach customized to the individual can work wonders in terms of maintaining health and strength. Studies of women and testosterone are few and far between, but so far the ones that have been done have yielded some surprisingly good news in this regard. They have shown that testosterone combined with estrogen has a more potent bone-sparing effect than estrogen alone. In one study, researchers gave postmenopausal women either a combination of estrogen and testosterone or estrogen alone for nine weeks. Estrogen has a particular effect on bone; although it can slow down the rate of bone loss, it has no effect on the formation of new bone. Therefore, although it can slow the progress of osteoporosis, estrogen is not a cure for this leading cause of death among older women. The good news is that women who took the combination estrogen/testosterone cocktail not only showed signs of a slowdown in bone loss (the estrogen effect) but, more important, also showed signs that *new bone was being formed,* an effect that could only be due to the addition of testosterone. I believe that the "cure" for osteoporosis may exist in simply following nature's blueprint by restoring the natural youthful balance of estrogen and testosterone that women lose after menopause.

Finally, there is another compelling argument for including testosterone as part of a woman's superhormone cocktail. It makes many women feel better and better able to tolerate the other hormones in their cocktail. Although some women swear by their estrogen/progesterone replacement therapy, many women do not like the effect of estrogen and progesterone, and often say they cause them to experience a lack of energy and zest for life. I think this unintended consequence occurs because their cocktail, which consists of only estrogen and progesterone, does not duplicate the normal hormonal state that existed prior to menopause. Some testosterone is necessary to help restore youthful levels. For many women, a small amount of testosterone can make a big difference.

PART III

Superhormones in the Vanguard

Introduction: Estrogen and Progesterone

ALTHOUGH ESTROGEN AND progesterone are regarded as female hormones, they are actually made in the bodies of both men and women. Interestingly, as we age, men's levels of estrogen and progesterone do not decline in the way that women's levels do, and therefore men do not need to boost them.

Although these superhormones are typically taken together, each has its own unique properties, and therefore I will be discussing them separately. You will notice, however, that at various points the two will overlap; this is because these two superhormones are very much interrelated.

Estrogen in combination with progesterone has been prescribed now for decades to millions of postmenopausal women. To my mind these women paved the way for the Superhormone Revolution that is now enabling us to take control of our lives and remain youthful, strong, and healthy all through our lifetimes. These millions of women were the first to put into practice the theory of hormone replacement therapy, which can be seen as the model for what is now being enlarged into the broader practice of superhormone replacement. Thanks to these women, scientists were able to see how effective and beneficial the replenishment of key hormones could be, and now they have the assurance as well, decades later, that the lives of these women have been significantly enhanced. Thanks to them the benefits can now be extended even further.

CHAPTER 5

Estrogen

MOTHER OF THE SUPERHORMONE REVOLUTION

Relieves menopausal symptoms
Protects against heart disease
Restores sexual function
Sharpens thinking
Enhances mood
May prevent Alzheimer's disease
Prevents osteoporosis
Reduces risk of colon cancer
Prevents tooth loss
Improves skin quality

Why do I take estrogen? I have an eighty-year-old mother who can keep up with me step for step. She's absolutely incredible—she can do almost anything that I can do. Her skin is smooth, she has lots of energy, and she looks great. No one can believe her age. Of course, she's been taking estrogen for thirty years. I've seen what estrogen can do for my mother, and I'm counting on the fact that it will do the same for me.

—KELLY M., 51, one of the 10
million women in the United
States currently taking estrogen

LONG BEFORE WE knew about the promise of superhormones, long before the discovery of the aging clock, long before scientists even had a clue about the power of DHEA and melatonin, women were taking estrogen.

More than forty years ago doctors prescribed estrogen for women who had undergone hysterectomies and suffered menopausal symptoms, such as hot flashes and insomnia, as a result. Estrogen worked so well for these women that within a few years many doctors were giving estrogen to women who were entering into normal menopause. Initially, women took estrogen to help them cope with this brief but difficult transition period. Many women felt so healthy and reinvigorated on estrogen, however, that they continued to take this superhormone even when their menopausal symptoms had long since ceased. As the years went by and the first generation of estrogen users progressed from their fifties to sixties and seventies, researchers started to notice something remarkable. Study after study documented the astonishing but inescapable fact that women who were taking estrogen were doing better, much better, in almost every way than women who were not taking estrogen. Here are some of the well-documented findings:

- Estrogen users stood taller and straighter than women who did not take estrogen and did not suffer the bone loss typical of osteoporosis.
- Estrogen users had half the risk of heart disease, the leading cause of death among postmenopausal women.
- Estrogen users had a significantly lower rate of Alzheimer's disease, a debilitating brain disorder that afflicts three times as many women as men.
- Estrogen users had half the risk of developing colon cancer.

As if the discovery that estrogen spares women from these and other serious illnesses was not enough wonderful news, researchers then discovered that estrogen also vastly improved the quality of day-to-day life for women. Women taking estrogen reported that they not only felt more youthful and energized, but they also clearly looked better. Women taking estrogen had better muscle tone, fewer wrinkles, and stronger, shinier hair. Moreover, estrogen also made it possible for them to enjoy a satisfying sex life after menopause.

A recent study confirms just how much better estrogen users are doing than non-estrogen users, and the results are nothing short of amazing. Researchers studied 454 women born between 1900 and 1925 who were members of the Kaiser Permanente Medical Care Program in Oakland, California. About half the women started using estrogen in 1969, which means that by the time of the study they had been using it for several decades. Knowing what you now know about the superhormone promise, you probably won't be surprised to know that the estrogen users not only lived *longer* lives, but they lived *healthier* lives. Among the non-estrogen users there were eighty-seven deaths from all causes, but among the estrogen users there were only fifty-three deaths. In other words, and to put these figures in proper perspective, *there was a 46 percent reduction in the rate of death for estrogen users.* Here is clear and dramatic evidence that a superhormone can extend life! It is no wonder that 10 million women take estrogen today and that it is the most widely prescribed drug in the United States.

Although the women who began taking estrogen decades ago did not know it at the time, they were in the vanguard of the Superhormone Revolution. These women are a living testimony to the power of estrogen in particular, and to the promise of superhormones in general. From their experiences we have learned about the specific powers of one superhormone and have also learned the secret of how to harness the age-reversing benefits of all the superhormones.

From the millions of women who have taken estrogen we have learned that the diseases of aging, such as heart disease, Alzheimer's disease, and osteoporosis, are not inevitable and can be prevented by restoring superhormones to youthful levels. In short, we have learned that superhormones not only can extend life but can greatly enhance the quality of life. Estrogen has also taught us something about the synergy of the superhormones and how they perform related and complementary roles in our bodies.

When estrogen was first used, it was used by itself, not as it is now: in combination with progesterone. Estrogen alone can cause the lining of the uterus (the endometrium) to grow. This can promote hyperplasia, a condition in which the endometrium grows excessively; it is considered a precursor to cancer. In fact, in 1975 a study of estrogen users revealed that these women had a higher risk of uterine cancer than did nonusers. Today, that risk has been virtually eliminated by the addition of synthetic progesterone (progestins) or natural progesterone to the superhormone regime. (Women who have had hysterectomies do not take progesterone, because there is no risk of hyperplasia.) By triggering periodic bleeding, much like a menstrual cycle, progesterone prevents the buildup of excess uterine tissue that could at a later date become cancerous. In fact, women who use the estrogen/progesterone combination actually enjoy a lower risk of uterine cancer than do women who do not use these superhormones. This brings home a very important point: Realizing the super-hormone promise means restoring the natural youthful balance of *all* superhormones as you need them.

Many of you may feel that you already know everything there is to know about estrogen. Trust me, you don't. As you read this chapter most of you will be in for a few surprises. I feel confident in saying this because, although estrogen has been used for years, the estrogen story changes daily as researchers continue to discover new ways that estrogen benefits a woman's body and mind. From these discoveries we learn even more about the power and potential of the other superhormones.

For instance, it was only recently discovered that estrogen is a potent antioxidant—like vitamin E and beta-carotene—and that it can protect against damage by free radicals. Free radicals, you will recall from earlier chapters, are those unstable molecules that can destroy a cell's DNA and—many scientists believe—accelerate the aging process. You may also be unaware of the newfound link between estrogen and brain function. Recent studies now show that estrogen levels can affect mood and mental performance. And, fi-nally, I suspect that most of you have not yet heard about new forms of estrogen that will soon be available, the so-called smart estrogens. These provide the same beneficial effects of regular estrogen but, in addition, protect against breast cancer. These and many other fascinating facts about this unique superhormone are the focus of this chapter.

What Is Estrogen?

Before I tell you more about the promise of this amazing superhor-mone, let me begin by telling you a bit about what estrogen is and where and how it is made.

In women, estrogen is produced in the ovaries, adrenal glands, and in the placenta of a developing fetus. In men, estrogen is produced in the adrenal glands from testosterone. Men, of course, have much lower levels of estrogen and much higher levels of testosterone. (As explained in chapter 3, women also produce a small amount of tes-tosterone in their ovaries and adrenal glands.) Estrogen is chiefly a female hormone, however; indeed, it is the chief female hormone. During fetal development, estrogen plays an important role in form-ing a girl's sexual identity. It is also believed to be instrumental in the development of the brain and in forming the subtle psychosocial characteristics that some say distinguish women from men.

Three types of estrogen are found in a woman's body: *estrone* and *estradiol beta 17* (*estradiol,* for short), which are both fairly potent, and *estriol,* the weakest. Estradiol is the main estrogen produced by the ovaries. Estrogen production is regulated by the hypothalamus, a tiny structure located just above the pituitary gland, the body's so-called master gland. The hypothalamus works in concert with the pituitary and pineal glands to control sexual development and behavior, and it also controls our ability to regulate body temperature. At the onset of puberty, hormones produced by the hypothalamus set in motion the monthly menstrual cycle. In the first part of the menstrual cycle, two hormones, luteinizing hormone (LH) and follicle stimulating hormone (FSH), stimulate the ovaries to produce estrogen and prepare for ovulation. Ovulation is the process in which the egg cell is released from the ovary to travel down the fallopian tube for possible fertilization. Estrogen stimulates the growth of the lining of the uterus to prepare to receive the fertilized egg. During the second half of the menstrual cycle, estrogen levels dip and progesterone levels rise. If the egg is not fertilized, progesterone levels drop, triggering the shedding of the uterine lining, or the menstrual flow.

Estrogen is not only instrumental in orchestrating the menstrual cycle, but it also controls the development of what are known as secondary sexual characteristics—that is, the physical traits we associate with femininity. Estrogen "rounds out" a woman's body, filling out her breasts and hips, softening her skin, and increasing body fat, which helps keep skin from sagging and becoming wrinkled. Estrogen also helps maintain muscle tone, especially in the breast and pelvic areas.

Like the other superhormones, estrogen levels begin a gradual decline as a woman reaches her forties, and then they begin a free fall as she reaches her late forties or early fifties. In premenopausal women, blood levels of estradiol average about 200 picograms per milliliter. After menopause that number drops to under 30 pc/ml, and the ovaries literally shut down.

Ironically, older men produce *more* estrogen and have higher levels of estrogen in their brains than postmenopausal women do. But there's more to this than mere irony. As mentioned earlier, women are three times more likely than men to develop Alzheimer's disease. Some researchers now believe that this higher estrogen level in older men may be the reason. Since older men produce such high levels of estrogen on their own, they do not need to include it in their superhormone cocktail.

Estrogen: The Antidote to Menopause

Recently, a great deal of attention has been paid to menopause, but when I was in medical school more than forty years ago, menopause was barely mentioned. And when it was, it was treated as purely a medical event. I remember sitting through a very dull and dry clinical lecture about the female "climateric" in which we were told that without estrogen, women lose their reproductive capacity and—oh yes—various of their organ systems begin to decline. That was it. End of story. Not one word about life after menopause was mentioned, nor was there even the slightest suggestion that a woman might have the capacity and the desire to maintain a sex life after menopause. There was no suggestion that a woman might have any kind of life for that matter. (Nor did it seem to occur to anyone that if a decline in estrogen is accompanied by a decline in a woman's organ systems, then that too might be treated with estrogen. Nor did this suggest to anyone that men and women might suffer other body system declines as other key hormone levels dropped. In other words, the superhormone promise was staring us right in the face, but we couldn't see it. But I'll return to that later.) At that time the message was clear: After menopause it was all downhill for women.

Fortunately, the attitude of the medical profession toward menopause has changed radically, and the change has been due in no small part to estrogen. From decades of observing women on estrogen, we now know that there is absolutely no reason for women to suffer any untoward or unpleasant symptoms during menopause, nor is there any reason that women cannot stay sexually active and vital before and after menopause. Estrogen is a super cure for the most common and obvious symptoms of menopause.

Why is restoring estrogen levels after menopause so important? Because the drop in estrogen that leads to menopause is abrupt and has profound effects that are felt throughout the body, and these can be avoided with estrogen.

The official definition of menopause is the last menstrual period, but the hormonal shift that sends many women on a roller coaster–like ride of shifting physical and emotional symptoms may begin two years earlier, at the stage known as *perimenopause*. During perimenopause, women may experience irregular periods, mid-period bleeding, and other symptoms characteristic of full-blown menopause, such as hot flashes, insomnia, vaginal dryness, bladder problems, difficulty concentrating, and anxiety. At one time physicians believed that there was simply nothing to be done for women during perimenopause, and they would only prescribe estrogen once menstruation had stopped completely. Today, more enlightened physicians are prescribing low-dose birth control pills (which contain estrogen and progesterone) to help ease the transition from perimenopause to menopause, and for many women this treatment completely eliminates the annoying symptoms.

One of the most common and unpleasant menopausal symptoms is the infamous hot flash, experienced by a whopping 75 percent of women. Some women try to put a positive spin on hot flashes by calling them "power surges," but no matter what you call them, they can be quite uncomfortable. Hot flashes are characterized by a sudden feeling of intense heat, followed by heavy sweating. Hot flashes are caused by the body's discharge of LH and FSH to stimulate ovulation at a time when the ovaries are winding down and are no longer able to produce an egg cell. Hot flashes rarely last more than a few minutes, but they can leave sufferers feeling absolutely drained. Some women experience them only occasionally, whereas others are bombarded with one intense hot flash after another. They are particularly problematic when they come at night. Being rudely awakened from a sound sleep by hot flashes is not only annoying, it can be debilitating. According to The Yale Mid-Life Study of 104 women, about 60 percent felt that the symptoms of menopause had adversely affected their ability to function in their daily activities. Although most women experience these symptoms most acutely up to two years after menopause, a good number will have symptoms for five years or more.

Most women also experience some degree of vaginal thinning after menopause due to estrogen loss. If declining levels of estrogen are not supplemented, the vaginal wall thins out, and there is a decline in the production of the secretions that lubricate the vagina. The vaginal tissue becomes less pliable, making sex uncomfortable.

Within a short time after beginning estrogen, however, the symptoms of menopause simply vanish for the vast majority of women. Hot flashes cease, the vagina is restored to its youthful condition, and women find that they can enjoy sex as much in the years following menopause as in the years preceding it. Most women feel reenergized and revitalized, and ready to get on with their lives. The anthropolo-

gist Margaret Mead referred to a phenomenon called "postmenopausal zest" that occurs once the roller coaster ride of symptoms end.
At that point a menopausal woman can feel truly recharged and can
devote her time to pursuing her goals and dreams.

I firmly believe that estrogen is the superhormone that can help a
woman reach this "zestful" period even earlier and equip her with
the strength and vigor she needs to achieve—and truly enjoy—her
full potential.

Should I Continue to Take Estrogen Once the Symptoms Subside?

Estrogen does a superb job of virtually eliminating the symptoms of
menopause and has made it possible for women to weather this
passage with comfort and grace. Many women feel that once the
acute symptoms of menopause abate, they no longer need to continue taking estrogen.

I think this is a mistake.

From the experiences of millions of women who have been on
estrogen for several decades, we have learned that estrogen does far
more than simply relieve menopausal symptoms, and to profit from
the full "estrogen advantage," a woman should continue to take this
superhormone for at least ten years.

Remember, the superhormone promise is not just about using superhormones to treat specific ailments, it is about maintaining a
strong, healthy body that prevents disease and debility from taking
hold. It is about maintaining the youthful state so that we preserve
(or recover) our youthful resilience. It is about keeping our bodies at
their peak physical condition and averting the downward spiral of
physical decline. As I will explain, estrogen does more than eliminate
the symptoms I have been describing. It also has an important role
in maintaining a woman's youthful resilience and resistance to the
diseases of aging. That is why women need to take it for a long
enough period—so that estrogen can do its job.

No More Broken Bones!

When physicians first began prescribing estrogen, they knew it gave
women immediate relief from menopausal symptoms, but they did
not yet know precisely what other benefits it might offer. Within a

decade after estrogen use became widespread, however, they discovered that it offered a surprising and unexpected benefit: It cuts a woman's risk of osteoporosis by half.

This was a big surprise, because the longstanding belief was that there was little hope for the one in four women who was at risk of developing osteoporosis. In other words, the prevailing view was that they were all destined to become bent, frail, little old ladies. Thanks to estrogen, the stereotype is outdated. Now the picture of a seventy-year-old woman standing straight and tall, exercising, playing tennis, and power walking in her spare time is commonplace. This superhormone not only changed the way that we think about women, but it also changed the way we think about hormones in general. Estrogen showed us that superhormones play a critical role in keeping us strong and disease free.

Osteoporosis, which means "porous bones," is caused by a thinning or wearing away of bone, making it vulnerable to breaks and fractures. Vertebrae, hips, and forearms are especially vulnerable. About 24 million Americans have osteoporosis, and four out of five are women. Nearly 40 percent of all postmenopausal women suffer from vertebrae fractures of the spine, and each year more than three hundred thousand women will suffer a broken hip. These are not trivial injuries; 25 percent of all women over fifty with broken hips die within a year of the injury due to complications. We do not think of osteoporosis as life threatening, yet at least indirectly it is a leading cause of death among older women. It is a disease that robs a woman of life, but long before it does that, it robs her of the opportunity to lead a full and active life.

As the years pass, it is normal to lose some bone as part of routine wear and tear, but women with osteoporosis lose bone at a much more rapid pace. Although osteoporosis is most often diagnosed in women who are in their sixties and seventies, the damage really begins immediately following menopause, long before there are any obvious signs.

In order to understand osteoporosis, you need to think of the human body as a factory that is constantly replenishing itself. If you think in terms of hair and nails, we are continuously growing new cells to replace old cells. This is true of our bones as well because they undergo a continuous process called remodeling, in which old bone is broken down and new bone is created in its place. The cells that destroy old bone are called osteoclasts. The cells that make new bone are called osteoblasts. During childhood and early adulthood, the osteoblasts, the bone builders, work faster than the osteoclasts, the bone destroyers. But then, at around age thirty, the situation becomes reversed. The bone breakers begin to work faster than the bone builders. In fact, after thirty-five, both men and women begin to lose about 1 percent of their bone mass each year. After menopause, however, the bone breakers begin to work overtime, and the average woman loses from 2 to 4 percent of her bone mass each year for about the next decade. After that the bone loss begins to level off, but much of the damage has already been done. By the time a woman is in her sixties or seventies, her bones may be so thin and brittle that even a minor fall can result in a significant fracture.

The rapid loss of bone after menopause has been attributed to the decline in the production of estrogen, which is essential for the utilizations of calcium, a mineral necessary for bone growth. Although we do not fully understand the precise role estrogen plays in bone formation, we do know that there are estrogen receptors in bone and that estrogen affects the activity of both the osteoclasts and the osteoblasts.

It is also important for women to understand that estrogen not only helps preserve bone but also helps prevent tooth loss, which is related to osteoporosis. One study showed that out of four thousand retirement-age women, those who had taken estrogen replacement therapy for more than fifteen years had half the risk of losing their teeth and needing dentures, compared to those who never took estrogen. Teeth are connected through ligaments to the jawbone, a fact which has led researchers to speculate that as the jawbone thins out, it sets the stage for tooth decay and loss.

Not every woman is at risk for osteoporosis. Both genetics and environment appear to be determining factors. Women who have dense bones to begin with, who don't smoke (smoking saps the body of estrogen), and who eat enough calcium-rich foods are considered to be at lower risk. Even if they lose some bone, they have enough remaining bone to offset the loss. Conversely, slim, small-boned Caucasian or Asian women, particularly those with a family history of osteoporosis, are considered to be at greatest risk.

Even a woman who is at high risk of developing osteoporosis can significantly reduce her risk by taking estrogen after menopause. Restoring estrogen to more youthful levels can very effectively prevent the damage caused by osteoclasts and help a woman conserve her precious bone mass. Even women who already suffer from osteoporosis can benefit from taking estrogen because it will help slow down further bone loss. *But in order for a woman to be protected against osteoporosis, she needs to take estrogen for at least ten years following menopause.*

I emphasize this point because, as mentioned earlier, too few women stay on estrogen beyond three years. Most women who use estrogen today do so simply to relieve menopausal symptoms, and once the symptoms abate, they stop taking the hormones. Many women believe that even a short time on estrogen is enough to save their bones, *but this simply isn't true.* In fact, for a woman who is at risk for developing osteoporosis, this could be a serious mistake. It is also important to note that in order to prevent osteoporosis, women need to maintain a blood level of estrogen above 50 pc/ml. I mention this because many physicians are giving women the absolute lowest dose of estrogen required to treat the hot flashes and are not measuring blood levels to determine whether the women are getting enough estrogen to protect their bones. There is a tendency to undertreat menopause and to give "cosmetic" doses of estrogen—that is, just enough to stop the obvious discomfort but not enough to make up for the true loss. What we're seeing is that ten years down the road at least one-third of the women whom we thought were being protected from osteoporosis will develop it because they didn't get enough estrogen.

The question that remains is, if you don't have symptoms of osteoporosis until you actually break a hip or an arm, how do you know if you should be taking estrogen after menopause as a preventive measure? There is an easy answer: Prior to menopause, every woman should have a bone density test to determine the condition of her bones, especially her spine and hip bones. The gold standard of these tests is the Dual Energy X-ray Absorptiometry, known as DEXA. For reasons that are mysterious to me, few doctors recommend that their patients have this test, and so very often it is up to women to request it. If I were you, I would prevail upon my physician to order a test and try to get my HMO or insurance company to pay for it. But even if you have to pay for this test directly, I still urge you to have it because the information it discloses could truly save your life. If, for example, you are in your late forties and just heading into menopause and the test reveals that your bone density is low, it's a safe bet that you will develop osteoporosis after menopause unless you start on estrogen as soon as you become menopausal.

There are other steps that you can take to save your bones, and when I say "steps," I mean this quite literally. Weight-bearing exercise, such as walking, jogging, running, and weight lifting, can also help preserve bone mass and strengthen muscles, which support the bones. Every woman should be doing some kind of exercise to maintain body strength. Getting enough calcium is also critically important. Since few women get enough calcium in their food, it is advisable to take at least 1,500 mg. of calcium daily along with 400 i.u. (international units) of vitamin D, which aids in calcium absorption. When combined with estrogen, these other measures can help keep your body sturdy, straight, and strong for your entire lifetime.

Matters of the Heart

As explained in earlier chapters, the drop in the levels of superhormones in both women and men corresponds to a sharp rise in their risk of developing heart disease, the number one killer of both women and men. Nowhere is this connection clearer than in the case of women and menopause. When a woman's estrogen levels drop, her risk of heart disease soars.

Heart disease rarely strikes young women. Few women in their forties or even fifties have heart attacks, compared to men of the same age for whom it is the leading cause of death. But as women age, heart disease becomes an equal opportunity killer. At about age fifty, the risk begins to rise steadily. By sixty and from then on, a woman's risk of dying of heart disease is equal to that of a man her age.

Why does a woman's risk of dying of heart disease increase so dramatically between the ages of fifty and sixty? What is happening in her body that creates an environment in which heart disease can take hold and flourish? By now the answer is probably obvious. Most women reach menopause during the fifth decade of life, and that means their estrogen levels plummet. Scientists believe that estrogen protects women from heart disease. This is very apparent in the case of women who have had hysterectomies. Not only do they experience menopause prematurely, they also experience a threefold increase in their risk of developing heart disease. This is a very sobering statistic, considering that one in nine women between the ages of forty-five and sixty-four have some form of blood vessel disease (although it may be in its earliest stages); this ratio soars to one out of three for women sixty-five years and older.

There is compelling evidence that by restoring estrogen to more youthful levels after menopause, we can protect the hearts of women in many different ways. In fact, estrogen may prevent the onset of heart disease in the first place. In one well-known study, the Nurses' Health Study, researchers monitored 120,000 women for more than a decade. The postmenopausal nurses on estrogen had about half the incidence of heart disease as the women who were not taking it. In other words, by taking estrogen these women managed to reduce their risk of heart disease by 50 percent! Given the fact that we physicians get excited when we discover that a drug can reduce the risk of heart disease by 10 to 20 percent, a 50 percent reduction should have us celebrating. Yet, for reasons that escape me, many women who are at risk of developing heart disease have not been informed about estrogen's protective effect.

Estrogen also seems to work wonders for women who already have heart conditions. Studies have shown that postmenopausal women with established heart disease had a 70 percent decrease in mortality over a ten-year period compared to women who did not take estrogen. This is very compelling evidence that estrogen can save lives, and I feel that any woman with heart disease or who is at risk of developing heart disease should seriously consider taking estrogen. If her doctor has not recommended it, I urge her to ask about it.

Estrogen Reduces Bad Cholesterol and Increases Good Cholesterol

What is particularly intriguing about estrogen's effect on the heart is that it seems to work in several different ways to keep the heart strong and pumping efficiently. We know that estrogen can lower total blood cholesterol and raise HDL, the good cholesterol. For women, a low level of HDL is considered a major risk factor for developing heart disease. There are very few known substances that can raise HDL, so estrogen is a very valuable weapon in the fight against heart disease.

Estrogen Is Now Known to Be an Antioxidant

Estrogen, like the superhormones DHEA and melatonin, is a potent antioxidant, and is also, like vitamin E, beta-carotene, and vitamin

C, a free radical scavenger. Free radicals are highly unstable oxygen molecules that bind easily with other molecules. The energy that results from this bonding can cause damage to the cells and tissues of our body, including our arteries. If arteries become damaged, they can develop deposits of plaque that in turn can block the flow of blood, causing a heart attack or stroke. Free radical scavengers such as estrogen interfere with the ability of these unstable molecules to bind with others, preventing this chain of events from occurring.

Estrogen Helps Strengthen Blood Vessels

Estrogen has other beneficial effects on arteries that could explain how it protects against heart disease. For example, within the endothelium, the lining of our arteries, special cells produce a substance called nitric oxide that helps keep the arteries dilated or relaxed. If the endothelium becomes damaged from oxidative stress, this can interfere with the production or effectiveness of nitric oxide. Researchers believe that by protecting against oxidative damage to the endothelium, estrogen helps maintain proper vascular reactivity. In other words, the arteries remain undamaged so that the blood can flow freely to the heart and other vital organs.

How Much Estrogen Is Enough?

Even if you are already taking estrogen, you may not be getting enough of it to protect your heart adequately. Researchers now believe that blood estrogen levels must be kept at 80 to 100 picograms per deciliter to prevent heart disease, and yet many women are receiving doses that are too low to maintain this level. Their doses are high enough to prevent the symptoms of menopause, but they are too low to raise HDL, cut cholesterol, or maintain healthy arteries (or, as discussed earlier, protect against osteoporosis). At low doses, estrogen is doing only half the job it could be doing. If you are at risk of developing heart disease—that is, if you have a family history of heart disease, have high cholesterol or high blood pressure, or have had a premenopausal hysterectomy—your physician needs to make sure that your estrogen levels are high enough so that you are getting proper protection. (For more information on how to take estrogen, turn to chapter 10, How to Take Superhormones.)

Estrogen and Your Brain

Until very recently it was commonly believed that the sex hormones —estrogen, progesterone, and testosterone—operated chiefly below the head. The brain itself was believed to be controlled by an entirely different group of hormones called neuroendocrines, which are produced inside the brain. We now know that this view is highly simplistic and that there is actually a delicate feedback mechanism between the brain and the sex hormones; in fact, sex hormones also function as neuroendocrines. Indeed, all the superhormones affect brain function in one way or another and are instrumental in maintaining mood, psychic energy, and memory. That is why restoring superhormones to youthful levels has such a profound effect on our body systems, on our psyche, and on our overall health.

For many women estrogen is a brain tonic. It is the fuel that keeps their brains running and keeps them happier, more focused, and more energetic. My friend Joan K., age forty-nine, who has a Ph.D. in mathematics and teaches calculus to college students, is typical of such women. Joan is not only smart, she is funny, attractive, and a wonderful teacher who prides herself on her ability to make such a formidable subject as calculus entertaining and easy to learn. After she became menopausal in her late forties, however, Joan found that she was struggling to teach her classes. "I found that I couldn't think straight anymore. I had a great deal of difficulty formulating my thoughts. I pride myself on my ability to explain complicated concepts in a simple, easy-to-understand way. But suddenly I found myself standing in front of the classroom grappling for the next word. I was unable to think clearly. Estrogen gave me my brain back. For me it is the difference between feeling smart and sharp and feeling completely out of it."

Given what we know about the way hormones behave, it is not surprising that estrogen has such a profound effect on mental function. Hormones are involved in literally every bodily process, and cognitive function is no exception. In fact, there are estrogen receptors throughout the brain. These are sites where estrogen binds to molecules in the cell, triggering a biochemical reaction. Wherever there are receptors, there is activity, and for estrogen, the brain is a virtual hotbed of activity.

From our earliest days estrogen helps shape the way the brain develops, and this is why researchers believe that the brains of men and women contain subtle but very real differences. You may recall the discussion in the chapter on testosterone concerning how men tend to perform better than women on certain kinds of tasks, including map reading and jobs that require visual spatial skills, such as darts and skeet shooting. As you might have guessed, women are better than men at other kinds of tasks, and this is believed to be related to their higher estrogen levels. For example, women typically outperform men in arithmetic calculation, are better able to alphabetize words, and are much more proficient at verbal recall. By verbal recall I mean that if you read a man and a woman a list of words and five minutes later ask them to recall the words, the woman will do better. Although men are better map readers, women are actually better at remembering landmarks along a route. In other words, if a man loses the map, he had better have a woman along in the car to guide him, or he won't have a clue! (And as we all know, even without the benefit of blind clinical studies, a man will certainly never ask for directions!)

Researchers have found that estrogen appears to have several interesting effects on the brain that could explain its role in mental function. For example, animal studies have shown that estrogen increases the amount of an enzyme necessary for the synthesis of acetylcholine, a chemical neurotransmitter in the brain that is involved in memory and Alzheimer's disease.

Estrogen also has a direct influence on the memory center of the brain, known as the hippocampus. Neurologist Dr. Bruce McEwen of Rockefeller University in New York has found that when estrogen binds to certain cells in the hippocampus, it stimulates the formation of small branches of nerve cells called dendrites; these dendrites form the network through which brain cells communicate. As we age, our ability to form dendrites declines, which may be one of the reasons memory begins to wane. Other researchers have shown that in animals there is a direct correlation between estrogen levels and the ability of cells in the brain to absorb nerve growth factor, a protein that is critical for the maintenance of brain cells.

Last but not least, estrogen is an antioxidant, as already noted, and in much the same way that it protects the cells of the coronary arteries from damage inflicted by those troublesome free radicals, it may also protect the cells of the brain from oxidative damage.

What all this means is that estrogen is involved in the formation and maintenance of precious brain cells. When a woman becomes menopausal and her estrogen levels take a nosedive, she may begin to experience some real and palpable changes in how well she can think, learn, and remember.

Numerous studies have shown that postmenopausal women on estrogen typically perform certain types of tasks better than women who do not take estrogen. For example, two distinguished researchers at McGill University in Montreal, Drs. Barbara B. Sherwin and Diane L. Kampen, tested twenty-eight women who were on estrogen and forty-three women who were not. The researchers read a short passage aloud to each woman and then, half an hour later, asked them to recall as much as they could about the passage. The women taking estrogen were able to recall more than the non–estrogen users could. In real-life situations this means that estrogen users may be able to remember facts more readily, such as phone numbers and names of new acquaintances. If this sounds like a benefit of little consequence, consider that these are precisely the kinds of tasks that we are called upon to perform daily, at home and on the job. If you consider how many times in a given day you are called upon to remember a name or a number or a fact, you will quickly see how having a more agile brain will not only improve your performance but will make the difference between feeling confident and competent, and feeling "over the hill."

If estrogen can help preserve memory, can it help prevent Alzheimer's disease? As we have said, AD is a degenerative brain disorder characterized by severe and progressive memory loss, mood changes, confusion, and serious physical problems. Tantalizing new evidence suggests that taking estrogen may indeed protect against AD. In one study, researchers at the University of Southern California School of Medicine in Los Angeles have since 1981 been tracking the physical and mental health of 8,877 female residents of a retirement community. Between the years 1981 to 1992, 2,529 female residents died, and of that group, 138 had AD, senility, or dementia listed on their death certificate. The researchers reviewed the menstrual history of each of these women and then checked to see if they had ever taken estrogen. They discovered that women who had taken estrogen had a 30 percent reduced risk of developing AD.

What is even more intriguing is that other studies have revealed that women with mild AD show marked improvement in memory and social behavior within a few weeks after being put on estrogen. In fact, women who had difficulty identifying the month or even the year recovered their ability to recall both shortly after treatment began. The results have been so good that some researchers are considering giving estrogen to men with AD.

More research will be required before we can say with any certainty what causes Alzheimer's disease and how it can be prevented. What is already becoming clear, however, is that in women the decline in estrogen levels plays a role, perhaps a major role.

Synthetic or Natural: Which Estrogen Should I Take?

I have previously outlined the many benefits of estrogen and how this superhormone can improve nearly every aspect of a woman's life. That estrogen can protect a woman against many of the diseases of aging and that postmenopausal women on estrogen typically feel better and stay healthier is beyond dispute. Most gynecologists and primary care physicians today prescribe estrogen to patients they feel will benefit from it.

As has already been said, estrogen is the most widely prescribed drug in the United States. When I said "estrogen," I was really referring to a form of estrogen sold under the name of Premarin. Premarin is a blend of more than ten different types of estrogens found in the urine of pregnant mares (hence its name, *pre*gnant *mare*'s ur*ine*). For more than fifty years, and particularly during the last decade, Premarin has been aggressively marketed, and it has achieved widespread name recognition. To many physicians Premarin is synonymous with estrogen, and when they write a prescription for estrogen, it is most often for Premarin.

The problem is that Premarin, which comes from horses, is not necessarily the best estrogen for humans. As mentioned earlier, there are three kinds of estrogens produced in a woman's body: estrone, estriol, and estradiol. The primary estrogen in a woman's body is estradiol. Premarin contains only a small amount of estradiol, and the balance consists of estrogens that are natural to horses but foreign to women. The estrogens used in Premarin are more potent than estradiol; they are therefore broken down in the body into compounds that are eliminated more slowly than natural estrogen and thus have greater estrogenic activity. In some cases the stronger estrogens in Premarin may cause side effects in some women, such as bloating or headaches.

Some doctors prefer to prescribe pure estradiol—natural estrogen

—because it is identical to the estrogen produced by a woman's ovaries; it may be better tolerated than Premarin and cause fewer side effects. (In this case the use of the word "natural" is misleading. In reality, both Premarin and estradiol are synthetic products in that they are both processed. The real difference between them is their chemical structure.)

Pure estradiol is available in a few products, including the Estraderm skin patch (which delivers estrogen through the skin) and Estrace tablets (which are taken orally), and vaginal cream. These products are not as well known or as widely used as Premarin, and they are not marketed with the same intensity.

There is yet another advantage to using the so-called natural estrogen over Premarin. Premarin is sold in .625-milligram tablets, and this allows little flexibility in terms of how a prescription can be written. Tablets can be halved or even quartered, but tailoring a dose to the needs of an individual patient can be difficult. Estradiol, on the other hand, is sold in powder form that can be made by a compounding pharmacist into capsules of virtually any size dose. This makes it possible for a physician to modify a dose by even a few milligrams and carefully adjust the amount of hormone to the needs of each patient, reducing the risk of prescribing a scant too much or too little. I believe that having the flexibility to make subtle changes in the estrogen dose can help reduce the incidence of common side effects, such as breast tenderness, headaches, and, in some cases, bloating, and thus eliminate a major reason that women who could benefit from estrogen don't take it or don't stay on it long enough.

If you are taking Premarin and doing fine on it, I want to stress that there is nothing wrong with using Premarin. Keep in mind that Premarin has been the hormone used in nearly all the studies that have shown estrogen to be beneficial. Premarin was used in the studies which showed that women who took estrogen had half the risk of heart disease and less than half the incidence of fractures due to osteoporosis. All I am suggesting is that estradiol may be a better choice, especially for those who have not had a good experience with Premarin or who are now starting on superhormones.

The New Estrogen

You have probably heard that some studies have shown that estrogen can slightly increase the risk of developing breast cancer. I want to make it clear that estrogen is not a carcinogen. Estrogen will not turn healthy cells into abnormal or malignant cells. On the contrary, given what we know about estrogen's antioxidant properties, there is good reason to believe that it may actually help prevent certain forms of cancer. We know, for example, that estrogen reduces the risk of colon cancer. Estrogen is, however, a trophic, or growth, hormone, and the significance in this context is that estrogen could stimulate the growth of an already existing cancer. That is why I recommend that any woman who goes on estrogen should first have a mammogram. (By the way, if you are fifty or older, you should have an annual mammogram in any event!) Women with a personal or family history of breast cancer are often advised to avoid estrogen altogether. I know many women with this particular risk profile who have taken estrogen safely, and I myself have given it to such patients because their quality of life was severely diminished by severe menopausal symptoms. I monitored them very closely, and there were no untoward effects.

Many doctors, myself included, have often thought wistfully that it would be wonderful to have a form of "safe" estrogen for women who either have had breast cancer or who are at high risk of developing it. Our wish may soon be answered. There may soon be a new type of estrogen available in the United States that virtually eliminates this small but nevertheless worrisome cancer risk.

Several pharmaceutical companies are testing new compounds that do everything estrogen does in the bones, the heart, and perhaps even the brain but, unlike estrogen, do not promote the growth of cancers in either the breast or the uterus; in fact, they may even help prevent them.

These new compounds are called "selective estrogen receptor modulators," or SERM, and they are popularly known as "smart estrogens." As their official name suggests, these compounds attach to estrogen receptors on cells throughout the body and act according to the kind of tissue involved. In bone tissue, for example, designer estrogens may slow down the loss of bone cells and perhaps even stimulate the formation of new bone, whereas in uterine and breast tissue, the same designer estrogen may block cells from reproducing, thus preventing cancerous growths.

Tamoxifen, the drug used in breast cancer therapy since 1978, was the first SERM used on women. Researchers discovered that tamoxifen not only thwarted the growth of breast tumors but also produced some unexpected benefits, including a reduction in bone loss and lower cholesterol. Tamoxifen has its downside, however. It does not relieve menopausal symptoms, and, in fact, can actually cause hot flashes. Moreover, in the very high doses used to treat breast cancer, it can promote uterine cancer in a small group of women. Nevertheless, tamoxifen showed researchers that it is possible to design a synthetic estrogen that can selectively turn on or turn off estrogen receptors, and the race to find the right synthetic estrogen was on.

The SERM of choice may be Raloxifene, an Eli Lilly drug that is now being tested on thousands of women around the world. So far the test results look promising. Raloxifene can lower cholesterol and prevent bone loss but does not promote uterine cancer. Eli Lilly expects Raloxifene to be available to women as early as 1998 and possibly earlier if the FDA gives its approval.

The one thing that designer estrogens don't do as well as the real thing is relieve menopausal symptoms such as hot flashes. Developers of these new estrogens anticipate that during perimenopause and immediately following menopause, women will still need to take real estrogen if they are experiencing these symptoms. For most women, however, the acute symptoms are over within two years following menopause, and at that point they may switch to a designer estrogen.

The Promise of Superhormone Estrogen

It is truly wonderful that women now have more options than ever when it comes to the type of estrogen they can choose from, yet I do not want the discussion over the merits of "natural" estrogen or a "synthetic" estrogen or even "smart" estrogen to obscure an important point: For the vast majority of women, estrogen—whatever kind they take—is a lifesaver and a life enhancer. This superhormone will not only protect women from the diseases of aging but will protect them from the underlying disease of aging itself. It will enable women to maintain a standard of physical and mental well-being that makes life worth living, which to me is the true embodiment of the superhormone promise.

CHAPTER 6

Natural Progesterone

THE FEEL-GOOD HORMONE FOR WOMEN

Protects against cancer
Natural tranquilizer
Promotes feelings of well-being
Enhances action of estrogen
Relieves menopausal symptoms
May stimulate new bone formation
Potential treatment for nerve disease

AS WE SAW in the last chapter, estrogen is a superhormone that reverses many of the ravages of aging and prevents and treats many of the conditions that can age women prematurely.

But estrogen is only part of the story!

There is another female hormone of equal importance to women, although it is rarely discussed. It is a superhormone that has been given short shrift by physicians, the research community, pharmaceutical companies, and the FDA, to the great detriment of women. It is a superhormone that in many cases can safely and effectively relieve menopausal symptoms, protect against cancer, and prevent osteoporosis. Yet, because it is so ignored, few women are taking it.

The superhormone is *natural* progesterone, with the emphasis on the word "natural." Today, most women take synthetic versions of progesterone, or *progestins,* with estrogen. Yet, as you will see, this is not what Mother Nature had in mind.

Natural progesterone enhances the action of estrogen, and according to Mother Nature's blueprint, these two superhormones were meant to work together. When women are in their youthful prime, and estrogen and progesterone are at their adult peaks, these superhormones work together to maintain the normal hormonal balance within their bodies. At midlife the levels of both these superhormones decline, leaving women vulnerable to diseases such as osteoporosis and heart disease, and to other changes in their bodies that can severely diminish their quality of life. The combination of natural progesterone and estrogen can prevent this downward spiral by keeping women vital, strong, and sexy, and that is why they are *both* superhormones.

In addition to enhancing the action of estrogen, natural progesterone is a potent anti-aging superhormone in its own right; it can do some things that estrogen cannot.

Before I tell you about the wonders of natural progesterone, let me first explain the difference between natural and synthetic products. When used in the context of superhormones, the word "natural" is actually a misnomer, since all the superhormone supplements are synthetic products that undergo some degree of chemical processing. Here, "natural" refers to the chemical structure of the superhormone. A natural hormone simply means one that is *identical* in structure to the hormone naturally produced by the body. By comparison, a "synthetic" hormone is one that has the same action as the hormone produced by the body but has a slightly different chemical structure.

The form of progesterone most commonly now used in the United States is the synthetic form, which is called progestin. The most commonly prescribed brand of progestin is Provera, or medroxy-progesterone. Progestin was developed in the 1930s from diosgenin, a compound found in wild yams, and was used as an ingredient in birth control pills. At one time progestin was considered superior to natural progesterone because the form of natural progesterone then available was not as readily absorbed by the body. This is no longer the case. Today's natural progesterone undergoes a process called micronization, which breaks it up into tiny particles that are easily absorbed, and micronized progesterone is now used in all oral preparations.

I am among a growing number of physicians who do not believe that synthetic progestins work as well for women as natural progesterone. Nor do I believe that they offer the same health benefits. There is another important reason that I prefer natural progesterone. I call natural progesterone the "feel-good" superhormone because most women feel better on natural progesterone than they do on synthetic progestins, for reasons that I will explain shortly. (Before continuing, I want to stress that there is nothing wrong with using progestin. My only objection to it is that I feel natural progesterone is a better choice. If a woman is taking progestin with estrogen and feels fine on it, however, there is no need for her to switch. If a woman does not feel well on progestin, however, or is just starting on estrogen, then I think that she and her physician should strongly consider using natural progesterone.)

Despite the growing evidence that natural progesterone is better for women, it has been extremely difficult to get the medical community to focus on it. The reason that natural progesterone has been overlooked is precisely the same reason that superhormones like DHEA, pregnenolone, and melatonin were, until recently, pretty much ignored. Natural progesterone is a natural substance that cannot be patented. Consequently, pharmaceutical companies have no financial incentive to study and market it. As I have said repeatedly, one of my goals in writing *The Superhormone Promise* is to "rescue" natural progesterone and other superhormones from neglect and to make sure they receive the attention and funding for the research they deserve.

What Is Progesterone?

"Pro" and *"gesterone"* mean *"for gestation."* As its name might suggest, progesterone is produced in huge amounts by the placenta during pregnancy. If a woman does not produce enough progesterone, she will have difficulty carrying her pregnancy to term, and this is why progesterone is often prescribed during pregnancy to women with a history of miscarriage. In fact, the so-called abortion pill used in France, RU-486, works by blocking the action of progesterone. This results in a spontaneous abortion of the pregnancy.

As most women know, hormones can have a profound effect on mood, and progesterone is no exception; it is a natural antidepressant. Progesterone is the hormone that gives pregnant women a sense of well-being and contentment. It is also a natural tranquilizer and, in high enough doses, can even be used as an anesthetic.

Progesterone plays a major role in the menstrual cycle, which could not occur without it. The menstrual cycle prepares a woman's body for pregnancy. The cycle involves a delicate interplay of several hormones, the most important of which are estrogen and progesterone. Estrogen levels rise during the first half of the menstrual cycle when the egg-forming cells in the ovaries, called follicles, are prepared for ovulation, which occurs around mid-cycle. During ovulation the follicle ruptures, and the mature egg cell travels down the fallopian tubes to the uterus or womb, where it can unite with sperm and become fertilized. The remaining portion of the follicle becomes the corpus luteum, a glandlike structure that produces progesterone. During the second half of the menstrual cycle, a woman's levels of progesterone rise steadily, stimulating the growth of the uterine lining in order to prepare it to receive the fertilized egg. If the egg is not fertilized, the levels of progesterone drop off, triggering the sloughing off of cells on the uterine wall. It is the decline in progesterone that triggers a woman's monthly bleeding.

Almost every woman (and by now most men) know about the condition called premenstrual syndrome, or PMS. PMS is characterized by a combination of symptoms, including moodiness, irritability, bloating, and headaches that occur seven to ten days before the onset of menstruation. PMS occurs during the time of the cycle when progesterone levels are supposed to be high, but many women who suffer from PMS have lower than normal progesterone levels. That is why one common treatment for PMS is to take progesterone supplements during the second half of the menstrual cycle to boost levels to normal. Although progesterone does not cure all cases of PMS, it has been used successfully to treat many.

Progesterone is produced primarily at three sites in the body: the corpus luteum (the ruptured follicle), the adrenal glands, and, in pregnant women, the placenta.

By the time a woman reaches her thirties, her progesterone levels begin to decline. Not only do her progesterone-producing adrenal glands begin to slow down, but she may also begin to have erratic menstrual periods, which will also affect her progesterone levels. It is not uncommon, in fact, for a woman in her thirties or forties to experience what are known as anovulatory cycles. During an anovulatory cycle, estrogen may stimulate the buildup of the uterine lining, but ovulation does not occur. As a result, there is no ruptured follicle to produce a corpus luteum, and no corpus luteum to produce progesterone. When estrogen levels fall, the uterine lining is shed, as in a normal period, but it is not a normal period. Anovulatory periods can become more frequent as menopause approaches. This means that there is no monthly surge in progesterone levels. After menopause, when ovulation stops completely, progesterone production is virtually nil.

The question is, since progesterone levels decline, do women need to boost their progesterone back to youthful levels? For years the medical community said no. The prevailing wisdom was that since menopause is an estrogen-deficient state, estrogen is the only hormone that should be replaced. And, when estrogen replacement therapy was pioneered in the 1960s, estrogen was routinely given alone —or, in scientific terms, unopposed—to millions of women. The problem with this practice was that it completely ignored what nature so clearly intended: that estrogen and progesterone should work in tandem. Unfortunately, the effect of ignoring nature's blueprint was disastrous. In the mid-1970s researchers discovered that women taking unopposed estrogen had an alarmingly high rate of uterine cancer, up to fourteen times the normal rate for women their age. Also very disturbing was the fact that up to a third of women who used estrogen were developing hyperplasia, a condition of the uterine lining that could presage cancer. Estrogen quickly fell into disfavor, and physicians and women steered clear of it. This was no solution, however, for the millions of women who were suffering from menopausal symptoms, who were losing significant amounts of bone, and who were becoming more likely candidates for heart disease.

Finally, researchers took a look at nature's blueprint and saw that there was a simple answer to the estrogen problem: If they gave progesterone along with estrogen, the progesterone would perform the same function that it had in the menstrual cycle. In other words, the progesterone would prevent the buildup of excess uterine tissue and, by doing so, protect against cancer.

Several major studies have since confirmed that progesterone in combination with estrogen does indeed provide remarkable protection against uterine cancer. As a result, women are no longer advised to use estrogen alone unless they have undergone hysterectomies (the surgical removal of the uterus). Today, most women who use estrogen take a small amount of a synthetic progesterone, called progestin, every day along with estrogen, or they take progestin for about twelve days each month following estrogen to prevent buildup of uterine tissue. If the progestin is used for only part of the month, it will trigger some bleeding, albeit usually lighter than a normal menstrual period.

The interdependency of progesterone and estrogen is a great illustration of the principle on which the superhormone promise is founded. That principle is not to boost any single superhormone to an artificially high level but rather to restore the youthful balance between key hormones. Nature provided us with a wonderful model and blueprint, and all we need to do is follow it as faithfully as we can.

You may have noticed that medical researchers decided to add progesterone to estrogen pretty much as an afterthought and solely because it moderated the effect of estrogen, and not because of any positive properties it might have. In the years since women started using progesterone, however, we have learned that, like estrogen, progesterone is a superhormone that has wonderful properties of its own.

The Feel-Good Superhormone

As explained earlier, natural hormones are identical in chemical structure to the hormones that our bodies produce naturally, and therefore they are less likely than synthetic hormones to cause side effects. Women who take synthetic progesterone sometimes complain of bloating, headaches, moodiness, or other side effects not usually experienced by women taking natural progesterone. Moreover, instead of causing irritability and mood swings, natural progesterone does just the opposite: It has a mild tranquilizing effect and enhances feelings of well-being. Indeed, most women using it report that they actually feel better during the time of month when they are taking natural progesterone. As one former synthetic progestin user put it, "When I was taking synthetic progestin, I felt as if I was between a rock and a hard place. I was ready to quit hormones altogether because I hated the progestin days. I felt tired, moody, and real jumpy. Since I have low bone density, however, I was afraid of getting osteoporosis, so I was reluctant to stop taking hormones. A friend recommended that I try using natural progesterone, but when I asked my doctor about it, she had never heard of it. She did a bit of research and then decided that it was okay to prescribe it. It was the difference between day and night. I don't get headaches, and I don't feel dragged out on the progesterone days as I did on progestin."

Although it is not marketed with the same vigor as synthetic progestin, oral forms of micronized natural progesterone in varying strengths are sold by prescription by compounding pharmacies such as the Women's International Pharmacy, the Medical Center Pharmacy, the Bajamar Pharmacy, and others listed in the Resource section of this book. Natural progesterone is also available by prescription in vaginal suppositories and skin creams. Progesterone creams in weaker strengths are sold over the counter in pharmacies and health food stores.

Few studies have compared women's reactions to progestin and natural progesterone, but one such study yielded results that should be of interest to every woman taking superhormones. Dr. Joel T. Hargrove and a group of researchers at Vanderbilt University Medical Center compared ten menopausal women using natural estrogen and natural oral progesterone with five women taking synthetic estrogen, Premarin, and synthetic progestin. The study showed that the women who used natural estrogen and natural progesterone daily fared the best. Their menopausal symptoms improved dramatically, and they had the fewest side effects. In addition, the natural progesterone offered the same protection against uterine cancer as did the progestin.

They also discovered some unexpected benefits related to the use of natural progesterone: The women on the natural hormones had a greater reduction in cholesterol levels and an increase in levels of HDL, the good cholesterol. Perhaps what is most telling of all is that at the end of the study, all of the ten women who were using the natural superhormones wanted to continue with them, whereas two of the five women taking the synthetic hormones wanted to quit.

The Vanderbilt study not only highlights the positive effects of natural progesterone but shows that no matter how beneficial a treatment may be, if it makes us feel bad, we will not stay with it.

Proof Positive: Natural Progesterone Is Better

There is other compelling evidence that natural progesterone is superior to progestin. When progesterone was first added to estrogen, researchers were concerned that it might interfere with estrogen's positive effects on cholesterol. We know that after menopause a woman's risk of developing heart disease rises dramatically and that 250,000 women die of heart disease each year. As we saw in the previous chapter, the belief is that there is a direct connection between falling levels of estrogen and the rising rate of heart disease. As we also saw, women who take estrogen cut their risk of dying from heart disease in half, in part because estrogen reduces levels of LDL, the bad cholesterol, and raises levels of HDL, the "good" cholesterol. Scientists feared that if women were given progesterone along with estrogen, it would negate estrogen's beneficial effect on cholesterol.

In January 1995 an article in the *Journal of the American Medical Association* reported some surprising results from the first major clinical trial to examine the effect of sex hormones on heart disease risk factors in postmenopausal women. The study to which the article referred was called "The Postmenopausal Estrogen/Progestin Interventions," or the "PEPI trials" for short. In the PEPI trials, researchers tracked 875 women aged forty-five to sixty-four for three years. The women were randomly assigned to one of five treatment groups, as described below:

1. One group was given a placebo.
2. One group was given daily estrogen (Premarin) alone.
3. One group was given estrogen (Premarin) daily and synthetic progestin for twelve days per month.
4. One group was given daily estrogen (Premarin) and synthetic progestin.
5. One group was given estrogen (Premarin) daily and natural oral progesterone for twelve days per month.

The PEPI trials found that estrogen alone had the most beneficial effect in that it increased HDL more than any of the other regimes. However, one-third of the women taking estrogen alone, or unopposed, developed uterine hyperplasia, which made this treatment unacceptable. That's the bad news. The good news is that there was a safe treatment that worked nearly as well as estrogen alone. By now you may have guessed that it is estrogen combined with *natural* progesterone, which came in a close second in terms of raising HDL levels but without producing the precancerous changes in the uterus. Although synthetic progestin combined with estrogen worked better than the placebo in terms of reducing risk factors for heart disease and protecting the uterus, it could not compete with the natural progesterone/estrogen combination.

To sum up, the PEPI trials clearly demonstrated that

- natural progesterone actually works better than progestin in terms of protecting the heart
- natural progesterone can protect against uterine cancer as well as synthetic progestin

Other studies have confirmed that women feel better on natural progesterone. Yet, inexplicably, this message has not yet reached the medical community. The overwhelming majority of doctors still write prescriptions for progestin, and most do not even know that there is a different, and in my view better, kind of progesterone available.

The situation appears to be changing, however. There is a grass-roots movement of knowledgeable women who have themselves undertaken to research the best superhormone strategies for menopause and who are now demanding that their physicians prescribe natural progesterone. The FDA has not yet approved natural progesterone for use during menopause, and because of this, some doctors are reluctant to prescribe it. And because no drug company stands to profit from marketing it, no one is undertaking the expensive kinds of studies the FDA needs before it approves a new drug.

Because natural progesterone cream is sold over the counter, some women have taken matters into their own hands. They use it along with estrogen instead of taking an oral progestin or natural progesterone. There is nothing wrong with using a progesterone cream, but the kind that is sold over the counter may not be strong enough to counteract the effect of estrogen on the uterus for some women. If you are using an over-the-counter progesterone cream along with estrogen, be sure that you are being monitored by your physician so that your physician can watch for signs of uterine hyperplasia. In some cases your physician may decide to take an endometrial biopsy, a sample of the endometrial tissue, to make sure that it is normal. When all is said and done, though, I think you are better off finding a doctor who will write a prescription for natural progesterone and make sure you are getting the proper dosage. Whatever superhormone strategy you choose, it is always best to work together with your physician.

Progesterone Is a Bone Builder

Up to this point I have been discussing natural progesterone as an adjunct to estrogen, but, as suggested earlier, it has some wonderful properties of its own. One is its role as a bone builder.

One of the primary reasons that doctors prescribe estrogen is to halt the progression of osteoporosis, the thinning or wearing down of bones that leaves them vulnerable to fracture. Let me briefly summarize the cause of osteoporosis and the role that hormones play in this process. Throughout our lives, our bones undergo a continuous process called remodeling in which old bone is broken down and new bone is created in its place. The cells that destroy old bone are called osteoclasts, and the cells that make new bone are called osteoblasts. As long as new bone is made at least as quickly as old bone is destroyed, our skeletons remain strong. After age thirty-five, however, the osteoclasts (bone breakers) outpace the osteoblasts (bone builders), and men and women begin to lose about 1 percent of their bone mass annually. After menopause, the destructive process speeds up, and the average woman loses from 2 to 4 percent of her bone mass each year for about the next decade. After that, the bone loss begins to level off, but much of the damage has already been done. By the time a woman is in her sixties or seventies, her bones may be so thin and brittle that even a minor fall can result in a major fracture, and major fractures often result in death from complications.

As we saw in the previous chapter on estrogen, the rapid loss of bone after menopause has been attributed to the decline in the production of estrogen, which is essential for the maintenance of calcium, a mineral necessary for bone growth. Although we do not fully understand the precise role estrogen plays in bone formation, we do know that there are estrogen receptors in bone and that estrogen affects the activity of the osteoclasts. Although estrogen can very effectively stop bone loss, it cannot promote the growth of new bone. Nor is it a cure for osteoporosis. Studies have shown that estrogen can prevent up to 50 percent of all fractures, but the flip side of that equation is the sobering fact that estrogen still does not prevent half of all fractures. Women who take estrogen are still at risk of breaking a bone, although they are at a greatly reduced risk.

Recent studies demonstrate that progesterone can halt the loss of bone at least as well as estrogen. Dr. Jerilynn C. Prior, of the University of British Columbia in Vancouver, has performed some groundbreaking studies on the role of progesterone in the maintenance of bone, and her work in both animals and humans has clearly demonstrated that it can arrest bone loss. But what is even more exciting is that Dr. Prior has shown progesterone can do something that estrogen can't: It can stimulate osteoblasts to form *new bone*. For example, in animal studies, progesterone administered with or without estrogen has been shown to not only stop bone loss but enhance new bone formation. In fact, some of these animal studies have shown that there are progesterone receptors, or binding sites, on osteoblasts, the cells that build bone.

Dr. John R. Lee, a California physician, is a well-known proponent of natural progesterone. For three years Dr. Lee followed the progress of one hundred postmenopausal women, aged thirty-eight to eighty-three, who were at risk of developing osteoporosis. In addition to putting the women on a healthy diet, which included supplemental calcium and vitamin D, Dr. Lee prescribed estrogen (Premarin) to women who could take it, along with a natural progesterone cream that was applied daily during the last two weeks of estrogen use each month. For women who could not take estrogen he prescribed a natural progesterone cream applied twelve days a month. The women were instructed to get regular exercise, forbidden to smoke, and told to limit their alcohol intake. At the end of three years, bone density studies of sixty-three of the patients revealed that the regimen had not only slowed down the osteoporosis but had reversed it. These women had an increase in bone density, which indicated that the patients had stopped losing bone and were actually gaining new bone. Dr. Lee notes that although some patients improved more than others, all the patients improved. Surprisingly, according to Dr. Lee, the patients taking the estrogen/progesterone combination did not fare any better than the patients taking progesterone alone. Dr. Lee, who has written several excellent books on natural progesterone, has come to the conclusion that osteoporosis is actually a disease of progesterone deficiency and that estrogen plays a minor role in osteoporosis if any. In support of his thesis, Dr. Lee points out that even when a woman's estrogen levels are relatively high, when she is in her thirties and forties, she is beginning to lose bone. As mentioned earlier, by the time a woman reaches her thirties, her progesterone levels (but not her estrogen levels) have begun to decline, and this is consistent with Dr. Lee's analysis. Dr. Lee's work is provocative, and his thesis certainly warrants further investigation. In fact, let me not mince words: Given the fact that 25 percent of all women are at risk of developing osteoporosis, I think it is unconscionable that progesterone's role in this disease has been neglected.

Progesterone Alone?

Countless numbers of women are now using over-the-counter natural progesterone creams to treat common symptoms of menopause, most notably hot flashes. Many report that these creams work well for mild menopausal symptoms, and they are content to use it. I can understand their position. Progesterone cream is easy to use (you simply rub it into your skin), you don't need a prescription to get it, and you can buy it at your neighborhood drugstore. I am concerned, however, that these women are cheating themselves because they are not following nature's blueprint and are not getting some of the benefits that only estrogen together with progesterone can offer.

We know that natural progesterone protects against uterine cancer, that it appears to arrest bone loss and may promote bone growth, and that it does not counteract estrogen's positive effects on the heart. What we don't know, however, is whether progesterone can do everything that estrogen does. Estrogen is, among other things, an antioxidant that can protect against damage inflicted by free radicals. Progesterone is not an antioxidant, and there is no evidence that it will offer the same protection against heart disease that estrogen does. As we saw in the last chapter, estrogen also appears to have a positive effect on memory and may even inhibit Alzheimer's disease. Although natural progesterone enhances mood, there is no evidence that it has any effect on memory and learning. Estrogen reduces the risk of urinary tract infections and can restore vaginal function. As far as we know, progesterone does not.

For me the key to the superhormone promise, as I've said before, is to follow nature's blueprint and recreate the same balance and harmony of superhormones as we enjoyed in our youth. That means replenishing, in this context, both natural progesterone and estrogen so that a woman will be able to realize the full benefit of the superhormone promise.

On the Horizon: An Exciting New Use for Progesterone

The more we learn about superhormones such as progesterone, the more we learn about their amazing potential. Progesterone is no exception.

In this regard, some of the most exciting work on progesterone is being done in France by a group headed by Dr. Etienne-Emile Baulieu, who is also a pioneer in DHEA research. Recently, Dr. Baulieu's team at the University of Paris found evidence that progesterone may be an effective treatment for certain nerve diseases, including multiple sclerosis.

It has long been known that progesterone is produced in the central nervous system and that it plays a role in helping nerves communicate with each other. That is why progesterone, like other superhormones such as estrogen and testosterone, are related to neurotransmitters, that is, substances that carry messages from nerve to nerve and help run the vast communication network within the body. The French researchers found that progesterone is produced in yet another site in the nervous system, in special cells called Schwann cells. These are found in the peripheral nervous system, the collection of nerves that branch off from the central nervous system. In the peripheral nervous system, progesterone may play a previously undetected role in the maintenance of nerves, i.e., touch and motor function.

The French researchers discovered that progesterone promotes the formation of the myelin sheath, the fatty substance that surrounds and protects nerve fibers. The myelin sheath is to nerves what plastic insulation is to electrical wires. They learned about progesterone's role in myelin formation by injuring nerves in the legs of male mice and monitoring the mechanism in the body that repaired the injury. These researchers noted that concentrations of progesterone were significantly higher near the damaged nerves than in the blood, suggesting that progesterone plays a role in the healing process. To test this theory, the researchers added supplemental progesterone near the damaged nerves and then noticed that there was a significant increase in the thickness of new myelin sheaths. When researchers administered a drug that blocked the action of progesterone, they noted that the thickness of the new myelin sheaths was decreased. Based on these experiments, it appears as though progesterone does indeed play a role in myelin production and in repairing nerve injuries.

The reason researchers are so excited about progesterone's newly discovered role in myelin formation is that several serious diseases can occur when myelin production is impaired, leaving the nerve tissues exposed. In fact, in multiple sclerosis, a disease of the central nervous system, the loss of myelin results in a breakdown of the nerve signaling system throughout the body. Symptoms of multiple sclerosis include muscle weakness or paralysis, vision problems, and lack of coordination. To date there is no cure and there are few effective treatments for multiple sclerosis. What is so exciting about the discovery of progesterone's role in myelin formation is that it may one day lead to a treatment for this disease and similar myelin-deficiency diseases.

PART IV

Superhormones for Special Circumstances

Introduction: Thyroid Hormone and Growth Hormone

THIS SECTION OF *The Superhormone Promise* is devoted to a discussion of two superhormones that not all of us will need to take, but about which all of us need to know.

For most of us the superhormone promise can be achieved through the use of melatonin, DHEA, and the rest of the superhormones discussed in the other chapters of this book. Yet there will be times when some of us need an added boost, and that is where thyroid hormone and growth hormone have a very important role to play.

A thyroid insufficiency is a fairly common problem, but it often goes undiagnosed in adults because physicians expect thyroid levels to decline as we age. They therefore fail to make the connection between falling thyroid levels and the effects, which include fatigue, arthritislike pain, mental fogginess, and increased susceptibility to colds and flu.

Growth hormone can revive a failing heart, stave off kidney failure, and reverse osteoporosis. It is a very potent superhormone with great potential, and it occupies a special place in the pantheon of superhormones.

The next two chapters tell you about these superhormones and the special roles they play in preserving and restoring health.

CHAPTER 7

Thyroid Hormone

The Energizer

Provides energy and "fuel" for all body functions
Enhances immunity
Maintains body temperature

CLOSE YOUR EYES and visualize someone who is in failing health.

Did you picture someone who is listless and slow? Someone who moves about unsteadily? Someone who is easily fatigued and easily chilled? Someone whose mind is fuzzy and who may even seem confused and "out of it" from time to time?

I have asked you to perform this simple exercise in order to illustrate two very important and closely related points that go to the very essence of the superhormone promise.

The first point is that this stereotypical image of someone in failing health conforms to the letter with a classic textbook case of hypothyroidism, which is a deficiency in the superhormone thyroid. The second point is simply to underscore that the textbook image of hypothyroidism bears an uncanny resemblance to our old-fashioned image of someone who is elderly. In other words, there is a strong resemblance between the symptoms normally associated with aging in the elderly and those at any age who suffer from abnormal thyroid function.

People who suffer from hypothyroidism—no matter how old they are—tend to experience fatigue and low energy, slowness in their speech and actions, forgetfulness and mental confusion, depression, loss of hearing, arthritis-like pain, chills, hair loss, and susceptibility to colds and respiratory infections. A younger person with these symptoms is more likely than an older person to be diagnosed and treated. In an older person, these symptoms are too easily dismissed as the standard signposts of what is erroneously perceived as the downward decline of normal aging. Some physicians are so locked into the belief that aging is an inevitable downward spiral that they are too quick to accept the abnormal as normal. To my way of thinking, this attitude is endemic in the medical profession and is, tragically, the chief reason that the downward spiral—which is merely the symptom of the disease of aging—often goes untreated. It is also the primary reason that hypothyroidism goes undiagnosed and untreated in adult patients who, as a result, "grow old" needlessly.

The good news is that we now know that thyroid hormone deficiency can be easily treated. If you are one of the many thousands of people who have a thyroid insufficiency, please take note: Thyroid hormone is an indispensable ingredient in your personal superhormone cocktail.

Like the other superhormones, thyroid hormone production declines as we age. The usual age-related decline in the production of thyroid hormone is not considered to be true hypothyroidism, however. In order to be diagnosed as suffering from hypothyroidism, your thyroid hormone levels have to drop below what is regarded as normal *for your age*. The prevailing philosophy in the medical community is that the drop in thyroid hormone production is a normal part of aging and that restoring thyroid hormone to youthful levels is unnecessary for most people.

I agree in part.

If you do not have any of the symptoms of thyroid hormone deficiency and are perfectly strong and healthy, then despite your declined production of this superhormone, you are probably making enough thyroid hormone to satisfy your body's needs and you don't need more.

On the other hand, many people have thyroid hormone levels that are "normal for their age" but are clearly suffering obvious symptoms of a thyroid hormone deficiency. These individuals present, as I said, the very image of the sick person that you pictured at the beginning of this chapter. Yet typically they are not being put on thyroid hormone because their doctors are too quick to accept their low thyroid levels—and the resulting symptoms—as part of the physical and mental decay we call aging. These people are quite literally being cheated out of their potential for good health.

Thyroid hormone deficiency is a fairly common problem. As many as one in ten women and one in twenty men over the age of fifty have some symptoms of hypothyroidism. (For reasons still not fully understood, thyroid disorders are more common in women than in men.) The risk of developing this problem increases with age, and by age sixty, nearly 17 percent of all women and 9 percent of all men will show some signs of low thyroid function. Thyroid problems also run in families, and if one of your parents or grandparents had either an underactive or overactive thyroid gland, that puts you at greater risk of developing a disorder of the thyroid gland. In fact, thyroid deficiency is one of the most common and overlooked causes of infertility in men and women. As noted earlier, many of the symptoms of thyroid deficiency can easily be mistaken for signs of aging, and consequently they are overlooked. The mother of one of us (Carol) exhibited classic symptoms of thyroid deficiency for more than a decade before—at age sixty-three—she was finally properly diagnosed and treated. Ironically, Carol's husband—a law school professor, not a medical school professor—made the correct diagnosis, and he did it within fifteen minutes of meeting her mother for the first time. Interestingly, he was sensitive to the condition because he had been treated briefly for hypothyroidism while a young child. After chatting briefly with Carol's mother, Ruth, he took Carol aside and said, "You know, your mother's very nice and bright, but I think you should have her thyroid checked." He said that her fatigue, slow speech, thin hair, and facial puffiness made him think she had a thyroid deficiency. Her new doctor performed the appropriate tests and confirmed the diagnosis. He prescribed a thyroid hormone supplement, and almost overnight, Ruth said, she felt "reborn." She found that she suddenly had the interest—and the capacity—to do the things that she had lacked the energy to do for a decade. She could go to the theater and museums, she could go shopping and out for dinner, and she could enjoy a long walk. Ruth snapped back so profoundly that she even took a job! Stories like Ruth's are gratifying, but I won't be completely satisfied until more of the people who are thyroid hormone deficient who would benefit by adding thyroid hormone to their superhormone ℞ are doing so.

Let me tell you a bit about thyroid hormone and the gland that produces it. The thyroid gland is a butterfly-shaped structure located at the front of the neck under the Adam's apple. It weighs less than an ounce but is critically important to virtually every activity in the body. This small but powerful gland produces less than a teaspoonful of hormone each year, and yet without this gland and the superhormone it produces, we could not live.

The production of thyroid hormone actually begins in the pituitary gland, located in the brain; this gland produces a hormone called thyroid stimulating hormone, or TSH. As its name suggests, TSH stimulates the thyroid gland to make thyroid hormone as the body needs it. The thyroid gland secretes three active hormones: *triiodothyrine* (known as T3), a very potent hormone; *thyroxine* (known as T4), which is a weaker version of T3; and *calcitonin,* which is necessary for calcium metabolism. When we talk about thyroid hormone, however, we're really talking about T3 and T4. Too little thyroid hormone can wreak havoc on the body, but so can too much. Although the condition is not as common as hypothyroidism, some people are *hyper*thyroid—that is, their thyroid glands pump out too much hormone. This can result in serious problems, including an abnormal heartbeat, hyperactivity, and irritability.

Iodine (which is sometimes added to table salt) is essential for the production of thyroid, and a deficiency of this mineral can result in an insufficiency in thyroid hormone. In the United States, where salt is readily available and consumed in abundance, iodine deficiency is rare, and few cases of hypothyroidism are attributable to a lack of iodine. But conditions are different in other parts of the world where iodine deficiency is still very much a problem. In fact, experts estimate that about one-fifth of the world's population, some 1 billion people, live in regions where iodine deficiency is a common cause of hypothyroidism.

Before we understood the important role that iodine plays in thyroid hormone production, thyroid problems were far more common in this country than they are today. One of the classic symptoms of a thyroid problem (too little or too much) is a goiter, a bulge in the neck. It is a sign of an enlarged thyroid gland and the need for immediate treatment.

The Importance of Thyroid Hormone

What makes thyroid hormone a superhormone? Simply put, T3 and T4 are critical for the production of energy in the body, and that process is key to our survival. We humans need a steady stream of energy to function well and normally. Without adequate energy supplies we would be unable to perform even the simplest tasks. We could not breathe, we could not walk, we could not digest food. In fact, our hearts would stop beating. You already know, of course, that we need oxygen in order to live. Well, the reason for this is that energy production begins with breathing. Oxygen in the air we breathe is essential to metabolism, the process by which our bodies convert food into energy. The production of energy in the body is controlled by microscopic structures inside our cells, called mitochondria. You can think of them as tiny little furnaces, and in fact they are popularly known as the "powerhouse" of the cell. Mitochondria burn oxygen to produce a substance called adenosine triphosphate (ATP for short), which is the fuel that actually runs the body. What is the stuff that tweaks the mitochondria into action? Thyroid hormone. Thus, as you can see, if there is not enough thyroid hormone available to keep the mitochondria going, they will not produce enough ATP, and the body will simply not have enough fuel to keep it running. When this happens, the consequences can be utterly disastrous. In fact, some scientists believe that the slowing down of the "mighty mitochondria" is what begins the downward spiral that we associate with the most destructive characteristics of aging.

Let me explain what I mean.

As noted earlier, mitochondria need thyroid hormone to burn oxygen and produce ATP, the fuel that runs the body. To be more precise, mitochondria need ample supplies of T3, the most potent form of thyroid hormone. As we age, however, we produce less T3, and this may result in an inadequate amount of T3 for the mitochondria. If the mitochondria are weakened due to an inadequate supply of thyroid hormone, they will not be able to burn up proper amounts of oxygen. What happens to oxygen in our body when it is not utilized properly? "Leftover" oxygen can form free radicals, which are highly unstable molecules that are bursting with energy. When they attach themselves to cells in our bodies, they transfer their energy to those cells, inflicting serious damage. Free radicals can inflict terrible damage on DNA, the precious genetic material inside our cells, impairing the ability of our cells to divide and repair themselves. This, in turn, can lead to a breakdown of our body systems, resulting in what we know as the aging process. Damage caused by free radicals is believed to be responsible for many diseases, including cancer, heart disease, diabetes, Parkinson's, cataracts, and arthritis. The cells within our bodies are subject to attack by free radicals every second of every day of our entire lives, and as we age we lose our ability to defend ourselves against these unruly molecules. If we are deficient in thyroid hormone, the damage inflicted by free radicals may be accelerated, resulting in premature aging.

In order to protect ourselves from the damage done by free radicals, many of us take vitamin and mineral supplements called antioxidants. These are free radical scavengers that basically gobble up free radicals before they can inflict their cellular damage. You may remember from other chapters of this book that other superhormones—notably DHEA, estrogen, and melatonin—are antioxidants. In a sense, thyroid works as an antioxidant in several ways. Antioxidants such as vitamins C and E and the superhormone antioxidants act by cleansing the body of free radicals after they are formed. Thyroid hormone intervenes earlier in the process. By keeping our mitochondria—our cellular furnaces—functioning efficiently, thyroid ensures that we burn oxygen up before it can form free radicals.

There is yet another way that thyroid hormone acts as an antioxidant. Recently, some new and exciting findings about thyroid hormone have shown that it, too, may be a free radical scavenger that not only reins in troublesome free radicals but actually helps stimulate the repair of DNA, the genetic material in each and every cell. When DNA gets injured, it can cause cells to mutate, to change in dangerous ways that can make us vulnerable to cancer and other degenerative diseases.

The problem is that as many of us age, our thyroid glands slow down and produce less thyroid hormone. One reason is that we become more susceptible to an autoimmune disease called chronic lymphocytic thyroiditis, or Hashimoto's disease, named for the doctor who identified it. Hashimoto's occurs when the immune system produces autoantibodies that attack the thyroid gland. Damage to thyroid gland tissue results, and the gland's ability to produce adequate amounts of hormone is impaired. We don't know why our bodies' own immune system turns against the thyroid gland, but we do know that autoimmune diseases in general are more common among people aged fifty and older, especially women, and that autoimmune diseases appear to be associated with declining levels of other superhormones, including DHEA and melatonin, which help keep our immune systems in balance. (For more information on autoimmunity and aging, see the chapters on DHEA and melatonin.) If we begin taking DHEA early enough in life, we may short circuit the process and actually prevent the autoimmune problems that lead to hypothyroidism. But for those of us for whom it is too late and who already have a thyroid deficiency, we can easily overcome it simply by including thyroid hormone in our superhormone cocktails.

Whatever the cause of the thyroid deficiency, the effect is the same. Being deficient in this superhormone means that you will neither feel nor look good. It means that you will gain weight no matter how hard you try to diet because your metabolism will have slowed down to a virtual crawl. It means that you will probably have a high cholesterol level because your body will be unable to properly metabolize lipids. It means that you will have little interest in sex. It means that you will be constipated because your digestive tract is sluggish. It means that you will have difficulty controlling your body temperature: You may be too cold in the winter and too hot in the summer. It means that you will feel tired all the time no matter how much sleep you get. It means that your hair will thin and your nails will be brittle. It means, in sum, that you will be energy starved, and so will every system in your body. That is why it is so essential for everyone to be tested for thyroid deficiency. And those who are thyroid deficient should make sure that thyroid hormone is a component of their superhormone cocktail.

How Do You Know if You Are Thyroid Deficient?

As I have said, because thyroid deficiency so often mimics the symptoms commonly associated with old age, many doctors tend to view the symptoms dismissively. More astute physicians, knowing that this can be a terrible mistake, will test for thyroid function.

There are several ways to diagnose thyroid deficiency. Typically, a physician who suspects a thyroid problem will order a blood test to determine the levels of the key thyroid hormones T3 and T4 as well as TSH, thyroid stimulating hormone. Low levels of T3 or T4 are a clear sign that you are not making enough thyroid hormone. But an elevated level of TSH is also a sign of trouble. When your TSH level is high, it means that the pituitary gland is trying to rev up the thyroid gland to get it to produce more hormone. A growing number of physicians feel that these tests do not tell the whole story and that further investigation is necessary before reaching a definitive diagnosis. Here's why: Thyroid hormone is carried through the bloodstream and brain on a substance called transthyretrin (also known as prealbumin), and even if the levels of all the other hormones are normal, a low level of transthyretrin could mean that although you are producing ample quantities of thyroid hormone, it is not being delivered properly to the cells. I believe, therefore, that it is imperative for physicians to check the level of transthyretrin as well. When transthyretrin levels are low, even if thyroid hormone levels are normal, restoring thyroid to more youthful levels may be called for. Thyroid transporting proteins should be monitored.

What about someone who is suffering from the classic symptoms of thyroid deficiency but has normal test results? I believe that too many physicians tend to rely excessively on "the numbers" and fail to take patients' symptoms into account when making a diagnosis. I strongly recommend that physicians take a careful medical history of a patient and then base their treatment on a combination of factors, including symptoms. Since thyroid hormone helps regulate body temperature, it is sometimes advisable to have patients take their basal temperature first thing in the morning to check thyroid function. To do this, simply place a thermometer under your arm for ten minutes immediately upon waking and before getting out of bed. If your morning temperature falls below 97.4 degrees Fahrenheit, it is a sign that your thyroid function is deficient and that you may need thyroid hormone added to your superhormone cocktail.

Replenishing thyroid hormone can have a truly rejuvenating effect. Within a few weeks, people who were once sickly and sluggish feel reinvigorated, imbued with energy, youthful vitality, and the feeling of good health. They can't imagine how they lived without their thyroid cocktail. But having said this, I want to add a word of caution: Thyroid hormone is strong stuff, and if you are taking it, you should be monitored by a physician. As I've said throughout, I recommend that you work with your doctor and be periodically monitored. But it is especially important for thyroid. If thyroid hormone is not taken properly, agitation and heart palpitations can result, so the dose should be carefully controlled.

Mind and Mood

When I described at the start of this chapter the stereotype of the person in failing health, I described a person whose thinking was dull and sluggish, a person who was unable to keep up mentally as well as physically. The fact is that we need sufficient supplies of energy to keep our brains functioning properly, and so thyroid—the energy superhormone—has a profound effect on our ability to think well and clearly. An infant born with a thyroid deficiency is at risk of developing cretinism, a severe form of mental retardation, because his brain cannot develop normally. Similarly, thyroid deficiency in older people can result in confusion and a loss of mental acuity. But again, all too often these symptoms are dismissed as part and parcel of the aging process. As a result, they go unnoticed—or if noticed, untreated—by physicians and family members. Instead of dismissing a deterioration in mental function as normal (as in "Well, she's getting older, and the blood just isn't getting to her brain anymore"), we should be testing for a decline in levels of thyroid hormone and other superhormones.

Feeling strong and energetic is also essential for mood. One of the signs of depression is low energy, but like the proverbial chicken and the egg, it is hard to say which begets which. If you have low energy, feel tired, and are unable to cope with life's daily tasks and travails, you will undoubtedly feel depressed. If you feel depressed, you will feel drained of energy. We also know that depression is another problem that often goes undetected among the elderly, and, in fact, older people often "treat" the problem on their own by turning to alcohol and tranquilizers.

I believe that much of this so-called depression is actually due to a thyroid deficiency and could be treated and cured with a superhormone cocktail—not the other kind, for not only will alcohol (and drugs) fail to solve the problem, they will actually exacerbate it.

Immune Function

Low thyroid function also means that you will be more vulnerable to disease. As we age, our immune system slows down, becoming weaker and less effective. That is why older people are more prone to illnesses of all kinds and why a child can shake off a sniffle that in a grandparent will turn into a serious cold or even pneumonia. Thyroid hormone plays an important role in immune function by stimulating the formation of lymphocytes. Lymphocytes are the immune cells that attack viruses, bacteria, fungal and other foreign substances that the body does not recognize as its own. Many scientists, I among them, have come to believe that the age-related decline in the production of thyroid hormone is instrumental in the weakening of immune function typical of old age.

In animal studies that I performed, I demonstrated that thyroid hormone and a thyroid analogue (a synthetic copy of the hormone) stimulated the ability of the liver to produce phagocytes, a type of white blood cell that functions as the "bouncer" or "bodyguard" of immune resistance. Phagocytes search out invading troublemakers, such as viruses and bacteria, engulf or grab hold of them, and in essence throw them out before they can penetrate cells and tissues where they could do great harm. Without these hardworking phagocytes, bacteria and viruses would run amuck, and we would sicken and die.

I first became intrigued by thyroid hormone's effect on immune function more than three decades ago when I read a paper written by physician and medical researcher Max Lurie of the University of Pennsylvania. Dr. Lurie's paper described some remarkable experiments involving rabbits and a particularly virulent and highly contagious form of tuberculosis that is spread through the air and is introduced into the body through the mouth and lungs. Dr. Lurie had noticed that when he infected two different breeds of rabbit with this tuberculosis bacteria, one strain, as might be expected, developed TB. Much to his surprise, however, the other breed of rabbit remained disease free. Why was one strain of rabbit able to resist the same infection that killed the other? The answer had to do with the function of the thyroid gland in both animals. The strain of rabbit that succumbed to the infection was characteristically hypothyroid; that is, it had low thyroid function. The strain of rabbit that stayed healthy was hyperthyroid; that is, it had a higher than normal thyroid function. TB is a particularly insidious infection in that it interferes with the ability of phagocytes to disarm the invading TB bacteria. With the phagocytes disabled, the TB bacteria runs rampant. Dr. Lurie showed us that thyroid hormone appeared to have a particularly protective effect against TB and was able to defeat the infection by strengthening the ability of the phagocytes to resist the TB bacteria.

Why am I bringing up this thirty-year-old study today? For two reasons:

First, I strongly believe that the time has come to investigate thyroid hormone as a means of "up-regulating" immune systems that are no longer as strong and vigorous as they should be. Obviously, I have AIDS patients in mind. But I am also thinking about the fast-growing population of people that are now age eighty-five and over who regrettably have not enjoyed the superhormone promise and whose immune systems have become worn out as a result, leaving them more vulnerable to diseases of all kinds.

Second, it so happens that United States hospitals today are confronting an antibiotic-resistant form of TB that is infecting both patients and staff. AIDS patients, who have compromised immune systems to begin with, are particularly vulnerable to this type of TB. In light of the fact that antibiotics are not effective against this form of the disease, we should try using thyroid hormone to "up-regulate" the immune systems of TB patients.

Synthetic or Natural?

There is an ongoing debate in the medical community over the use of so-called natural versus synthetic hormones, and the debate over thyroid hormone has recently heated up. As is most often the case, physicians routinely prescribe the synthetic form of this superhormone, sold under the name of Synthroid. Synthroid contains T4, only one kind of thyroid hormone. The second most prescribed thyroid hormone is a synthetic version of T3 marketed under the name of Cytomel. A small but growing number of physicians, however, are now prescribing the desiccated thyroid, an animal-based product that was used long before the synthetic versions were available. Desiccated is a combination of T3 and T4, which is more in keeping with the way the thyroid gland produces thyroid hormone. I personally feel that a patient should use desiccated thyroid. I am convinced that it will not only be more effective but will restore thyroid hormone in a more natural way, and I believe that many patients do feel better on it. If, however, you are already taking synthetic thyroid hormone and it's working for you, I see no reason to switch.

Thyroid hormone is not a superhormone that everyone will need to add to their superhormone cocktail, but for those with a deficiency, it is an important weapon in our arsenal of anti-aging agents. For the people who need it, thyroid hormone can make an enormous difference in their physical and mental well-being. It can literally bring people back to life, infusing them with the energy they need to live full, active lives.

It is heartening to note that as this book goes to press, an article appearing in *The Journal of the American Medical Association* (July

24, 1996) by researchers at Johns Hopkins University who urge physicians to include testing for an underactive thyroid gland as part of routine physicals for patients after age thirty-five. The article notes that low levels of thyroid hormone, which can lead to high cholesterol levels, as well as weight and depression problems, often go undiagnosed.

CHAPTER 8

Human Growth Hormone

THE RESTORATIVE SUPERHORMONE

Builds muscle
Enhances immune function
Strengthens the heart
Helps control stress-induced damage
Aids kidney function

OF THE EIGHT superhormones, growth hormone is by far the most controversial and, in my opinion, the most misunderstood.

Supporters say that it is a panacea for virtually all that ails us and a veritable fountain of youth. They say that its effects on health and well-being are so remarkable, and its age-reversing properties are so great, that it is well worth the $9,000 to $12,000 a year it costs to use it.

Detractors say that it is overhyped and overpriced. They point to studies that show growth hormone doesn't pump up muscle nearly as well as a good old-fashioned exercise regimen, and they point out that in many cases the side effects are sufficiently problematic to outweigh any benefit.

As is often the case, the truth lies somewhere in between.

I have never used growth hormone in my practice, nor do I take it myself. This is due in large part to the fact that I believe it is possible to obtain many of the same beneficial effects of growth hormone by using the other superhormones, particularly DHEA, melatonin, estrogen, and testosterone, all of which are inexpensive and easily available, and have no untoward side effects. I have, however, studied growth hormone extensively through the years and believe there is a place for growth hormone in the superhormone pantheon of age-reversing agents. Growth hormone can do specific things that the other superhormones cannot. Growth hormone has a very special role to play, and its benefits will be most acutely felt by those who are in greatest need and who are suffering from more severe problems. For these people I think the risk of side effects is minimal compared to what they stand to gain.

As I have said repeatedly, growing weak, growing frail, and getting sick is not an inevitable part of the aging process, and by restoring our superhormones to their youthful levels, we should be able to prevent the diseases of aging. For most people, the standard superhormones should be enough to maintain the youthful state. Yet there are special circumstances when some of us may need an added boost to restore a failing organ or stave off a serious illness. That is when I believe that the power of growth hormone will be put to its highest and best use. Growth hormone can revive a dying heart, stave off kidney failure, and reverse severe osteoporosis. It is strong medicine indeed and not, in my opinion, something for standard use.

The use of growth hormone in its current form will be limited by both its expense and its potential side effects, but, as I will explain, this doesn't mean we will never benefit from growth hormone. Now in development are some new and exciting substances called Growth Hormone Releasing Agents that actually stimulate the body's own production of growth hormone, offering the benefits of growth hormone without the cost or the side effects.

Growth Spurts

Growth hormone is made in the pituitary gland, which is located just under the brain and is known as the body's master gland. Growth hormone, as its name implies, triggers growth in the young, and a child who is deficient in growth hormone will not reach his or her normal adult height and may not develop fully in other important ways. Growth hormone triggers the onset of sexual maturity in adolescents, increases the size of their muscles, and stimulates their bones to grow. It is released slowly but steadily by the pituitary throughout the day, and the levels change continuously, with peak production occurring during sleep. As the father of six, I have noticed that when adolescents are undergoing a "growth spurt," they often require a great deal of sleep. Getting them out of bed in the morning can be difficult, and they are prone to nap after school. This is not due to laziness; rather, it is due to the fact that their growing bodies need to replenish their supplies of growth hormone. Interestingly, vigorous exercise also stimulates the production of growth hormone, and some researchers believe that the benefits we derive from exercise are actually due to an exercise-induced "spiking" of our own growth hormone levels. We know that restoring estrogen to youthful levels in women enhances growth hormone production, and so does restoring testosterone in men. This is one of the reasons I believe that most people who are already taking these other superhormones may not need to take supplemental growth hormone.

As is the case with the other superhormones, our levels of growth hormone decline dramatically as we age; they drop at a rate of roughly 14 percent for each decade of adult life. Our pituitary glands continue to pulse growth hormone throughout the day, but the peaks do not get as high. By age sixty most of us produce very little growth hormone on our own. Extreme stress and illness can also interfere with normal growth hormone production.

There is a great deal that remains unknown about growth hormone. For example, scientists still do not fully understand how it works. We do know that growth hormone triggers the production by the liver of another hormone called "insulinlike growth factor," or "IGF-1." Most likely the effects of growth hormone are actually due to the action of IGF-1. As you may recall from chapter 1, the superhormone DHEA also increases the production of IGF-1, so DHEA's strengthening effect on the immune system may relate to its ability to promote the production of IGF-1. This shows yet again how the superhormones work in synergy.

One thing we know for sure about human growth hormone is that if a child is deficient in it, he or she will not grow. Since the 1960s, children with low levels of growth hormone have been given the hormone to help them reach normal height. For more than two decades the only growth hormone available was extracted from the pituitary glands of cadavers, but that practice was banned in 1985 when some young adults who had been treated with growth hormone in the 1960s began developing Creutzfeldt-Jacob disease (also known as Mad Cow disease) a fatal neurological disorder caused by a "virus." The growth hormone that is used today no longer poses that threat because it is synthesized, and that is why it is so expensive. Unlike the other superhormones, for very complicated reasons having to do with molecule size, growth hormone is far more difficult to synthesize than the other superhormones. Recent breakthroughs in genetic engineering led to the development of a new technology that makes it possible to grow growth hormone in a test tube from cell cultures using recombinant DNA. The result is that growth hormone is once again available, but because this new technology is so expensive, the cost is very high.

Not Just for Kids

Until quite recently it was commonly believed that although growth hormone was essential for growth and development in children, it had no role in the adult body. That is why to date the FDA has only approved the use of human growth hormone for children who are either deficient in it or who are suffering from kidney failure, which can cause stunted growth. We now know, however, that growth hormone is an important factor in maintaining adult health. Today, growth hormone deficiency is recognized as a clinical syndrome in adults who suffer from a malfunction of the pituitary gland. This condition is called pan hypopituitary syndrome, and much of what we know about growth hormone's effect on adults is from studying people who suffer from this disorder. We have learned that adults who are deficient in growth hormone will suffer from very specific symptoms, including the loss of muscle strength, a weak immune system, the loss of bone, high cholesterol levels, loss of sexual function, depression, sleep disturbances, thin skin, and excess body fat. If these symptoms sound eerily like the "normal" changes that we have to come to regard as part of "normal aging," it is because they are. What is truly remarkable is that when these growth-hormone-deficient adults are given growth hormone supplements, their symptoms can be reversed. These adults become stronger, lose weight, have improved immune function, and sleep better; their skin becomes thicker, and their mood improves. In a sense they are "rejuvenated."

Growth hormone's potential as an age-reversing agent captured the hearts and minds of the scientific community in 1990 after a paper appeared in the *New England Journal of Medicine*, reporting on a study headed by the late Daniel Rudman, M.D., of the Medical College of Wisconsin. Dr. Rudman and his research group designed an experiment to test whether or not the declines in growth hormone and IGF-1 were responsible for the increase in fat tissue and the decrease in lean body mass or muscle that occurs as we age. In their study, they selected twenty-one healthy men aged sixty-one to eighty-one who had low blood levels of IGF-1. Growth hormone injections were given to twelve of the men three times a week for six months. The rest of the men were untreated and served as a control group. At the end of the six months, Dr. Rudman reported some amazing results. The men on growth hormone had an 8.8 percent increase in lean body mass, a nearly 15 percent decrease in fat tissue, a 7 percent increase in skin thickness, and a 1.6 percent increase in lower spine bone density. Based on his study, Dr. Rudman concluded that the decline in growth hormone was indeed responsible in part for the loss of muscle, the increase in fat, and the thinning of skin that occurs in old age. In Dr. Rudman's own words, the men who received six months of growth hormone experienced a reversal of the "equivalent to the changes incurred during ten to twenty years of aging."

Thanks to Dr. Rudman's study, many good and serious scientists and physicians outside of the anti-aging field began to think about aging in a different way, not as inevitable but as a "condition" that could be treated—and, yes, even reversed. It sparked a new interest in research on aging, and for that reason I feel Dr. Rudman's study on growth hormone will always have a very special place in history.

Dr. Rudman's study also created a mystique about growth hormone. The media seized on growth hormone as the "fountain of youth," and soon people were clamoring to get it. Some American and European physicians began making it available, at least to patients who could afford it. Intrigued by Dr. Rudman's findings, the National Institutes on Aging has sponsored several clinical studies to determine if growth hormone can be useful in helping the elderly remain strong and vigorous. These studies have looked at whether growth hormone replacement therapy can help prevent loss of muscle strength and osteoporosis. As of this writing, the studies are still in progress and results are inconclusive. Some of the preliminary results have been negative, due primarily to the large number of patients who have suffered side effects. In fact, in a report that recently appeared in the *Annals of Internal Medicine,* researchers said that they were so discouraged by the discomfort from sore joints and swollen legs and ankles suffered by older people taking growth hormone that they did not believe it should be used by the general population. Moreover, although this study did show that growth hormone reduced fat and increased lean body mass (muscle), it curiously did not show that the people taking growth hormone were actually any stronger than they were before they began taking the hormone. Nor could the researchers confirm that growth hormone had any special effect on mental function or mood.

Other studies have investigated whether growth hormone can enhance the effect of exercise in older people. As previously mentioned, it becomes increasingly important for people to maintain muscle strength as they age. (This is one of the reasons I urge people to begin their superhormone program long before they begin this "downward slide." Several of the superhormones, notably testosterone, DHEA, and estrogen, specifically help preserve muscle.) The loss of muscle can be a problem even for older people who exercise regularly. The reason is that the stem cells in the bone marrow which are responsible for the replacement of muscle tissue run out of steam and are not able to keep up with youthful exercise levels. This is why the careers of most professional athletes end by the time they are in their forties, why marathon races tend to be won by people in their twenties, and why older golfers often complain that they need to swing a lot harder. Several studies have investigated whether growth hormone could make a difference in terms of helping older people who exercise retain muscle mass. So far the answer is no. As of yet, there is no evidence that growth hormone can enhance the effect of vigorous exercise. Despite this, I have heard that bodybuilders are using—or, to be more accurate, abusing—growth hormone because they think it will help them pump up their muscles. They should save their money. If you are able to pump up, you don't need growth hormone. If you don't believe me, just read the studies.

I noted that growth hormone cannot enhance the effect of exercise, and to my way of thinking there is no reason that anyone who is strong enough to get to the gym should require growth hormone. What about people who are sick or too weak to work out? Studies show that growth hormone can indeed increase muscle mass in people who are sick, frail, and suffering from what is called "wasting syndrome." This merely confirms what I said earlier: The effects of growth hormone will be most keenly felt by those who truly need it.

Despite the negative studies, some people who can afford the steep price are already using growth hormone as part of their superhormone cocktails. Doctors who prescribe growth hormone say that it is a "true rejuvenator." According to Dr. Edward Chein of the Palm Springs Life Extension Institute in California, the results have been nothing short of amazing. "It is the only hormone that can reverse all the parameters of aging. DHEA and melatonin can slow down the aging process, but from what I have seen with my patients, only growth hormone can actually reverse biological aging," says Dr.

Chein, who has prescribed human growth hormone to more than a thousand patients, including many physicians. Dr. Chein recites a long list of the benefits that growth hormone has conferred on his patients: "Lung capacity improves, body fat decreases, muscle mass increases, cardiac function improves, kidney function improves, bone density increases, fingernails and toenails grow faster, the skin is more resilient, the immune system improves—antibody production goes up, natural killer cell activity is restored."

Dr. Chein's belief that growth hormone can turn back the clock, revitalizing every major bodily system, is echoed by Sam Baxas, M.D. Dr. Baxas, an American-born, Swiss-trained physician, is the founder of the Swiss Rejuvenation Centre, an upscale anti-aging clinic in Basel, Switzerland. (The Centre may open an offshore facility near the United States soon.) Dr. Baxas, too, includes growth hormone in the hormone cocktail he prescribes for his patients. "We can take people back at least twenty years," according to Dr. Baxas, who adds that growth hormone has some unique properties that cannot be duplicated by the other superhormones. "As we age, the organs in our body shrink. The heart, the liver, everything shrinks in size. Growth hormone brings you back to a youthful state in which the organs are returned to their normal size, that is, the size they were at age twenty-five or thirty. The liver will regain its normal size, the kidneys become larger, all the organs in the body come back to normal size. Nothing else can do this."

Their patients heartily agree. They say that they have never felt better or looked better. For example, one man who has been using growth hormone for two years says he has lost thirty-two pounds, has lowered his cholesterol by more than fifty points, and has fewer wrinkles; he is happier, healthier, and stronger in virtually every way. It is true that growth hormone can improve immune function and enhance the size and function of organs and organ systems. It also helps reduce fat, lower cholesterol, and build muscle. However, despite some obvious benefits and the rave reviews that some patients and their doctors give growth hormone, its use as a treatment for reversing aging remains controversial for several reasons. Numerous studies have shown that growth hormone can cause serious side effects, such as carpal tunnel syndrome, diabetes, and severe fluid retention. Clinical studies of growth hormone have a fairly high dropout rate because so many of the participants cannot tolerate these side effects. This has led many researchers to conclude that growth hormone has a limited application as a therapeutic agent, and still others say that it has no useful purpose in the treatment of adults.

On the other hand, the doctors who prescribe growth hormone counter such challenges by saying that when the dose is properly tailored to the individual and the case is managed properly, the effects are nothing short of miraculous. Many of the growth hormone users with whom I spoke agreed.

Frankly, I don't see any point in a healthy forty-, fifty-, or even ninety-year-old spending money on growth hormone and risking the side effects if they are able to get a comparable result from the other superhormones, and I am confident that most of them will.

We know that for men, testosterone can enhance muscle strength, reduce fat, increase energy, reduce cholesterol, and prevent bone loss. We know that for women, estrogen and progesterone can protect against heart disease and osteoporosis, improve mental function, and make them generally feel better. We know that for both men and women DHEA has many of these same benefits. Melatonin, of course, has its own rejuvenating effect on many body systems and enhances the power of the other superhormones.

So, for whom and for what is growth hormone good? The answer is that despite its drawbacks, growth hormone can be good in special circumstances. Growth hormone can play an important role in the practice of age-reversal medicine, but it is important to understand the special circumstances in which its use is appropriate.

Important Uses for an Important Hormone

When should growth hormone be added to our superhormone cocktail? In my opinion the people who will benefit the most from growth hormone are the sickest. If we begin a superhormone program when we are in even reasonably good health, employing the other superhormones as appropriate, we can maintain our health for many years, with the result that many of us will never need growth hormone.

But having said that, I also need to point out that insofar as our health is concerned, we were not all created equal. Some people were born with an underlying weakness that may make them prone to certain diseases such as kidney disorders and heart failure, or another ailment that may confine them to bed for an extended period of time.

I believe that in cases involving "special circumstances" like these, growth hormone may be the superhormone that can help tip the odds back in their favor by helping to restore some of the natural strength and capacity that illness has stolen away.

SAVING MUSCLE

I have often said that people who do not consider aging a disease should look at people who are severely ill and confined to their beds. I am often shocked at how patients who are confined to bed can quite literally age overnight. Their hair can turn gray and wrinkles can appear on their face, and they appear to put on years. It is almost as if the clock has been fast-forwarded, and each week of illness inflicts a decade's worth of damage. Even very young people who are seriously ill look old and wasted. When older people break a hip or suffer a serious illness that immobilizes them for a long period of time, they experience a rapid physical decline. Studies have shown that even a few days of bed rest can result in a significant loss of muscle strength for people of all ages, and that several weeks or months of inactivity can be especially devastating to an older body that simply cannot repair itself as well. Within a short time, muscles begin to atrophy, bones become brittle and vulnerable to breaks, and there is a striking loss of lean body mass; before too long, the body becomes frail and weak.

In order to understand how growth hormone can help turn back the clock for these people, you need to understand a bit about what is happening inside their bodies.

When we are sick or subjected to stress, our bodies respond by pumping out high levels of corticosteroids, or stress hormones. As explained in earlier chapters, stress hormones are part of the "flight or fight" response that revs our bodies up for defensive or evasive action. Stress hormones increase our levels of blood sugar and speed up our heart rate to prepare us for a sudden burst of physical activity. Stress hormones can also dampen the activity of other systems (such as the immune system) so that the body can direct its energy to evading danger. The flight-or-fight response was designed to help our ancestors survive in a rough and unpredictable world where they were often at the mercy of predators, and this mechanism works extremely well for those extreme conditions. The problem is that our bodies don't distinguish between an attack by a tiger, our boss at the office, or an illness. Any kind of "stressor," including chronic illness, causes the stress response to kick in. In this situation, we do not "use up" the stress hormones by taking physical action. As a result, they linger in our bodies. Exposure to stress hormones can, over time, cause serious damage to body tissue and organs.

In order to maintain muscle strength, we need, as the saying goes, "to use it or lose it." When we are ill and unable to exercise, we suffer a double blow. Not only are we "losing" muscle because of inactivity, but stress hormones generated as a result of the illness can themselves cause severe damage to muscle. Here's how: In order to maintain muscle, you need to be able to replace muscle cells faster than you lose them; that is, you need to be *anabolic*.

Anabolic means that you have the capacity to build muscle. You may have heard the word *anabolic* in connection with the term anabolic steroids, which are hormones that can bulk up muscle and that are sometimes abused by bodybuilders. (Anabolic steroids are very potent muscle builders, but they can also cause severe health problems, including diabetes, cancer, and some other serious side effects and can be abused if taken in excess. That is why we recommend only replacement levels that restore us to our natural peaks.) As we age, or when we are sick, we become the opposite of anabolic. We become *catabolic;* that is, we lose muscle. This happens for several reasons. One is nutrition, which plays a big role in the maintenance of muscle. We need to be well nourished to stay anabolic, and many older people simply do not get enough food or the right kind of food. But it's not only the food that we eat that helps build muscle. Much depends on the ability of our bodies to maintain the proper protein balance. When we are sick and stressed out, or when we are very old, we do not properly assimilate the amino acids that we obtain from food. As a result, we lose nitrogen, a substance that is essential for the production of protein, or lean body mass. Studies have shown that stress hormones can accelerate the loss of nitrogen and, in so doing, promote the loss of muscle. In chronically ill people there is often a wasting away of muscle that makes it very difficult for them to climb stairs, walk, or even get up out of a chair. Without strong muscles to support their bones, they are more likely to fall and break a hip or suffer a spinal injury, and complications from orthopedic injuries are actually a leading cause of death among these people. Such complications are also the major reason that older people end up hospitalized or in nursing homes.

Can anything stop muscle wasting? There are a few drugs that can reverse muscle loss in the chronically ill, and I believe that growth hormone may prove to be one of the best. We know that growth hormone can help increase muscle mass in healthy people who don't exercise and who would ordinarily lose muscle. Several excellent clinical studies have also shown that growth hormone can prevent nitrogen loss in sick and malnourished people, and this, too, can help maintain muscle. It makes sense that growth hormone should be used as a treatment for people who are rapidly losing muscle and who need a quick and effective boost. Granted, growth hormone is expensive, but if a short-term course of growth hormone can prevent further deterioration and hasten the ability of a patient to get out of a hospital or nursing home and back on his or her feet, the treatment could actually save money. This is precisely the role that many leading researchers in the United States believe that growth hormone will eventually play. "Right now, the focus of our research is to help the frail and elderly," says Dr. David B. McLean, who is conducting some of the clinical studies on growth hormone for the National Institutes on Aging. "In theory, if growth hormone could really help the frail elderly and reduce the nursing home population, that is something you could put a real dollar value on and justify the cost."

The purpose of extending life is to enjoy it. We should be able to play with our grandchildren, go out for dinner and a movie, and enjoy lovemaking. Extending life so that we can spend it in a nursing home is, to my way of thinking, rather pointless. The superhormone promise is not just about living longer; it is about living stronger and living better. Administered to the right people at the proper time, growth hormone can be an important part of the superhormone promise.

SAVING YOUR KIDNEYS

The kidneys remove nitrogenous waste and other waste products from the blood and also help the body maintain the proper balance between salt and water. If kidney function is impaired—that is, if the kidneys fail—we cannot survive without the aid of a dialysis machine, a mechanical device that takes over for the kidneys. With age, the kidneys do not function as efficiently, and we become more prone to kidney failure. Studies have shown that growth hormone can decrease the amount of nitrogenous waste that passes through the kidneys, thereby reducing the load on the kidneys. Moreover, if kidney function is impaired, growth hormone may stave off the need for dialysis or reduce the frequency of dialysis treatments. Not only is kidney dialysis an ordeal for the patient—they need to be attached to dialysis machines at least three times a week for several hours—but it is very expensive. If growth hormone could reduce the need for dialysis, it would be a real boon. Dr. Bengt-Ake Bengtsson, of the Research Center for Endocrinology and Metabolism at Sahlgrenska University Hospital in Sweden, is currently investigating the use of growth hormone on a small group of patients suffering from renal failure. According to Dr. Bengtsson, growth hormone has yielded excellent results. More studies are needed to determine if growth hormone can be used routinely for these patients, but if growth hormone could postpone or reduce the need for dialysis, this would certainly be another circumstance in which it would be well worth the expense.

SAVING YOUR HEART

Growth hormone has unique properties that set it apart from the other superhormones, and, as a result, there are particular situations in which it may be invaluable. For example, I think growth hormone may prove to be a highly effective treatment for heart disease and, in fact, may even help prevent the decline in heart function that results from decades of "wear and tear." We tend to forget that the heart is basically a muscle. The older we get, the harder it has to work. As a result of "overwork," the heart muscle begins to thicken, and its capacity to pump or squeeze out blood declines. In the words of cardiologists, we experience a reduction in cardiac output. The heart has an increasingly difficult time pumping blood throughout the body, and if the heart becomes too sluggish, heart failure may result.

These very same changes can also occur in younger people who have a severe heart condition called cardiomyopathy. This is characterized by the destruction of heart muscle, which can result in the inability of the heart to pump blood properly. Cardiomyopathy is usually treated with medication, such as digitalis, which increases the pumping action of the heart. In severe cases—that is, when a large portion of the heart muscle has been destroyed—the only hope for survival is a heart transplant. Medical researchers have known for quite some time that young people who are growth hormone deficient are at high risk of developing cardiomyopathy and other heart abnormalities and that these conditions can be reversed by taking growth hormone supplements.

In light of this, researchers began to wonder whether growth hormone could also help other people who, though not growth hormone deficient, nonetheless suffer from cardiomyopathy. In a study reported in the *New England Journal of Medicine,* researchers gave young people with cardiomyopathy growth hormone injections. The results were quite impressive. Not only was there a dramatic improvement in cardiac function, but the heart patients were able to cut down on the use of digitalis, a drug that strengthens the action of the heart. What I found particularly notable about this study is that it clearly shows that growth hormone has a restorative effect on the heart, and for this reason I feel that growth hormone shows great promise also as a treatment for older people with cardiomyopathy. Again, I believe this is an area that truly deserves further research. Considering that heart failure is the leading cause of death in the United States and that it exacts a severe toll in terms of human suffering and medical and financial resources, it is imperative that we investigate growth hormone's potential as a treatment.

Growth hormone may also protect against heart disease in other important ways. It can dramatically lower cholesterol, and it appears to be a more effective cholesterol "buster" than even the other superhormones. Growth hormone will lower both total cholesterol and LDL, or bad cholesterol. It does not raise HDL, or good cholesterol (as estrogen does in women), but by lowering LDL it automatically improves the ratio between the good and bad cholesterol, and that can be very beneficial.

People who take growth hormone often say that they have not only lost weight but that it has been redistributed so that they have a more youthful appearance. This is not merely wishful thinking on their part. Solid scientific studies have shown that growth hormone can actually mobilize body fat and change body shape. This is not just of cosmetic benefit, for it may also reduce the risk of heart disease. As we age, our weight tends to settle around the midriff, and we carry more fat in the abdominal area. This is not only unattractive, but it is a potentially serious threat to our health. Studies show that those who are round in the middle or shaped like apples are at greater risk of having a heart attack than those who carry their weight on their bottom half, in their hips and thighs, and are shaped like pears. Interestingly, younger people who are growth hormone deficient also tend to be "apple-shaped." Studies also show that mid-center obesity—the so-called spare tire—is more common in men, and this could help explain why men are more likely than women to get heart attacks at a young age. For reasons not well understood, abdominal or midriff fat is much harder to lose than fat deposited in other parts of the body, although aerobic exercise can help. Studies have shown that growth hormone supplements can help reduce midline obesity, possibly by enhancing the effect of exercise. Researchers are hopeful that growth hormone will also have a residual effect on midline obesity; that is, it may not only help get rid of the fat but help keep it off. Several studies are currently under way to determine whether growth hormone is indeed a cure for midriff bulge, and whether it can be used as a short-term therapy to help restore a more youthful and healthier body shape.

The Future of Growth Hormone

The point to remember about growth hormone is that it has some amazing powers, but its benefits must be carefully weighed against its cost and potential side effects. Down the road it may be possible to gain all the benefits of growth hormone at a fraction of the cost and with virtually no side effects! If you could just get your body to produce more "homegrown" growth hormone on its own . . .

A number of scientists are now working to develop a drug that can do just that. They are developing a substance that can stimulate the body to produce more growth hormone naturally. These substances are called growth-hormone-releasing agents or growth-hormone-secreting hormone or secretogogues. I believe that if growth hormone is ever to be used widely, it will be in this form. I think this is the case because one of the problems with taking growth hormone by injection is that to do so is not in keeping with normal physiology —or nature's blueprint. Growth hormone is pulsed out into the bloodstream in small amounts throughout the day with a nocturnal peak, and many researchers believe that the side effects of growth hormone result from the fact that users are receiving concentrated bursts of artificially high quantities. The theory is that if the pituitary could be "tweaked" so that it would stimulate growth hormone production, the hormone would be delivered in a more natural manner that is more easily tolerated by the body.

There are several growth-hormone-releasing agents in the works, and some are already undergoing clinical tests. For example, researchers at the University of California at San Diego have studied the effect of growth-hormone-releasing hormone over a four-month period on men and women aged sixty-six to seventy-one. The participants injected themselves nightly with the drug. The researchers were particularly interested in seeing the effect on two areas: immune function and metabolism, including its effect on lean body mass and fat.

According to researcher Dr. Omid Khoramm, growth-hormone-releasing hormone had a significant effect on immune function that amazed the participants themselves. Although many of the participants had been exposed to cold and flu viruses during the study period, none fell prey to viruses, and only two caught colds, and minor colds at that. The effect on metabolism, however, was not as clear. Dr. Khorram said that this growth-hormone-releasing hormone did decrease fat mass and increase lean body mass in men, and also in women who were not also taking estrogen. In women who were also taking estrogen, however, the growth-hormone-releasing hormone actually appeared to increase body fat. For a woman who is too thin and suffering from a compromised immune system—the classic "wasting" syndrome—this combination might actually be a true lifesaver.

Several pharmaceutical companies are currently developing oral agents that will help stimulate the production of growth hormone. For example, Merck is testing a growth-hormone-releasing agent for use by people with immune problems and diseases such as cancer. It will be several years before these growth-hormone-releasing factors are available, and whether or not they work remains to be seen. Researchers who are most optimistic believe that by the year 2005 these growth-hormone-releasing factors will be an ingredient in just about everyone's superhormone cocktail.

PART V

The Age-Reversing Superhormone

Introduction: Melatonin

MELATONIN, THE MIRACLE superhormone, not only slows down the aging process but reverses it as well.

I regard melatonin as the cornerstone of the superhormone promise because it was our discoveries about melatonin and the body's aging clock which taught us that the progressive disease and debility we have come to regard as normal aging can be prevented.

This chapter relates how melatonin can help you "grow young," remain disease free, get a restorative night's sleep, and enhance the quality of your life in a number of ways.

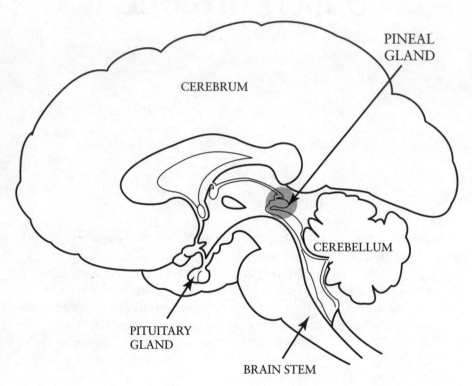

PINEAL
GLAND

CEREBRUM

CEREBELLUM

PITUITARY
GLAND

BRAIN STEM

Diagram of the brain, highlighting the pineal gland which produces melatonin

CHAPTER 9

Melatonin

AN UPDATE

Extends life
Maintains youthful health and vigor
Enhances sexual vitality
Strengthens immune system
Is a potent antioxidant
Protects against stress
Protects against cancer
Prevents heart disease
Restores normal sleep patterns
Cures jet lag

IN THIS CHAPTER I will recap the story of the melatonin miracle and will also report on the latest melatonin research, including important new findings on melatonin being made in laboratories all over the world.

In a very real sense, melatonin is the linchpin of the superhormone promise because melatonin and the pineal gland—the body's aging clock—first brought us to the discoveries that launched the Superhormone Revolution. These exciting scientific breakthroughs called attention to the fact that aging—and by aging I mean progressive disease and debility—can be prevented. It was our work with melatonin over two decades that showed us that the role superhormones play in our health actually extends far beyond the mere ability to cure obvious deficiency syndromes, such as hypothyroidism, or specific symptoms, such as hot flashes. Our work with melatonin helped us see that superhormones actually have the much larger role as *agents of rejuvenation*.

Our landmark experiments with melatonin demonstrated that it is possible not only to halt the downward spiral that far too many of us have come to accept as a normal part of aging, but also to actually extend the length and to improve the quality of our lives. In short, our work with melatonin revealed the secret of how we can "grow young" in a healthy, strong body that remains in the youthful state no matter our age. The lesson that melatonin taught us is that we can prevent the degenerative diseases associated with aging by curing the underlying condition that allows them to take hold in the first place. In other words, melatonin revealed that aging itself is a disease, and by virtue of and understanding of that disease, we now have a cure at hand. The superhormone promise is precisely that, the power to "cure" the disease of aging by restoring our superhormone levels to their natural, youthful values.

One of our goals in writing *The Melatonin Miracle* was to focus public attention on melatonin and the aging clock and to encourage other research organizations to undertake studies of this superhormone. At that time the distinguished National Institutes on Aging was only studying melatonin's role as a sleep aid, and although we regard melatonin's ability to give us a good night's sleep as important, we also knew it was only one small chapter in the larger melatonin story. I am deeply gratified to announce that as this book goes to press, the National Institutes on Aging is convening a special meeting on melatonin to which experts from all over the world have been invited. We will be there, as will many distinguished colleagues.

As you know from the earlier chapters in this book, each of the superhormones works in its own way to keep our bodies resilient and strong. By restoring these superhormones to their peak levels, we can preserve the proper functioning of these rejuvenating agents whose work keeps our bodies primed and ready to rise to the challenges that life throws our way. But there is only one superhormone that can actually reverse aging by resetting the body's aging clock—and that superhormone is, of course, melatonin.

Through the groundbreaking work of my good friend and coauthor of *The Melatonin Miracle*, Walter Pierpaoli, the discovery was made that the pineal gland is the body's aging clock, the internal timer that controls the aging process. A pea-sized structure located deep within the brain, the pineal gland releases the hormone melatonin, which transmits instructions to other body systems telling them how and when to age. We age because our pineal glands tell us to. This makes perfect sense in hindsight, since nearly all of our vital bodily functions—including the production of all the other superhormones—are tied to and under the control of the pineal gland.

Ancient Hindu mystics called the pineal gland the body's third eye, and in a sense that is exactly what it is. The pineal gland watches, monitors, and keeps us attuned to the daily and seasonal changes in our environment, helping us to adapt to and live in synchrony with nature. The pineal gland, for example, regulates the body's sleep/wake cycle, helping us to adapt to the earth's cycle of night and day. The pineal gland does this through its chief messenger, the superhormone melatonin. Here's how: The pineal gland, which sits deep within the brain, does not have direct access to light but contains light-sensitive cells. Light enters the eye through the pupil and is focused on the retina, the light-sensitive layer that lines the interior of the eye. From the retina a message is sent through the optic nerve to the middle brain to a cluster of nerve cells in the hypothalamus, an important gland. Special cells in the hypothalamus tell the pineal gland whether it is light or dark. The amount of light that is registered on the pineal through the eyes determines how much melatonin the pineal gland produces. Light suppresses the production of melatonin, and dark stimulates the production of melatonin. Thus, peak melatonin production occurs at night while we are sleeping, and, in fact, blood levels of melatonin at night are ten times what they are during the day. Melatonin influences when, how, and how well we sleep. When melatonin levels rise, we become drowsy and fall asleep. When melatonin levels begin to level off at daybreak, we wake up.

Controlling the body's sleep/wake cycle is just one small task assigned to the pineal gland. In reality, the pineal gland performs a vastly larger role. To get a sense of the role that the pineal gland plays in regulating our body systems and the production of other superhormones, imagine a symphony orchestra. In one section are the string instruments, in another area the woodwinds, and in another the brass horns, and so forth. If you play the violin, you sit with the other violinists and play your part. If you play the clarinet, you sit with the other clarinetists and play your part. Since your parts are very different, they might seem totally unrelated and independent of one another. But we know this is not true. All we have to do is stand in the position of the conductor to see that the performance of each orchestra section is interdependent on the others, and when the musicians follow the directions of the conductor, they produce beautiful music.

We have discovered that the pineal gland is to our bodies what the conductor is to the orchestra. The job of the pineal gland is to regulate and harmonize the functioning of a number of our bodily systems. One of these systems is our endocrine system, which is made up of many glands that produce the hormones that control our growth from childhood to adulthood. They also control our sexual development. Another of these systems is the immune system, which protects us against disease. These systems and the hormones they produce regulate virtually every bodily function, from breathing to reproduction to fending off disease. That is why we refer to the pineal gland as the regulator of the regulators and why the pineal gland also has come to be seen as the body's aging clock. When the pineal begins to run down, so do all the systems under its control. As a result, superhormone production is disrupted and our superhormone levels drop. To return to our analogy, it is as if the orchestra conductor has become too tired to lead the orchestra. The musicians become disorganized and unable to play in concert. Instead of synchrony and harmony, the musicians are now out of step with one another. The performance breaks down and finally stops altogether.

I call melatonin a *buffer* hormone because, unlike other hormones that target and directly affect specific organs, it operates indirectly to affect all organ systems. Its job is to maintain the homeostasis or balance of the body and thereby help the other hormones do their job more efficiently. To borrow an expression from Buddhism, there is a yin-yang relationship between melatonin and its cousin superhormones. This is what I mean: Rising melatonin levels stimulate the production of certain hormones and dampen the production of others. If the pineal gland is the conductor of the endocrine system, melatonin is its enforcer. Melatonin transmits the conductor's instructions to other hormones and makes sure that they are following those instructions—or, to return to the orchestra metaphor, that they are all playing the same tune.

Melatonin's influence on our lives begins even before we are born: It is passed from mother to developing fetus through the umbilical cord. Even in these earliest stages, melatonin is encoding us with life's daily rhythms, letting us know when it is time to wake, to eat, and to sleep. It is interesting to note that the pineal gland and melatonin have an equally profound impact on members of the animal kingdom. Through its messenger, melatonin, the pineal gland tells animals when to migrate, when to mate, and when to hibernate. Newborn human infants do not begin cycling melatonin on their own until they are several days old, but it continues to be passed from mother to infant via breast milk. Melatonin levels continue to rise steadily in children until age seven, and it is no coincidence that the greatest growth spurts in children occur during the period of their lives when melatonin levels are the highest. Melatonin induces sleep, and it is during periods of sleep that the pituitary gland pumps out high quantities of growth hormone, which stimulates growth and development. At around age seven, melatonin levels begin their first gradual decline. By adolescence the blood levels of melatonin have reached a new low which signals the pituitary gland that it is time to pump higher levels of the luteinizing hormone (LH) and follicle-stimulating hormone (FSH). This is the switch that turns on puberty.

At about age forty-five, when our aging clock strikes middle age, melatonin levels begin another decline, their steepest yet. Not only do melatonin levels begin to drop sharply, but the pineal gland itself begins to shrink and lose pinealocytes, the cells that produce melatonin. Indeed, at this point, for many of us, the pineal gland actually starts to harden or calcify, a sign of further deterioration. Production of melatonin becomes erratic, and our nighttime melatonin peaks are not as high as they once were. By age sixty we produce half the amount of melatonin that we produced in our twenties. And once we lose the ability to properly cycle melatonin, we begin "aging" in the bad sense of the word. The drop in melatonin alerts the other glands and organ systems of the body that the time has come to wind down. In women, the ovaries stop functioning, levels of the superhormone estrogen drop, and women enter menopause. In men, the testes slow down, and although men remain fertile, their production of the superhormone testosterone declines, and they, too, experience signs of diminished sexual function. In men and women alike the immune system begins to decline, leaving us more vulnerable to diseases ranging from infections to cancer to autoimmune ailments. Our other organs and body systems follow suit, and we begin the "downward slide" associated with aging. Returning again to the orchestra metaphor, it is as if the conductor dropped his baton and walked off the stage, leaving the orchestra to fend for itself. For a while the musicians may be able to play in sync, but before too long the tune would collapse in disharmony. Without our "conductor," the pineal gland, and its superhormone, melatonin, our bodies cannot run properly. The production of other superhormones is disrupted and we age.

But enough talk about "downward slides, "diminished sexual function," and "growing old." With superhormones we now know how to stop the clock and to maintain our bodies in the "youthful state," whatever our age. By now we all know that this bleak scenario

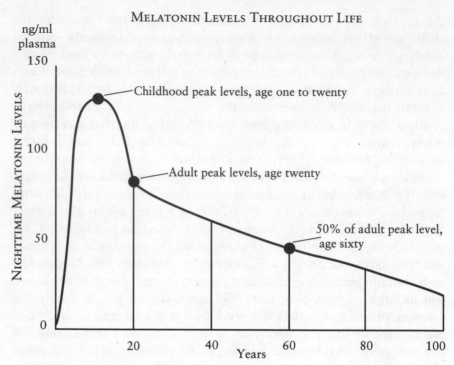

MELATONIN LEVELS THROUGHOUT LIFE

Childhood peak levels, age one to twenty

Adult peak levels, age twenty

50% of adult peak level, age sixty

At age sixty, we produce half of the nighttime melatonin that we did at age twenty, our adult peak

need not take place and that it is possible not only to stop the aging process but to reverse it once that process has begun. We know how to extend life and how to maintain life in a strong, healthy body by literally resetting the body's aging clock.

This knowledge did not come easily. Walter Pierpaoli's research on the pineal gland and melatonin took place over a period of thirty years and involved hundreds of experiments. Nor did the experiments end with the publication of *The Melatonin Miracle,* so let me take you to a laboratory in Ancona, Switzerland, where Walter Pierpaoli first began his remarkable work with melatonin and where more recently he has made some exciting new discoveries that confirm and supplement our original findings.

The Melatonin Miracle

Before I tell you about Walter's latest work and about the remarkable discovery we made together, let me tell you a bit about Walter Pierpaoli, the indisputable founding father of the Superhormone Revolution. Walter began his career as a physician and an immunologist, the latter being a scientist who specializes in the study of the immune system. Early on in his research, Walter recognized that there was a link between the immune system, which helps the body fight against disease, and the endocrine system, the glands that produce hormones. Today, a connection like this probably strikes you as obvious. We now know that our emotional state has a profound effect on our health, and, indeed, many distinguished scientists have devoted their careers to studying the so-called mind/body connection. You have seen examples of these links in this book already. For instance, when discussing the superhormone DHEA, I explained in considerable detail how corticosteroids, stress hormones produced by the adrenal glands, dampen the immune system, and I described experiments which showed that cancerous tumors grow faster in animals that are subjected to stress. I also described how DHEA counteracts the lethal effects of stress hormones. (So does melatonin, as I will shortly explain.) But what you should also know is that Dr. Pierpaoli's work was instrumental in establishing this mind/body connection early on. At the time Walter initiated his groundbreaking work, scientists generally still believed that each system in the body operated independently. In other words, they believed that every gland and every organ system performed solo, wholly independent of other glands and systems. Through a series of elegant experiments, Walter proved that the glands of the endocrine system were in constant communication with the cells of the immune system and that, in fact, an animal could not develop properly if the communication between these systems was severed. Once he had proven that the systems of the body were linked and interdependent, this led him to conclude that there must also be some overarching agency in the body, probably located in the brain, that was in charge of coordinating the exchange of information to carry out the operation of all these functions.

In the early 1980s, articles began appearing in scientific journals about melatonin and how it controlled the sleep/wake cycle in animals. Researchers also had discovered that melatonin levels decline as we age, although they did not understand the significance of that discovery at the time. Walter was struck by several facts. The first was that melatonin regulated a bodily function—the sleep/wake cycle—that is critical to our survival. The second was that levels of the hormone melatonin decline precipitously as we humans begin the slide into physical and mental disability that was associated with aging. The third was that melatonin is produced by the pineal gland, which is located in the brain. This led Walter to develop a hunch that melatonin played a far more important role in the body than anyone had ever imagined, and he devised an ingenious experiment to test his theory.

Melatonin and Water: The First Superhormone Cocktail

If you want to test the effect of a hormone or a drug on many different organ systems within the body, there is no better testing ground than a living, breathing animal. That is why, when Walter decided to study melatonin, he chose several breeds of mice as his subjects, all of which cycle melatonin. (Unless you are a research scientist, you probably don't know that there are literally hundreds of strains of mice, many of which have been specially bred for scientific study. All the mice that Walter chose to study—including strains that bear the unlikely names of BALB/c, C57BL/6, AKR, C3H/He, and hybrids of the F1 gene generation—cycle melatonin and display a peak of melatonin at night around 1 and 2 A.M., in a manner similar to melatonin cycling in humans.)

In the first of many studies, Walter selected healthy male mice that were nineteen months old. Since this breed typically lives to be around twenty-four months, nineteen months is the human equivalent of about sixty-five years of age. Walter divided the mice into two groups. The first group was given melatonin in its nightly drinking water. The second group was given regular tap water. Other than the fact that one group of mice was drinking a "melatonin cocktail," there was no difference between the two groups. Both groups of mice ate the same food, lived in the same type of cages, and received exactly the same kind of care. When Walter began his experiment, he was unsure what result, if any, it would yield. No one had ever done anything quite like it. Walter suspected that perhaps the mice on melatonin would show an improvement in immune function and stay healthier longer, but he had no clear preconception of what might occur. In fact, at the early stages of his experiment, Walter could perceive little difference between the two groups of mice. By the fifth month, however, the difference between the two groups of mice was nothing short of astounding.

The mice that had not been given melatonin (the untreated mice) had begun to show the normal signs and symptoms of old age. Their fur was pocked with bald patches, their eyes were cloudy with cataracts, their digestion had slowed down, and their muscles had grown weak and toneless.

In comparison, the mice who had been served the melatonin cocktail still looked like the mouse equivalent of teenagers. Their coats were thick and shiny, their eyes were cataract free, their digestion had improved, and they had maintained their strength and muscle tone. What was fascinating was that these mice even behaved as if they were young; they exhibited the level of physical activity typical of mice half their age.

The untreated mice reached their expected life span of twenty-four months and died on schedule. The melatonin mice not only did not die but showed no signs of winding down until some six months later when they finally began to die. Six months may not sound like much in human terms, but in mice it is considered one quarter of a lifetime. In human terms, the melatonin mice lived to be well over one hundred years old, and what was even more remarkable, their bodies remained strong and youthful to the end.

Walter would want me to stress at this point that the youthful appearance of the melatonin mice was more than a matter of looking good. Rather, it reflected a change from within—true physiologic rejuvenation of virtually every organ system in the body. Walter's research group performed a battery of tests on these animals, and the results were quite remarkable:

- The melatonin mice had strong, vigorous immune systems, resembling those of much younger mice. The melatonin mice had much higher levels of lymphocytes—the disease-fighting immune cells—than did untreated mice.
- The melatonin mice had more youthful levels of another super-hormone, thyroid. As explained in chapter 7, thyroid provides energy for every cell in the body, and the increase in thyroid hormone could also explain why these mice had so much more energy than the untreated mice.
- The melatonin mice stayed healthy up until their last days. Most significant, some strains of mice used in experiments typically fall prey to cancer as they age, but this was not the case with the melatonin-treated mice.

Walter repeated the experiment several times to make sure that it could not be dismissed as a fluke or aberration. Each time, the melatonin-treated animals lived much longer—30 percent longer, or the equivalent of twenty-five years in human years—and stayed healthier and more vigorous throughout their extended lives. In one of his experiments where he used male and female mice, he discovered something else: The melatonin mice were not only stronger and healthier than the untreated mice, but they maintained sexual activity right up to the end of their lives!

In more recent studies involving mice and rats performed after the publication of *The Melatonin Miracle,* Walter and his colleagues in Ancona have been able to identify why melatonin has such a profoundly rejuvenating effect on the reproductive systems of both male and female animals. As animals (including we humans) age and their sexual organs are no longer needed for reproductive purposes, the sexual organs tend to shrink and atrophy. But Walter found that in both the male and female melatonin-treated animals, the sexual organs retained their youthful size. The testes of melatonin-treated male mice were twice the size of the testes of untreated mice. The ovaries of the melatonin-treated female mice were twice the size of the ovaries of the untreated mice. Walter theorized that inasmuch as sex hormones are produced in the testes and the ovaries, the youthful sexual behavior of the mice was likely due to higher, more youthful levels of sex hormones. When Walter checked the levels of sex hormones in male mice, he found that they were indeed significantly higher in the melatonin-treated mice than in the untreated mice. Although the testosterone levels are not as high as they are in young male mice, Walter believes that the testosterone boost provided by melatonin accounts for the heightened level of sexual interest and activity. Walter has not yet completed similar tests on melatonin-treated female mice to determine estrogen levels, but he is planning to, and strongly suspects that estrogen levels will also prove to be higher in melatonin-treated mice than in untreated mice.

Walter recently made another important finding that I would like to share with you now. You may recall that in the chapter on testosterone I described how the production of sex hormones is regulated by the brain. In the case of testosterone, a site in the brain called the hippocampus produces luteinizing hormone-releasing hormone (LH-RH), the hormone that stimulates the pituitary gland to produce luteinizing hormone (LH), which, in turn, stimulates the testes to produce testosterone. As we age and testosterone production by the testes winds down, our cells experience a corresponding decrease in the number of LH receptors. These receptors are the sites on cells to which LH can bind. The decrease signifies that the testes are "tuning out" and no longer "listening" to commands from the pituitary gland. At the same time there is also an *increase* in the number of LH-RH receptors in the hippocampus, a sign that the brain is trying to compensate for the loss of receptors in the testes. In other words, as the testes are trying to cut testosterone production, the brain is trying to rev it up. Eventually the brain loses the battle and can no longer compensate, and testosterone levels begin to decline. In his latest study, Walter discovered that the melatonin-treated mice had a more youthful level of LH receptors in both their testes and their hippocampus, clearly demonstrating that their testes were again functioning at a more youthful level. What makes this new finding so important is that it demonstrates that the melatonin operates not only at the surface to treat the symptoms of aging but at a much deeper root level to treat the causes of aging. At the very highest levels in our bodies, melatonin alters the very environment that allows the aging process to take hold.

The implication for humans is that melatonin may help maintain more youthful testosterone levels, thereby postponing the necessity of adding testosterone to your hormone cocktail. I believe that for some men the combination of DHEA (which is converted into testosterone) and melatonin may postpone the need for testosterone indefinitely! Since we do not yet have data on melatonin's effect on estrogen levels, we cannot say at this point whether it will postpone the need for women to take estrogen. In the chapter on DHEA I also mentioned that since DHEA is converted into estrogen, it is quite possible that it will help relieve some of the symptoms of menopause and may reduce or postpone the need for estrogen. The combination of DHEA and melatonin may postpone it even further.

The suggestion that melatonin actually restores the function of the testes so they again produce higher levels of testosterone—and that the same may hold true for women and the production of estrogen—poses some very exciting possibilities for what this might mean in terms of human reproduction. Although this is still at the point of speculation, these recent experiments suggest to Walter that the implications could signal a breakthrough of great significance for women. He not only believes that this means melatonin will forestall the need to take estrogen but that there is now good reason to think it will actually extend the time during which a woman is fertile and capable of bearing children.

Along with an associate in Zurich, Walter is currently supervising

a study to test the effect of melatonin on perimenopausal women—
that is, on women who are in the earliest stages of menopause. As
Walter explains, "By keeping the body in the juvenile condition, the
whole function of the body will be more juvenile, including reproductive function." Walter further says that he believes "if menopause
is not already too advanced, we will be able to reverse it with melatonin. We should be able to postpone the infertility period and increase
the time in which women will be able to bear children."

Given the fact that these days so many women are pursuing careers
and marrying later, the ability to extend fertility through their forties
and possibly fifties would be quite a boon for women who want
children. As Walter puts it, "This could prove to be a true revolution
for women."

Since Walter performed the first of his melatonin cocktail experiments in 1985, he has duplicated his findings many times over in
scores of experiments, each one shedding more light on the important role melatonin plays in our bodies. What is so extraordinary
about his work is that it accomplished what up until now was considered impossible. For the first time he has shown that it is not only
possible to extend life but we can also reverse the ravages of aging.
It is possible, by taking melatonin, to rejuvenate the various organ
systems in the body so that we can remain strong, healthy, and
sexually vital. Walter's work with melatonin laid the foundation for
a series of truly incredible experiments that we performed together
which further proved the power of the pineal gland and its role as
the body's aging clock.

The Power of the Pineal

In the 1980s I helped organize a foundation, The Fund for Integrative
Biomedical Research, or FIBER, an organization of scientists devoted
to encouraging and funding innovative research in the field of aging.
FIBER brought Walter to the United States so that we could learn
more about his fascinating work and so that we could introduce him
to others in the scientific community. Walter and I became fast
friends, and I soon went to visit him at his laboratory in Switzerland
so that I could see and study the melatonin miracle firsthand.

Walter's experiments with melatonin had convinced us both that
melatonin was no ordinary hormone and that the pineal gland which
produced it was no ordinary gland. We had seen that melatonin

could stop the aging process, rejuvenate the body, and extend life. This meant, in human terms, the potential for adding decades to our lives. But what gave melatonin its remarkable powers? Walter strongly believed that the age-reversing effect of melatonin resulted from the relationship of melatonin to the pineal gland. It was clear to Walter that the pineal gland controlled the aging process, and in his experiments when he restored melatonin to youthful levels, he believes he had "tricked" the pineal gland into believing that the animals were still young. The pineal gland, in turn, told the glands of the endocrine system to function at youthful levels, which in turn resulted in the production of other hormones at more youthful levels, which in turn helped rejuvenate each of various bodily systems. This was a bold, fascinating theory, but a theory nonetheless. It still needed to be proven, and Walter devised precisely the right experiment to prove it.

It was elegantly simple in design but would require extraordinary patience and skill in execution. Walter proposed that we transplant a pineal gland from a young mouse into an old mouse. This is no easy feat. The pineal gland of a mouse is about the size of the dot at the end of this sentence. Nevertheless, it was the only way to provide positive proof that the pineal gland controlled aging. Walter reasoned that if the young pineal could rejuvenate an old mouse in the way that the melatonin rejuvenated an old mouse, then it would prove without a doubt that the pineal gland controlled aging. Walter and I decided to transplant the young pineal into the thymus gland, a small gland located at the back of the breastbone. The thymus gland is critical for immune function in young animals and is where the immune system's all-important disease-fighting T cells are stored. The thymus gland is also connected to the same nerve center in the brain as the pineal gland, and it seemed a natural place to graft the new pineal. In our experiment we removed young pineals from mice who were three to four months old (or the equivalent of a human teenager) and transplanted them into six mice who were twenty-four months (about sixty-five to seventy in human years). We also transplanted pineal glands from young mice into older female mice who were sixteen, nineteen, and twenty-two months old (or fifty, sixty-five, and seventy in human years).

The mice that received the young pineal glands, like the melatonin-treated mice in the earlier experiments, appeared to grow younger. Their fur improved, they became friskier, and their immune response and thyroid function were equal to those of much younger animals.

Interestingly, the thymus glands of the transplanted mice, which are usually atrophied and shrunken in older animals, were restored to their youthful size and condition. Since the thymus gland is essential for immune function in younger animals, this suggested that melatonin's positive effect on the immune system was achieved by rejuvenating the thymus.

The mice that received the young pineal glands lived an average of three months longer than normal (about ten to fifteen human years). But what was striking to us was the fact that while they lived longer than average mice, they did not live as long as the mice who had received the melatonin cocktail. Why the difference? You may have noticed that when we transplanted the young pineal glands into the old mice, we did not remove the existing pineal gland. To explain why the transplanted mice did not live as long we theorized that the transplanted mice were actually getting mixed messages: One signal from the old pineal gland was telling the mice to age, while the new pineal gland was simultaneously telling them not to. We speculated that the young pineal gland was able to override the signal of the old pineal gland, but only up to a point.

Walter devised the next series of experiments to question these results and proved conclusively that the pineal gland was the aging clock. Working with Vladimir Lesnikov, a young Russian researcher, he devised a complicated surgical procedure in which he would cross-transplant the pineal gland from a young mouse into an old mouse, and from an old mouse into a young mouse. The new pineal gland would be transplanted into precisely the right spot in the brain, and the old pineal gland would be removed, leaving only one pineal gland in each mouse. Only by doing such a cross-transplantation of pineal glands could we see what effect, if any, an old pineal would have in a young animal, while also seeing the effect of a young pineal in an old animal.

The transplantation operations began in the spring of 1990. Walter and Lesnikov exchanged the pineal glands of mice aged four months (the human equivalent of twenty years) with the pineal glands of mice aged eighteen months (the human equivalent of about sixty years). For the control group they performed sham operations on groups of four-month-old and eighteen-month-old mice. Walter and Lesnikov removed the pineals from these control mice and then put them back in the same mice. From the control group they could determine whether the surgery itself, rather than the transplanted pineals, was somehow producing the amazing results.

The operations went well, and within a few months there were several cages of cross-transplanted animals living side by side. Each mouse was tagged, and each cage contained two mice that were four months old and two mice that were eighteen months old. Each week the mice were carefully examined and their vital signs checked. Several weeks passed, then one morning Walter entered the lab, glanced at the cages, and was positively alarmed by what he saw. The mice in several of the cages all appeared to be the same age. This was impossible. After all, he had personally housed the young mice together with the old mice so that he could see more precisely any contrasts in behavior and appearance that occurred. Walter at first assumed that one of the other lab technicians had accidentally mixed them up. Yet, on closer examination—after checking all their identification tags—he realized that the mice were indeed in the right cages.

The reason the mice all appeared to be the same age was that the experiment had actually worked! The old mice had been rejuvenated by the young pineals!

What was even more startling to discover, however, was the fact that the young mice with the old pineals were aging rapidly, long before their time. Both groups of mice looked precisely the same age. Walter took pictures of those mice, and to look at them is to see two mice standing side by side, one fifteen months old and the other thirty months old, both looking exactly the same age. In human terms that would be the equivalent of a forty-year-old standing next to an eighty-year-old—and passing as twins.

But soon after that, the age difference between the two groups of mice dramatically emerged. The young mice implanted with the old pineals began to age rapidly, wither, and die about 30 percent earlier than normal. The old mice implanted with the young pineals, however, lived on average 30 percent longer and maintained their youthful, vigorous bodies until the very end of life, which was about 33 months or, in human terms, around 105. Later examinations would reveal that the thymus glands of the old mice which had received the young pineals had regenerated, whereas the thymus glands of the young mice which had received the old pineals had withered.

What happened to the control mice who underwent the "sham" operations? Nothing out of the usual. They lived out their lives quite normally, fulfilling the life expectancy of the average mice.

From this experiment Walter had his long-sought proof that he had found the true aging clock and had finally unlocked the mysterious mechanism that determines not only *how* we age but *why* we age. A young pineal sends a youthful message throughout the body, keeping the body healthy and strong. Once the pineal ages, however, it sends quite a different message, telling the body that we are old and that it is time to wind down. One by one the various systems follow the pineal's lead until we grow old and die. By restoring melatonin to youthful levels, we are bringing the pineal gland back to its youthful state, and in doing so, we alter the message that it sends out to the rest of the body.

Further Confirmation

In science, corroboration is the key to credibility. It is imperative that results achieved by one research group in one laboratory be duplicated by another group in another laboratory. This is the proof positive that the research was not tainted in any way, either by bias, human error, or carelessness. I am delighted but not surprised to report that in March 1995 scientists from Israel's Tel Aviv University and the Hebrew University–Hadassah Medical School, and Spain's University of La-Laguna announced that they had reproduced the results of Walter's earlier experiments in which he extended the lives of mice by putting melatonin in their nighttime drinking water. These researchers gave older adult male rats melatonin in their drinking water and found that the rats not only lived significantly longer than rats who did not get melatonin but the melatonin-treated rats had higher blood levels of testosterone. Let me quote directly from this study that was published in *NeuroReport* (volume 6, 1995, pages 785–86):

> The melatonin-treated animals had a higher survival rate, and higher circulating testosterone levels, and their body weight tended to be lower than their aged-matched-vehicle treated controls. The results are compatible with previous reports demonstrating a significant increase in longevity, a postponement of the onset of aging symptoms by melatonin treatment, and appearance of pathological changes resembling senescence in pinealectomized mice.

The "previous reports" to which the scientists referred were the studies published by Walter and me. Thus, we have our corroboration that melatonin can extend life and help prevent the age-related decline in physical and mental function that we call "senescence." Melatonin does this by bolstering every system within the body, restoring youthful function and vigor.

Melatonin Enhances the Immune System: Nature's Own Bodyguard

When it comes to aging, many of us tend to focus on the outward physical manifestations of growing older. We worry about wrinkles, gray hair, weight gain, and other such external signs. I don't want to minimize the importance of looking well. How we look is unquestionably important to our self-esteem and sense of self. In fact, elsewhere in this book I have explained how certain of the superhormones—including DHEA, estrogen, and testosterone—actually do help with such cosmetic improvements. I still chuckle and also take pride in the fact that one magazine writer described me as a "living advertisement" for my cause. But even at the risk of sounding clichéd, I want to emphasize that what is going on inside our bodies is of vastly greater importance than how we appear on the outside, and if we take care of what's going on inside our bodies, that care will be reflected in how we look. Improving our looks from the inside out is the only way to achieve a real rejuvenation.

This is especially so when it comes to our immune system. As we age, our immune systems get weaker and less able to fend off foreign invaders. As a result, we are more vulnerable to viral and bacterial infection. Illnesses such as colds and flu that are easily sloughed off by youngsters can be perilous for older adults. As we age, our immune systems become less capable of distinguishing friend from foe, and for no apparent reason, our immune cells may begin to attack our bodies' own tissues. As a result, we are more susceptible to autoimmune disorders such as rheumatoid arthritis, lupus, and Hashimoto's disease, which interferes with the production of thyroid hormone. Ironically, these same cells that so vigorously turn against our bodies' own tissues become lax about destroying cancer cells. Instead of disarming potentially troublesome cells, they allow them to flourish. That is why our risk of developing cancer increases steadily as we age, and why cancer is very much a disease of aging.

Thus, you can see that maintaining a youthful immune system is vital to maintaining health. Extensive research has shown us that melatonin bolsters immune function, strengthening our resistance to infection and cancer. It does this in several key ways.

MELATONIN RESTORES THYMUS FUNCTION

One of the reasons that we lose our ability to fight disease is that, as we age, we lose our thymus gland. This is the small gland, located behind the breastbone, where the immune system's infection fighting T-cell lymphocytes are stored. There is compelling evidence that melatonin restores and preserves thymus function. When melatonin was placed in the nighttime drinking water of older animals, it had a rejuvenating effect on their thymus glands: They grew back to their youthful size and more actively produced T cells. Other tests showed that the "memory" of the T cells was also restored. In other words, they were better able to identify invading enemy cells and repel them.

MELATONIN STRENGTHENS ANTIBODY RESPONSE

Melatonin also strengthens the body's antibody response to unwanted invaders. When we are exposed to an infection, our immune system produces antibodies against the infection. Once antibodies are produced against a foreign protein, our immune system has a built-in memory for fighting this invader if it should attack again. "Immune memory" is the principle behind inoculation, in which a small amount of virus is introduced into the body so that the immune system can begin to develop antibodies against it. As we age, our immune system begins to lose its memory and does not "remember" a potential troublemaker from years or even months past; it therefore may respond weakly to an immune challenge. This is why inoculations against various diseases do not "take" as well in older people as they do in younger people. And this is why an older person is more susceptible to certain infections. Studies have repeatedly shown that melatonin can improve immune memory and strengthen antibody response. When given melatonin, older animals were able to produce antibodies against a foreign protein with the same vigor as a young animal.

MELATONIN FIGHTS VIRUSES

By enhancing T-cell production, melatonin helps strengthen our defense system against viruses. This has particularly important ramifications since, as of yet, science has not found a cure or an effective treatment for viral infections. As a result, our best line of defense is to bolster our resistance to viruses, and melatonin more than ever appears to have the power to help us achieve that aim. Since last fall when *The Melatonin Miracle* was published, there has been exciting new work in the field of immunology that confirms melatonin's potent antiviral properties. In one study, researchers from the Israel Institute for Biological Research and the Center for Experimental Pathology in Switzerland tested the effect of melatonin against viral encephalitis, a lethal disease. The researchers injected mice with a potent strain of encephalitis virus (the Semliki Forest virus), which invades the central nervous system and eventually destroys the brain, leading to death. The researchers found that the mice given melatonin injections were more resistant to the virus. The melatonin not only postponed the onset of the disease but also helped them weather the disease. While all the mice not treated with melatonin died of the disease, only 44 percent of the melatonin-treated mice succumbed. In other words, while all the untreated mice died of the disease, the majority of the melatonin-treated mice survived.

Melatonin Blocks the Damage Caused by Stress

When we are ill, we are under stress, and as a result, our adrenal glands pump out more stress hormones. Stress hormones can destroy immune cells, and this can interfere with the body's ability to heal itself. Several studies have shown that melatonin can counteract this effect by restoring levels of disease fighting T cells.

Chronic exposure to stress hormones can also throw the entire immune system out of whack, with even more far-reaching serious consequences. Some studies suggest that unrelenting stress may be a cause of autoimmune diseases, in which the body wages war on itself. We don't yet know the exact cause of autoimmune diseases or why they are more likely to develop as we age, but we do know that they are often preceded by stressful events such as emotional traumas or viral infections. In both situations, the body may be pumping out higher levels of stress hormones, called corticosteroids, which over time can inflict severe damage to immune cells. By inhibiting the harmful effects of stress hormones, melatonin may indirectly help prevent autoimmune diseases from taking hold. Melatonin not only bolsters the immune system against the ill effects of stress by controlling corticosteroids but actually works with special stress-relieving chemicals that are produced by the immune system. These chemicals are called endorphins; they are our body's own natural painkillers and are produced by both the brain and immune cells. Endorphins help relieve pain and can also help reduce anxiety and promote a feeling of euphoria. Melatonin has been shown to enhance the effect of endorphins and, by doing so, help the body withstand the stress of illness.

Chronic exposure to corticosteroids endangers our immune system and can inflict harm on nearly every body organ and system. For example, we know that if an animal is subjected to extreme stress, portions of its heart muscle will die—even if it had no previous signs of heart disease. Stress kills heart cells, and if enough heart cells die, so do we.

Stress damages the cardiovascular system in other ways as well. Corticosteroids appear to injure arteries, the "hoses" through which blood flows to the heart and from the heart to the rest of the body. If our arteries become so impaired that they can no longer deliver an adequate blood supply, a heart attack may result. If the blood supply to the brain is impaired, it can cause a stroke. Stress can also increase blood pressure, which can also inflict damage to the heart.

Melatonin has been shown to blunt the negative effects of corticosteroids. It does this by normalizing levels of corticosteroids in our body, preventing them from becoming too high. Thus, melatonin can protect our hearts and blood vessels against the damage inflicted by stress.

Prolonged exposure to corticosteroids can raise blood sugar levels, increasing the risk of diabetes. Indeed, medical science has long known that people with diabetes have higher than normal levels of corticosteroids. Diabetes is not only a serious disease in its own right, but it can increase the risk of developing heart disease, stroke, and blindness. Once again, melatonin appears to help prevent stress-induced diabetes by curbing the effect of corticosteroids, thus preventing the continual rise in blood sugar levels.

We do not think of osteoporosis as being a stress-related disease, but continual exposure to stress hormone, which interferes with the absorption of calcium, can weaken the bones and leave them vulnerable to breaks and fractures. Corticosteroids have also been shown to block the growth of special cells on the ends of bones that are necessary for the formation of new bone cells. By controlling the levels of corticosteroids, melatonin can help prevent this insidious disease.

Stress hormones can also damage the brain and even affect our capacity to think clearly and remember information. Corticosteroids have been shown to injure cells in the hippocampus, the portion of the brain that controls short-term memory. As we age, we typically lose some of our ability to retain new information. For example, it becomes harder to remember names and faces of people with whom we have been recently introduced, and it may take longer to process and absorb new facts. Perhaps this loss of short-term memory is due to a lifetime exposure to stress. Some researchers even suspect that Alzheimer's disease may be due to damage to the hippocampus, which, in turn, may be linked to severe stress and the prolonged exposure to corticosteroids. Here again, melatonin's buffering effect on corticosteroids can help protect our brains from stress-induced damage.

Anyone who has been subjected to serious stress—whether in the form of working for a difficult boss, going through a nasty divorce, undergoing one's own illness or the illness of a family member, losing a loved one, being fired from a job, or any one of the hundreds of stressful situations that life occasionally hands us—already knows that stress saps our energy, disrupts our living patterns, and takes the joy out of life. Since the publication of *The Melatonin Miracle,* we have heard from many people that melatonin has helped them cope with particularly stressful times in their lives. For example, Eric, a prominent New York lawyer, told us that his round-the-clock work schedule, combined with community service obligations and the day-to-day demands of family life, had put him under such unremitting stress that he feared he was en route to a nervous breakdown. "I couldn't sleep. I was jumpy and irritable, and I felt exhausted all the time. I felt unhappy and out of control," he recalled. He sought help from his doctor, who initially prescribed tranquilizers, but Eric discontinued them because he hated the lethargic, drugged way they made him feel. At his doctor's suggestion he tried biofeedback, but felt no improvement. One night, while on a business trip to Europe, at the suggestion of a friend, Eric took 5 mg. of melatonin to help combat jet lag. As has now been much publicized, melatonin is a "time-tested" cure for jet lag. Overnight, Eric felt better. For the first time in months, Eric had a good night's sleep and woke up feeling refreshed and revitalized. After a few more nights on melatonin, Eric noticed that he felt, in his words, "more relaxed, more centered, and more in control." He added, "I feel 100 percent better. I no longer feel 'stressed out.' I am sleeping well, and I am happier and more productive."

It's gratifying to hear stories such as Eric's, but not surprising. We know that melatonin can blunt the harmful effects of stress hormones, and that is probably one of the ways in which it helps keep us more youthful. Given the fact that melatonin is beneficial in so many other ways, it makes sense that it should be used as a treatment for stress-related ailments. It is certainly safer and easier on the body than standard tranquilizers, but, of course, the problem here is that few doctors are aware of this. Once again, the lack of attention given melatonin by the medical community is due to the fact that it is an inexpensive natural substance that cannot be patented, and the pharmaceutical houses have no interest in promoting melatonin when they can promote more expensive drugs from which they will reap a much bigger profit. Doctors are bombarded with promotional material on tranquilizers from pharmaceutical companies, and many view these drugs as *the* antidote to stress. I can assure you that there is no one sending doctors fancy brochures on melatonin, desk calendars or note pads embossed with melatonin's name, or free videos; no one is taking full-page advertisements in medical journals or sponsoring educational seminars at Caribbean resorts. That is why it is often necessary for you, the patient, to provide your doctor with the necessary information.

Melatonin as a Cancer Treatment

When the immune system is strong and doing its job, abnormal cells are rooted out before they can do damage. That is why cancer is so rare in children and young adults whose immune systems are functioning optimally, and so common in older adults whose immune systems are weakening. When it comes to cancer, prevention is the key, and the more we can fortify ourselves against this disease, the better we will be able to resist it.

In *The Melatonin Miracle,* we discussed at length the ability of melatonin to protect us from cancer and how it accomplishes this feat on many different fronts. For example, several studies have shown that melatonin can thwart the growth of breast cancer cells and prostate cancer cells in both test tube cultures and living, breathing animals. The odds of a woman getting breast cancer or a man getting prostate cancer increase exponentially as they age and as their melatonin levels decline. But by restoring melatonin to its peak, we can recover the "youthful advantage" that helped keep these diseases at bay when we were younger.

Some of the most innovative work with melatonin as a cancer therapy is being performed at the San Gerardo Hospital in Monza, Italy, by Dr. Paoli Lissoni, a true pioneer in the field. In many different studies, Dr. Lissoni has used melatonin supplements in patients along with conventional chemotherapy, often achieving remarkably good results. Dr. Lissoni's work is of particular interest because he often works with advanced cancer patients, many of whom have been given little hope, and many of whom have the types of cancers that are considered very difficult to treat or even incurable. Due to the nature of these cancers, he uses a particularly potent immunotherapy drug, Interleuken 2 (IL 2), which is known for its effectiveness but also its harsh side effects. In several studies, Dr. Lissoni has shown that when he combined IL 2 with melatonin, patients were better able to tolerate the IL 2. For example, in one study, Dr. Lissoni combined low-dose subcutaneous (administered by injection) Interleuken 2 plus 40 mg. of melatonin each day, six days a week for four weeks, in colon cancer patients who had not responded to the usual chemotherapy regimen. He compared their progress to that of similar patients who were given only supportive care; that is, they were made comfortable and were given antidepressants and painkillers but no further cancer therapy. At the end of one year, survival was significantly higher in the patients who had received the combined IL 2/melatonin treatment than in those who had received supportive care alone. (Nine of the twenty-five patients receiving the treatment were still alive, whereas only three of the twenty-five patients receiving supportive care were still living.) What is remarkable is that three out of the twenty-five survivors in the treatment group had actually shown some improvement in their condition in terms of tumor regression, whereas none of the people in the supportive care group showed any improvement.

In another study involving advanced cancer patients with incurable disease (including thyroid cancer, carcinoid, and endocrine pancreatic tumors), the researchers in Monza achieved similar results. Not only did some of the patients show improvement, but melatonin appeared to substantially reduce the toxic side effects associated with the chemotherapy. Reports of these and other studies conducted by the Italian group are contained in the bibliography. If you or a loved one is a candidate for IL 2 therapy, I encourage you to refer your physician to them. But please do not misunderstand the meaning of this research. Melatonin is not a cure for these difficult cancers, but it may make a difficult form of treatment more tolerable. And that treatment, at least in some patients, actually appears to help reverse symptoms.

Melatonin Protects Against Heart Disease

As our levels of superhormones, including melatonin, decline, our risk of developing heart disease rises. By age sixty, heart disease is the number one killer of both men and women. As stated before, this is no coincidence. The decline in superhormones creates an environment in which heart disease can flourish. I have repeatedly called your attention to the link between declining levels of superhormones and increasing risks of heart disease because the research amply demonstrates that seven of the eight superhormones play important roles in the prevention of heart disease. (The role of progesterone in maintaining cardiovascular health has not yet been adequately studied, but my intuition tells me that it, too, is important in this respect, and ultimately we will see how progesterone and all eight of the superhormones are instrumental in preventing heart disease.)

I mention this here to make a point—indeed, a point that is central to the theme of this book: *The diseases of aging—including heart disease—can be prevented, and by restoring levels of superhormones to their youthful levels, we can achieve a long, healthy life, and we can keep our hearts well functioning and disease free.*

Melatonin helps prevent heart disease in the following ways:

- Melatonin lowers high blood cholesterol levels, reducing our risk of developing atherosclerosis, or "clogged arteries," which can lead to a heart attack and stroke.
- Melatonin lowers high blood pressure, cutting our risk of heart attack and stroke. I have heard many anecdotal reports of melatonin lowering high blood pressure to the point that people were able to stop taking or reduce the dosage of high blood pressure medication. If you are taking medication for high blood pressure, do not stop taking it without consulting your physician.
- Melatonin prevents the formation of blood clots, cutting the risk of heart attack and stroke.

- Melatonin helps control stress hormones, which can actually injure arteries and heart muscle.
- Melatonin protects us from the damage caused by free radicals. Such damage is believed to trigger the formation of plaque in the arteries that can block the flow of blood to the heart, causing a heart attack, or to the brain, causing a stroke.

What is so interesting about melatonin is the fact that it knows how to correct what is wrong, yet does not interfere with what is right. If you have high cholesterol, melatonin will lower it, but if your cholesterol is normal, melatonin will not significantly affect it. If your blood pressure is elevated, melatonin may bring it down, but it will not lower a normal blood pressure. This is why Walter and I call melatonin a "smart" hormone: it knows what to do and when to do it.

Melatonin and Sleep

Melatonin is still probably best known for its effect on sleep. Melatonin and the pineal gland, as we have seen, regulate the body's sleep/wake cycle. As we get older and our melatonin levels decline, most of us experience a marked change in sleep patterns. We may begin to suffer from a wide range of sleep disorders, including insomnia, frequent night waking, and waking too early. About 50 percent of all Americans over the age of sixty-five suffer from some form of sleep disorder. Very often, sleep problems surface earlier in women, usually around the time of menopause.

The ability to get a good night's sleep and wake up feeling refreshed and invigorated is critical to our physical and emotional well-being. Disrupted sleep can make us feel irritable and depressed, and impair our ability to function. Sleep is also essential for good health. If we miss even one night's sleep, we experience a disruption in immune function, including a significant noticeable decline in "killer cells," the special cells that fight viral infections.

Most people with sleep problems suffer in silence and assume that there is nothing that can be done for them. Or if they tell their doctors about their sleep disorder, more often than not their doctors will prescribe sleeping pills, which can actually make the problem worse. Some sleeping pills raise blood pressure, others produce hangoverlike effects, and others are addictive. When combined with other medications, such as drugs to lower blood pressure, some sleeping pills can be downright dangerous.

There is a better solution, and one that is more in keeping with your body's natural rhythms. Taken before bedtime, melatonin can produce natural sleep patterns that result in a refreshing night's sleep. (A dose of 0.5 to 5 mg. is all it takes to restore normal sleep patterns. For more details see chapter 10, How to Take Superhormones.) Melatonin is nonaddictive, and if you are taking the proper dosage, it does not result in daytime grogginess. Given the fact that melatonin is so safe and effective as a sleep aid, I would be very surprised if it does not become the sleep aid that doctors recommend to their patients.

Sleep disorders are no more a necessary or "normal" part of aging than heart disease, Alzheimer's, or cancer. A lack of sleep can leave us more susceptible to mental and physical disorders. With melatonin, there is absolutely no reason why we can't get a good night's sleep every night.

In this chapter we have seen how melatonin helps restore normalcy and balance to our bodies, and how it can help preserve our youthful strength and vigor. Melatonin turns back the body's aging clock, rejuvenating the various bodily systems and organs. Melatonin is also the superhormone that helps regulate the other superhormones and works in tandem with them to help us maintain the youthful advantage. Melatonin's effectiveness is broad in scope. It can be seen in literally every system of the body, from the immune system to the reproductive system to the cardiovascular system. Thanks to melatonin and its sister superhormones, a longer and healthier life is within the reach of us all.

PART VI

Making the Superhormone Promise Work for You

Introduction: How to Get Started

THE GOOD NEWS for those who want to begin their superhormone regimen is that superhormones are more readily available now than ever before. Half of the superhormones are being sold over the counter and can be easily purchased in health food stores, pharmacies, or through mail order. The other half are sold by prescription, and a wide variation is available so that you can decide which form you prefer. For example, most of the superhormones come in a range of forms: pills, transdermal skin patches, gels, and lotions.

In this chapter, I will assist you in sorting through all the options so that you and your doctor can choose the superhormone regimen that is right for you. I will walk you through the various forms in which superhormones are currently available as well as explain the appropriate dosage levels for each superhormone. As I said earlier, however, I recommend you work with your doctor to determine the superhormone combination that will be of greatest benefit to you.

CHAPTER 10

How to Take Superhormones

THE RIGHT DOSAGES AND
WHERE TO FIND THEM

To FULFILL THE superhormone promise we need to refer to the personal blueprint that nature has provided each of us. All you need to do is find out the current levels of each of your superhormones and then, by learning which ones have declined, as well as taking into account any symptoms that you may be experiencing you will have your own personalized blueprint for what superhormones you should be replenishing. All that is required to make superhormones work for you is to locate where you have a deficiency and then replenish it so that the level is restored to its youthful peak. By doing this you can remain in a youthful body and maintain health, energy, and vigor even as the years tick by.

Because levels of superhormones vary from individual to individual, not all of us will need to replace every superhormone at the same time in our lives. Indeed, some individuals may never need to replenish certain superhormones because their levels will remain sufficiently high on their own. Also, as you'll remember from previous chapters, some superhormones, such as thyroid hormone and growth hormone, are required only under very special circumstances. The point is that each of us is different, and that is why the concept of the personalized superhormone cocktail is so essential. The guiding principle of the superhormone promise is to have a personal superhormone ℞ that is tailored to your specific needs. With the help of your doctor you can evaluate the deficiencies and get a full picture of your superhormone levels, and then you can put together a superhormone cocktail that is individually tailored to you and targeted to your needs.

As I have said before, I believe that anyone who is taking medication on a regular basis, whether it is aspirin, antacid, or superhormones, should be monitored regularly by a physician. I also want to stress that whether you are regularly taking any medications or not, once you are past the age of forty you need to have a complete physical examination every year. All individuals over forty, including those who are taking superhormones, should be including in this exam certain basic medical tests, which will be reviewed in the discussion that follows. If you have a family history of a particular medical problem or you yourself have had a medical problem in the past, your doctor may recommend additional tests as well.

For Men: The Basics

As part of his routine annual physical examination, every man should have a digital examination for both prostate and colon cancer. In addition, all men should have a CBC, or complete blood count, to check for anemia and signs of infection; a Prostate Specific Antigen (PSA) test to detect latent prostate tumors; a serum blood lipid profile to check cholesterol levels, including a breakdown of HDL and LDL; a baseline liver function test; a blood sugar test (to check for diabetes); a fecal blood occult test to check for blood in the stool; and a thyroid function test. Since tuberculosis is on the rise, I also recommend an annual chest X ray.

For Women: The Basics

As part of her routine annual physical examination, every woman should have a thorough gynecological examination, a manual breast examination, Pap smear, and a digital examination for colon cancer. Every woman past the age of forty should also have a mammogram every two years, and every woman past the age of fifty should have a mammogram annually. Women also should have a CBC, or complete blood count, to check for anemia or signs of infection; a serum blood lipid profile to check cholesterol levels, including a breakdown of HDL and LDL; a baseline liver function test; a blood sugar test (to test for diabetes); a thyroid function test; and a fecal blood occult test to check for blood in the stool. Given the fact that tuberculosis is on the rise, I also believe it is wise for women to have a chest X ray annually.

What Is the Best Way to Take Superhormones?

Today, most of the superhormones are available in many different forms: pills, capsules, injections, new transdermal skin patches, and even newer percutaneous skin gels, whereby superhormones are absorbed through the skin. You and your doctor will decide, based on your particular needs and preferences, which is best for you. Here is some information that will help you to choose.

When you take a superhormone orally (via tablets or capsules) it is broken down by the liver and then delivered into the bloodstream. The advantage of the oral forms over the others is convenience. Pills and capsules make it easier to control the dose. The disadvantage is that pills and capsules may be inappropriate for people who have liver problems.

The transdermal skin patch looks like a large round plastic Band-Aid and delivers the superhormone through a reservoir in its center. The advantage of the skin patch is that it delivers the superhormone directly to the bloodstream via the skin, bypassing the liver and in a more natural, steady stream. The disadvantage of the skin patch is that it must be worn continually, and some people, over time, especially in warm weather, may develop a skin rash or irritation.

In Europe, superhormone creams and skin gels are very popular, and they are beginning to gain more popularity in the United States now that compounding pharmacies are offering them. Creams, which are applied to the skin once or twice daily, need to be measured out carefully, and it is not always easy to get the precise dose. Gels are applied to the skin once a day; they dry rapidly and leave no visible trace or smell. Gels are sold in pump bottles that make it somewhat easier to control dose. Like the patch, creams and gels provide a continuous, more natural flow of superhormone directly into the bloodstream. For the sake of convenience, you can even ask your compounding pharmacist to combine several superhormones into a single cream or gel.

I do not recommend superhormones for women during pregnancy and lactation (unless directed by a physician), since Mother Nature does an excellent job of helping women maintain their normal balance of superhormones during this important time in their lives.

Similarly, healthy children will already have the appropriate levels of superhormones, so I do not recommend superhormones for them unless required to treat a professionally diagnosed deficiency.

HOW TO TAKE DHEA

Now that DHEA is being sold over the counter, there undoubtedly will be a great deal of interest in the hormone that I refer to as the superstar of the superhormones. When you restore DHEA to youthful levels, you will feel more energetic, happier, and even healthier. DHEA has a very palpable revitalizing effect.

Everyone should be tested to determine his or her DHEA level. Two types of tests are available for this. The most common is a simple blood test in which a small amount is drawn and then sent to a laboratory for analysis. If, as is likely for adults, the test reveals that your DHEA level is below the level considered normal in a twenty-year-old (for men that is 3,600 nanograms per deciliter of plasma; for women it is 2,600 nanograms per deciliter of plasma), I believe it is appropriate for you to take DHEA. (Standards may vary among laboratories. See chart, page 43.) Your physician may prefer to employ what is called a salivary hormone profile in which a small amount of saliva is sent to a laboratory and assayed for hormone levels. The comparison is basically the same, however.

There has been some disagreement over whether to check for DHEA or DHEA sulfate, which is what DHEA gets converted into in the body. Frankly, I don't think it matters which form of DHEA you measure since either one will give you the information you need.

If you are in your late forties and beyond, the dose normally given to return your DHEA to its twenty-year-old peak levels is between 25 and 50 mg. daily or every other day, depending on your particular requirements. For ten years I have been taking 50 mg. of DHEA every other day and have achieved an excellent result; however, every other day may not be enough for you. Although everyone's DHEA values will decline—and in our forties, we have roughly half the level of DHEA we had at age twenty—in some people the drop is faster and harder than in others. If your DHEA levels are relatively high for your age, you may need to take only 25 mg.–50 mg. every other day to restore youthful values. If your levels are on the low end, however, you will need to take 25 to 50 mg. daily to restore youthful levels. I also recommend that DHEA be taken in the morning since that is more in keeping with our natural pattern of production.

About a month after beginning your DHEA regimen, your doctor should once again run a test to confirm that your DHEA level is neither too low nor too high. Depending on the results, your doctor may adjust your dose up or down or leave it as it is. After your appropriate DHEA level is restored, you should be checked every six months to ensure that the level is being adequately maintained. In addition, your doctor needs to monitor you for other changes. DHEA can cut cholesterol, for example, so if you have elevated blood cholesterol levels and are already taking medication to bring them down, DHEA may reduce the amount of medication you need or eliminate your need for cholesterol-lowering medication altogether. Or, since DHEA may enhance the action if you are a diabetic who is using insulin, you may be able to use less insulin.

There are times when you may need to increase your dose, particularly if you are under extreme stress. As explained in the chapter on DHEA, there is an inverse relationship between stress hormones and DHEA, which is to say, as one goes up, the other goes down. If you are under extreme stress, your need for DHEA may increase, and your doctor should check your levels during times of stress to see if you need to increase your dose.

As discussed in chapter 1, DHEA is being studied as a treatment for lupus in women, and early studies have yielded promising results. The dose that has been used successfully on lupus patients is 200 mg. daily. Any woman who has or suspects she has lupus should be under the supervision of a physician who closely monitors her treatment. In some cases, women who take other lupus medications, such as prednisone, may need to take less if they are also taking DHEA.

DHEA is sold over the counter at health food stores and pharmacies in 25 mg. strength capsules. A pharmacist can compound any dose of DHEA, however. You need to be aware that some products sold over the counter that purport to be DHEA are not. The makers of these products contend that although their product is not DHEA, it converts to DHEA in the body. I recommend that you buy only a product that clearly states it is pure pharmaceutical-grade DHEA—that is, 98.8 to 99 percent pure DHEA.

Some pharmacies offer DHEA capsules in micronized form: The DHEA powder is finely ground for better absorption. DHEA capsules are also available in a time-release formula, which some people say releases it in a more naturally rhythmic way, but I do not feel that it makes much of a difference. The key is to try different products and see which one works best for you.

DHEA is also sold in a sublingual pill form—it is placed under the tongue and dissolves.

Compounding pharmacies offer DHEA in a cream or gel that can be rubbed directly on the skin. If you use a DHEA cream, you will need to measure out the cream carefully with a tiny measuring spoon to ensure that you are getting the correct dose.

Several compounding pharmacies now sell DHEA percutaneous gels that come in convenient pump bottles so that you can easily get the right dose simply by counting the number of pumps. The gels work like the creams. You can rub the gel on the skin, through which it is absorbed.

How to Take DHEA Eyedrops for Dry Eye

Dr. Michael Zeligs, who is the inventor of these eyedrops and has conducted the studies on them, cautions that his protocol is still experimental and should be used under the supervision of a personal physician. DHEA eyedrops can be obtained from any pharmacy that has experience compounding eyedrops. Ask your physician for a prescription based on the following:

The formulation is a DHEA ophthalmic suspension at a concentration of 0.25–0.5 (weight of DHEA to volume of vehicle). This is to be prepared using sterile pharmaceutical-grade microfine crystals of DHEA suspended in Tears II Naturale lubricant eye drop (Alcon Ophthalmic) or other bacteriostatic natural tear product.

To use the eyedrops, shake thoroughly before each use and administer two drops to each eye on rising, before bed, and at least one hour before inserting contact lenses.

How to Take Pregnenolone

Pregnenolone, the superhormone for your brain, is regarded by many as the most potent memory enhancer of all time. Studies have shown that pregnenolone enhances our ability to perform on the job while heightening feelings of well-being. It is the superhormone that will make us feel smarter and happier. It has also been shown to be an effective treatment for arthritis.

At around age forty-five, our pregnenolone levels begin to decline. By the time we are seventy-five, we are making 60 percent less pregnenolone than we did in our thirties. How do you know if you need to restore pregnenolone to youthful levels? First, have your doctor perform a blood test or a salivary hormone profile to verify that your pregnenolone level has, in fact, declined. Second, watch for specific signs of pregnenolone deficiency. If you find that you are not thinking as well as you used to, that you are not as smart and sharp as you once were, it may be time to replenish your pregnenolone levels to their youthful peak.

The good news is that pregnenolone is now very convenient to find since it is now being sold over the counter in pharmacies, health food stores, and also through mail order. It can be found in capsule form, and compounding pharmacies offer it in capsules and a sublingual pill form that is placed under the tongue and dissolved.

The usual dose for pregnenolone is 50 mg. daily. I recommend taking pregnenolone in the morning.

If you are taking pregnenolone to help improve mental function, you should notice a modest improvement within hours after taking this superhormone. Since the effect of pregnenolone is cumulative, however, the true beneficial effects will be felt over time.

If you are using pregnenolone to treat arthritis, you will need to be more patient. Studies show that it can take several weeks before you will begin to feel appreciably better. Still, I think it is worth the wait. Unlike other arthritis treatments, pregnenolone is safe and has no known side effects.

How to Take Testosterone

Testosterone is the hormone for sex and strength for both men and women. In men, testosterone can stop and reverse the physical decline that saps them of their energy, their strength, and their libido. Testosterone also restores muscle tone and improves stamina. In women, testosterone can rev up a sluggish libido as well as improve energy and stamina.

Although both men and women may need to replenish their testosterone levels, the approach will vary according to sex.

Testosterone for Men

At around age fifty, testosterone levels begin to decline in men, and for many men, the decline is discernible by how they feel. As a man at about this age, if you begin to experience a negative change in libido—that is, if you are no longer interested in sex—and notice a change in energy or mood, you should have your testosterone level checked. As in the case of DHEA, your doctor will use either a standard hormone blood assay test or a salivary hormone profile (which tests your saliva) to determine your testosterone levels. Getting an overall measure of total testosterone is not enough; as previously explained, in chapter 3, your doctor must check your level of free or unbound testosterone because this is the way to measure the amount of testosterone actually available for use in your body.

Testosterone is available by prescription only.

Many different forms of testosterone are available for men. I, and most physicians, do not recommend that testosterone be taken orally because, over time, oral testosterone may cause liver damage.

A better choice is to take testosterone by injections of 200 mg. testosterone enanthate; depending on need, these are given every two to four weeks for men who have been diagnosed with low testosterone levels. Testosterone injections are very effective, and it is the method most often used in the research studies that have documented the benefits of testosterone replacement. The problem with injections is that some men complain the effect is not consistent. They say that they feel a tremendous burst of energy during the first week following the injection but that this feeling begins to wear off within a week or two. Recently, a transdermal testosterone patch has become available in the United States that can be worn on the back or buttocks. (At one time, the only patch approved for use by the FDA had to be worn on the scrotum, which was not nearly as comfortable as these new patches.) The patch should be applied to clean, dry skin and must be changed according to directions. Some men prefer the patch because it offers a steadier delivery of testosterone than do testosterone injections and, as a result, there are no highs and lows.

Testosterone creams and gels come in varying strengths and are sold by compounding pharmacies, and are growing in popularity because they are both effective and relatively easy to use. Care must be taken to apply the right amount of cream in order to obtain the recommended dose. This is somewhat easier in the case of gels, which are supplied in pump bottles that produce a measured flow.

Compounding pharmacies offer testosterone in a sublingual pill form that is placed under the tongue and dissolved. The sublingual form is absorbed directly in the bloodstream, bypassing the liver. Hence, it does not have negative effects on the liver.

Before beginning to use testosterone, and periodically thereafter, a man should have an examination of his prostate and a Prostate

Specific Antigen (PSA) test to detect the risk of latent prostate tumors. Although testosterone is not carcinogenic, it may stimulate the growth of a preexisting tumor. Men should also receive periodic blood tests, because testosterone increases the number of red blood cells (which is one of the reasons men feel so energized on this superhormone), and it is not advisable to allow the red blood cell count to get too high. As noted earlier, all men should have these tests anyway as part of their annual physical, but men taking testosterone should have them more frequently.

TESTOSTERONE FOR WOMEN

The loss of libido that may occur in some women after menopause is a common sign of testosterone deficiency. Any postmenopausal woman who notices a decline in sex drive and energy should ask her doctor to check her testosterone levels. If her level of free testosterone is lower than normal, she may need to add testosterone to her superhormone cocktail.

For women who need testosterone supplementation, the trick is to use as little as possible to achieve the desired result. The dose for women will therefore be significantly lower than the dose for men. As in the case of men, I do not recommend oral testosterone for women because long-term use can cause liver damage. Many physicians do prescribe oral testosterone, however, because they believe the dose given to women is too low to cause any problems. In addition, women do not need to take testosterone daily; they may need it only a few days each month. Very often, oral testosterone is combined with estrogen and progesterone. Still, I personally believe that there are safer and better alternatives to oral forms.

Women may take testosterone via injection or, in some cases, by slow-release subcutaneous skin pellets that are surgically implanted under the skin.

Although the testosterone skin patch should not be used by women because it delivers too high a dose, compounding pharmacies offer a wide range of testosterone creams and gels that can be rubbed directly on the skin (arm, thigh, or abdomen); these are quite effective and easy to use.

A woman will usually feel the effects of testosterone in three to five days.

At the right dose, most women can use testosterone safely with no adverse side effects. As a rule, it is best to start with the lowest dose and then increase the dosage gradually to achieve the desired result, rather than start high and cut back.

Since testosterone can raise cholesterol and lower HDL, or good cholesterol, levels in some women, it is important that women have their cholesterol monitored while taking testosterone. This is something that all women should be doing in any case.

HOW TO TAKE ESTROGEN

Estrogen (alone or in combination with progesterone) has been prescribed now for decades to millions of postmenopausal women. Although estrogen was first prescribed to treat the symptoms of menopause, we now know that it does much, much more in terms of helping a woman remain youthful, strong, and healthy throughout her entire life. Among other things, estrogen can prevent osteoporosis, significantly reduce the risk of heart disease, enhance mental function, and stave off Alzheimer's disease. It even helps prevent wrinkles!

Estrogen is available in many different forms, which will be reviewed below. All forms of estrogen are available by prescription only.

So many physicians prescribe Premarin, a form of conjugated estrogens made from the urine of pregnant mares, that it is the number-one prescription drug in the United States. Premarin pills are sold in .625-mg. strength. The advantage of Premarin is that it is tried and true. It has been used for fifty years with good results. The disadvantage is that it allows for little flexibility in dosage. In order to adjust the dose, the pill must be broken into smaller pieces, which is not easy to do.

Today, a growing number of physicians are prescribing natural estrogen or estradiol, which more closely resembles the form of estrogen produced by the human ovaries. Estrace, a form of micronized estrogen, is the most well known brand of estradiol.

Oral estrogen is typically taken daily, although if a woman has severe symptoms, her physician may recommend that she divide up her dose and take it once in the morning and once at night. This method more closely resembles the way estrogen is normally produced in the body.

One advantage to using estradiol is that compounding pharmacies can make estradiol capsules into virtually any dose. I think this is a real plus. Several adjustments may be required before a woman finds the right level of estrogen for her, and clearly, the more flexibility her doctor has to alter the dose, the better.

Estrogen is also available in a transdermal skin patch (Estraderm) which delivers estradiol in .05-mg. and .1-mg. doses. The patch is applied to the abdomen or buttocks; it is worn every day and is changed twice a week. Some women develop an irritation from the adhesive, but this may be avoided by alternating where the patch is placed. The patch is the preferred method of estrogen for women with liver or gallbladder disease because the superhormone is absorbed directly into the bloodstream through the skin, bypassing the liver. In addition, women with high blood pressure and a history of blood clots may do better on the patch since oral estrogen might aggravate these conditions.

Compounding pharmacies offer a wide array of estrogens in creams and skin gels which are very popular. A weaker form of estrogen, estriol, is used in a skin cream that can be applied directly to the vagina and is excellent for helping to treat urinary tract and vaginal problems that may arise due to estrogen deficiency. In some cases, even if a woman is using the patch or taking the tablet form, she may occasionally need to use a vaginal cream in addition. To treat vaginal problems, women typically use the creams three times a week until the problem is resolved.

Estrogen creams and gels work well to relieve symptoms for many women. Estrogen creams are usually inserted into the vagina with an applicator. Gels can be rubbed directly on any area of the skin. There have been no adequate studies to determine whether creams and gels are as effective as oral estrogen in terms of preventing osteoporosis and protecting against heart disease, so we don't yet know whether it is more difficult to get a sustained blood level of estrogen topically.

Studies of the estrogen patch—which also delivers estrogen through the skin—do show that it can prevent bone loss and has a beneficial effect on cholesterol. The key here is that no matter what form of estrogen you use, you must have your blood levels checked periodically to make sure you are getting enough of this superhormone to not only relieve specific symptoms but also protect against osteoporosis and heart disease.

Before any woman begins estrogen, she should have a mammogram and manual breast examination to make sure that she does not have any previously undetected tumors. Although estrogen is not a carcinogen and even protects against colon cancer, it can promote the growth of existing breast tumors. Some studies suggest, however, that unlike estradiol or the conjugated estrogens, estriol, which is a very weak estrogen, does not stimulate the growth of preexisting breast tumors. In fact, these studies have suggested that estriol may actually inhibit the formation of breast tumors. In some cases estriol cream may be prescribed for women who have had breast cancer and who are suffering from vaginal atrophy and other problems associated with menopause.

Some compounding pharmacies offer estrogen combinations, notably estradiol, estriol, and estrone, in capsules and gels. This formulation is known as "Tri-estrogen" and championed by people who feel that since a woman's ovaries produce these three types of estrogens, it is important to replace them all. Some pharmacies offer a combination of just estriol and estradiol. Frankly, I am not sure that the type of natural estrogen makes that big a difference, and I think that the real point here is to find the prescription that makes a woman feel her best. Since no two women are exactly alike, each woman may need to try a number of different types of estrogen before finding the one that is right for her. I believe the more options that are available, the better.

Estrogen in the form of natural estradiol is also available from compounding pharmacies in the form of a subcutaneous skin pellet; surgically implanted under the skin, it slowly and naturally releases estrogen into the body. The estrogen pellet may be used by women who do not respond well to the other forms of estrogen.

At one time, women taking oral estrogen or using the patch were advised to use estrogen for three weeks out of the month and then skip a week. This approach was modeled after the way oral contraceptives were used. This is no longer the preferred method of treatment because many women complain of feeling poorly during the week they are off estrogen, and there is no reason for women to spend a week out of every month in discomfort. Today, we recommend that women use estrogen every day to sustain a more normal, natural level. (We recommend that women use estrogen even during the days that they are taking progesterone, as I will explain below.)

If you are using estrogen in any form, and you have not had a hysterectomy, you must also use another superhormone: progesterone.

If I Smoke, Can I Use Estrogen?

I don't advise it, and in fact, it's one of the best reasons for a woman to quit smoking before reaching menopause. A woman who smokes and uses estrogen is prone to develop blood clots, which can be very dangerous. Smoking also increases the odds of a woman's developing osteoporosis and heart disease, two diseases that estrogen can help prevent. If you smoke, the best thing you can do for yourself is to stop. When you are cigarette free, you can look forward to beginning your superhormone regimen and not only regaining your health but extending your life and increasing your vitality!

How to Take Natural Progesterone

Natural progesterone is a superhormone that works with estrogen to help maintain the normal hormonal balance within a woman's body. Because estrogen stimulates the growth of the uterine lining, progesterone is prescribed with it to prevent the lining from developing hyperplasia, a potentially precancerous condition. Progesterone also offers some benefits of its own, and together the two are important ingredients in a woman's superhormone cocktail.

The most commonly prescribed brand of progesterone is the synthetic version, Provera, or medroxyprogesterone. The usual dose is 5 to 10 mg. for ten to fourteen days of each month. After the progesterone is discontinued, there is usually a short and light menstrual period, at least for the first few years on estrogen/progestin until the uterus stops functioning completely. To avoid the monthly period, some physicians prescribe very low doses of progestin daily. This prevents the growth of the uterine lining. Many women, however, find that they do not like taking progestin every day, and so this method is becoming less and less popular.

Because progestin can have some unpleasant side effects, such as moodiness, bloating, and headaches, more and more doctors are turning to natural progesterone, which is virtually indistinguishable from the progesterone produced in the ovaries. Natural progesterone is not only less likely to cause any side effects, but women actually feel good on it! (That's why I call it the feel-good superhormone for women.)

Natural progesterone is available by prescription in capsules, creams, and gels. (A weaker progesterone cream is also sold over the counter.)

Micronized progesterone capsules are available from compounding pharmacies. The only problem with oral natural progesterone is that it is broken down very rapidly in the body, and therefore women who use it must take it twice daily—once in the morning, once at night, usually for ten to fourteen days each month. Some compounding pharmacies offer progesterone in a sublingual pill form that is placed under the tongue and dissolved.

Progesterone creams, gels, and suppositories are also available in varying strengths at compounding pharmacies. These pharmacies offer every conceivable combination of estrogen/progesterone and every possible dose. This enables a doctor to customize the prescription for each patient.

Over-the-counter progesterone body creams are growing in popularity as treatments for menopausal symptoms. The amount of cream that is normally used is one-fourth to one-half teaspoon applied twice daily (morning and night) to the abdomen, back, shoulders, neck, arms, and face. But over-the-counter creams may not be strong enough to prevent the growth of the uterine lining, and if you are using a weak progesterone cream with estrogen, you must be certain that your doctor is carefully monitoring your blood levels to make sure you are getting enough progesterone.

HOW TO TAKE THYROID HORMONE

I call thyroid hormone the "energizer" because this hormone provides the energy and "fuel" for literally every cell in the body. The main symptoms for hypothyroidism—a thyroid deficiency—are fatigue, low energy, lethargy, forgetfulness, mental confusion, depression, and susceptibility to infection. Since thyroid hormone helps to regulate body temperature, sensitivity to cold is also a sign that this essential superhormone is lacking. When people whose thyroid levels are too low replenish their levels back to normal, they feel recharged, and their energy and health is restored.

Although thyroid hormone levels decline as we age, not everyone is going to experience the decline acutely. Some people will need to take thyroid supplements, and some won't. How do you know if you are deficient in thyroid hormone? Here are several ways to diagnose thyroid deficiency. A doctor who suspects a thyroid problem will order a blood test to determine the levels of key thyroid hormones,

T3 and T4, as well as levels of thyroid-stimulating hormone, known as TSH. Low levels of T3 or T4 are a clear sign that you are not making enough thyroid hormone, and an elevated level of TSH is also a sign of trouble; it means that the pituitary gland is trying to rev up the thyroid gland to produce more hormone. Thyroid hormone is carried through the bloodstream on a protein called transthyretrin. It is also advisable to check the levels of transthyretrin, or thyroid antibodies, especially if the other tests are normal and the patient is showing classic signs of thyroid hormone deficiency.

Since thyroid regulates body temperature, another simple way to check for thyroid function is to measure your basal temperature first thing in the morning. To do this, simply place a thermometer under your arm for ten minutes immediately upon waking and before getting out of bed. If your morning temperature falls below 97.4 degrees Fahrenheit, it is a sign that your thyroid function is deficient and that you probably need thyroid hormone added to your superhormone cocktail.

Thyroid hormone is available only by prescription and must be monitored by your physician even more closely than some of the other superhormones. If the dose is too high, it can cause agitation, irritability, and, more seriously, heart palpitations. A patient on thyroid hormone who experiences any of these symptoms should call the doctor immediately. A dose that is too low, however, will not be effective. Even a patient who is showing the right blood levels of thyroid hormone may need to have the dosage increased if symptoms do not improve. The key is to find the right dose for each patient, which is another reason that the patient should work closely with his or her doctor.

Thyroid hormone is available in pill and capsule form, and is always taken orally.

Physicians routinely prescribe the synthetic form of this superhormone, sold under the name Synthroid, which contains T4, one kind of thyroid hormone. In some cases your physician may prescribe a synthetic version of T3, called Cytomel.

Compounding pharmacies offer a natural form of thyroid, an animal-based product used long before the synthetic versions were available. These are once more growing in popularity. It provides the combination of T3 and T4, which is similar to how the thyroid gland produces thyroid hormone.

There is no one best form of thyroid hormone, and treatment will vary, depending on each person's needs.

HOW TO TAKE HUMAN GROWTH HORMONE

Like the other superhormones, levels of growth hormone peak at around age twenty and begin a slow but steady decline throughout our adult lives. Not all of us will need to replenish growth hormone. In fact, as previously explained, in chapter 8, most healthy people who are already taking other superhormones probably will not.

There are people, however, who will need to use human growth hormone, and for them this superhormone can be a true lifesaver. I call growth hormone the "restorative" superhormone, and I believe that its positive effects will be best felt by people who need it the most—those suffering from specific ailments such as kidney disorders, heart failure, or wasting syndromes. Human growth hormone is available only by prescription and is quite expensive. A year's worth of treatment can cost between $9,000 and $12,000.

Doctors who prescribe human growth hormone to their patients as an anti-aging tool typically give patients premeasured syringes that they must self-inject. Although regimens vary from doctor to doctor, a typical regimen may be four to eight IUs of growth hormone a week taken in twelve doses over six days. A growth hormone user will typically give himself a shot in the morning and a shot at night.

Growth hormone can cause side effects such as swelling of the feet and ankles, carpal tunnel syndrome, and diabetes. It is essential therefore that anyone who is using growth hormone be carefully monitored by a physician.

I believe it is possible to obtain many of the benefits that growth hormone offers by using the other superhormones, particularly DHEA, melatonin, pregnenolone, estrogen, and testosterone, all of which are inexpensive and easily available, and have no untoward side effects. Vigorous exercise (running, weight training, or aerobics) performed at least three times a week will also stimulate the release of growth hormone in the body naturally.

HOW TO TAKE MELATONIN

Melatonin is the "miracle superhormone" that can help us grow young in a healthy, strong body that remains in the "youthful state" no matter what our age. It is the only superhormone that has been proven in animal studies to stop the aging process and extend life. By restoring melatonin to youthful levels, we will not only live longer but will live healthier, more fulfilled lives.

Melatonin is also a wonderful sleep aid and a proven cure for jet lag, and I will tell you how to use melatonin to achieve a good night's sleep and prevent jet lag.

The question of when you should take melatonin and how much to take will depend on the problem that you are seeking to correct; therefore, I will break down the guidelines into separate sections for dosage information and instructions for taking melatonin according to each of the specific problem areas that melatonin addresses.

Age reversal Our melatonin replacement strategy is to restore our melatonin levels to what they were when we were in our twenties. After that, the levels drop off very gradually until we reach our mid-forties, when a dramatic decline in our melatonin production occurs. Our basic strategy therefore is to reverse this downward curve and maintain our melatonin levels at their constant, youthful peak. Doing this is not complicated. All that is necessary is to take a sufficient amount of melatonin to bring our melatonin level up to its youthful baseline. Thus, we take a small dose in our forties, a slightly larger dose in our fifties, more in our sixties, and so on. By restoring our melatonin to youthful levels we restore the function of our body's aging clock—the pineal gland—and help maintain our body in the youthful state.

To maintain our melatonin levels at their youthful peaks, we recommend the following doses at the following ages. These doses are based on normative levels of melatonin in adults as they age and the amount of supplement required to restore levels to their youthful peaks. Recently, salivary testing has become available that may provide even more precise measurement of your melatonin levels and what dose of supplementation you require.

AGE	DOSE OF MELATONIN
40–45	Take .5 mg. to 1 mg. at bedtime
45–55	Take 1 to 2 mg. at bedtime
55–65	Take 2 to 2.5 mg. at bedtime
65–75	Take 2.5 to 5 mg. at bedtime
75-plus	Take 3.5 to 5 mg. at bedtime

You will notice that I consistently recommend that melatonin be taken at bedtime and also that there is some variation in dosage, that the range increases with age. In many people melatonin induces drowsiness. Some people who are highly susceptible to melatonin's sleep-inducing properties may find that the recommended dose is making them too groggy in the morning. I therefore recommend that you reduce your dose by approximately .5 mg. at a time until you find the right level for you.

You will find at your health food store or pharmacy that melatonin comes in capsules and tablets, typically in strengths of 1.0, 1.8, 2, 2.5, and 3 mg. If the right dosage for you is lower, simply do the following: If you are taking tablets, break a tablet to the size that you need. For example, if you have a 2-mg. tablet and you want a 1-mg. dose, break the tablet in half. If you want a .5-mg. dose, break the tablet into quarters.

Or, if you are using capsules and you have, let's say, a 3-mg. capsule and want to take a 1-mg. dose, empty the contents of the 3-mg. capsule into a small dish. For the first dose, mix approximately one third of the contents with an ounce of liquid. (Store the remaining contents in a small, covered dish in the refrigerator.) For the second dose, mix approximately half of the remaining melatonin with an ounce of liquid. For the third dose, mix the remaining melatonin with an ounce of liquid. (Compounding pharmacists can make any concentration available to you in capsule or sublingual tablet.)

Melatonin is also available in a sublingual form that dissolves under the tongue and may be absorbed by the body more rapidly.

Melatonin should be taken at night only, around a half-hour before bedtime. After taking melatonin, don't engage in activities that require a state of alertness, such as driving or operating machinery. Although melatonin will not make you feel "drugged" in the way that a narcotic sleeping pill does, you may feel relaxed and drowsy and ready for sleep. Beware of enhanced drowsiness with tranquilizers, antihistamines, alcohol, or narcotics.

There are two forms of melatonin on the market: the synthetic form and the so-called natural melatonin made from the extract of animal pineal glands. We prefer and recommend synthetic melatonin. Your pharmacist or shopkeeper will help you select the correct product.

For better sleep   For sleep disorders, we recommend taking between 1 and 5 mg. at bedtime to restore normal sleep patterns. The effect of melatonin will vary among individuals. Some people find that the smaller dose is sufficient to achieve a good night's sleep. Others need a higher dose. To determine the exact dosage that is right for you, we recommend that you begin with 1 mg. at bedtime. Even if you are sleeping well, we recommend that you take melatonin for two weeks to "reset" your body clock and reestablish your natural sleep schedule. After that time, you will probably find that your internal clock has been corrected, and you may not need melatonin to sleep. If you are unable to fall asleep, however, you can continue to take your usual dose of melatonin at bedtime.

If your sleeping problem is not solved—if, for example, you find that you are still waking up frequently at night—increase the dose the next night by 1 mg. to 2 mg. Continue to increase the dose each night by 1 mg. (to 5 mg. or more) until you are sleeping properly and feel refreshed in the morning.

If your problem is insomnia and you are unable to fall asleep within a half-hour after taking melatonin, increase your dose from 1 to 2 mg. the same night. If 2 mg. doesn't work within ten minutes, increase your dose by another 1 mg. (to 3 mg.). If you still aren't falling asleep (which is doubtful), you can continue to increase your dose by increments of 1 mg. every twenty minutes until you reach a maximum of 5 mg.

If you find that after taking melatonin at night you wake up feeling groggy in the morning, this is a sign that your bedtime dose is too high and you need to reduce it. For you, as little as .1 to .5 mg. may be adequate for inducing sleep.

Jet lag　Jet lag is caused by a disruption in circadian cycles caused by flying across time zones. Melatonin is a proven cure for jet lag. By taking melatonin you can "reset" your body clock so that you quickly adjust to the time change. Here's what you need to do. If you are taking a trip that involves travel across time zones, simply take 3 to 5 mg. of melatonin prior to bedtime once you reach your new destination. Continue to take melatonin at bedtime for about four nights, until your body clock is completely reset. If you find yourself waking too early in your new destination, you can take another 3–5 mg. of melatonin to help yourself fall back to sleep. When you return home, readjust your body clock by taking 3 to 5 mg. of melatonin before your normal bedtime and do so until you have readjusted to the time change. Many people claim that by taking melatonin they experience none of the symptoms normally associated with crossing time zones.

Note　Those of you on antidepressants, antihistamines, antihypertensives and other agents that affect mood and sleep should consult your physician.

Afterword

FULFILLING THE SUPERHORMONE PROMISE

FOR THOUSANDS OF years, scientists have assumed that the process of aging is as inevitable as the passage of time itself. They have regarded aging as synonymous with the physical and mental deterioration that all of us have come to accept as a normal function of growing older. We hope *The Superhormone Promise* will help inspire readers with its life-affirming message, that they will be heartened by what it means for their future, and, finally, that it will encourage a change in the way most of us, including physicians and the medical profession generally view aging.

A new model of aging is overdue, one that keeps up with the new reality. Gerontologists have been trained to see aging as a random collection of isolated diseases. Physicians are struggling mightily and with the best of intentions to treat older patients as they present with such degenerative diseases as osteoporosis, which may lead to vertebral collapse and hip fracture; adult onset diabetes; coronary artery disease and congestive heart failure; stroke; Alzheimer's; and cancer.

Eventually we must see that this approach is not enough. It misses the proverbial forest for the trees, because these are but symptoms of the underlying disease—indeed the ultimate disease—which is aging itself. A cure is already at hand, but now we must seize it.

We do not develop these degenerative diseases because time has worn us down. The enemy does not, it turns out, come from without; it strikes from within. We fall prey to the diseases associated with old age because our bodies cease to produce the adequate superhormones that keep our body systems primed and balanced. What makes us so vulnerable in our later years has little to do with new or different challenges from the external world. It has to do with an interior change that undermines the integrity of our body systems and thereby weakens our first line of defense.

The good news is that we now know we can intervene in that process. As we've tried to show in *The Superhormone Promise,* by following nature's blueprint to restore superhormones back to their adult peak, you can extend your youthful vitality and the length of your life. The promise of superhormones is that you will not only add years and possibly decades to your life, but just as importantly, you will live stronger, with bodies and minds that have not been enfeebled by the ravages we used to associate with aging. You can spare yourself from the diseases of aging that would otherwise rob you of the quality of life that is your due, by staving off the disease of aging itself.

Time will not stop. The years will still pass. But, as they do, you can remain happy, sexually active, vital, and strong, pursuing your hopes and dreams, unfettered by physical or mental deterioration. In sum, you will not have to experience the decline in mental and physical function that for too long we were forced to accept as normal aging.

I find it ironic that despite the obvious debility and dependency that is associated with aging, the medical establishment is reluctant to call it a disease. More alarming is the tendency of physicians and researchers alike to dismiss physical ailments as "normal" if the patient voicing the complaint is of a certain age.

Once you cross the threshold into middle age, your complaints to your doctor of fatigue are likely to draw responses like, "Well, what do you expect at your age?" Or if you complain about a flagging tennis game, you will probably hear, "Well, you're forty, and they say the legs go first." Worse, if an older person has an elevated blood sugar level or complains of minor memory problems, she will most likely be told, "Well, that's normal for your age." In other words, what is likely to be viewed as a sign of illness in young people is all too often just written off as part and parcel of the "normal" aging process in older people. I can assure you, these symptoms are not normal at any age. Indeed, to my way of thinking, there is nothing "normal" about the aging process because there is nothing normal about the process of disease.

This kind of ageism should not be tolerated by (or from) health care professionals. In the past this was perhaps understandable since there was no choice but to accept this fate with stoic fortitude. But today, we do have a choice, and our expectations should and must change as a result. With superhormones, we now have the knowledge and the tools to intervene in a meaningful way with the aging process. We no longer must sit by passively as our bodies, minds, and spirits decline. Today, we know why we age, and most importantly, we know how to stop it.

Twenty years of scientific research have shown me that the reason we age, the reason we experience the precipitous decline known as "senescence," is because of the breakdown of our body's aging clock. When the aging clock begins to wind down, it leads to a decline in our superhormone levels that, in turn, leads to the breaking down of virtually all our vital body systems. By restoring our superhormone levels to their adult peaks, we prevent this process from taking hold. Superhormones will enable us to fulfill our potential at any age, whether we are in our fifth decade or our twelfth.

The power of superhormones is already being felt throughout the medical community, in doctor's offices and research labs around the country and throughout the world. Doctors are already prescribing superhormones for their patients, and now that four superhormones —DHEA, melatonin, pregnenolone, and natural progesterone cream —are available over the counter, more and more people will want to get in on the anti-aging revolution that is rocking the country.

I also sincerely hope that the power of superhormones will soon be felt in the halls of the National Institute on Aging (NIA) and by the appropriate agencies in government. By the year 2030, there will be 52 million Americans over the age of seventy, placing a tremendous burden on our Social Security Agency and other government programs that benefit older people. Keeping people healthy and economically independent is also in our national interest. If we do not take steps to cure the disease of aging, an aging population will become an increasingly difficult financial burden on our children and their children.

Fulfilling the Superhormone Promise is ultimately about much more than simply restoring superhormones to youthful levels as a tool of rejuvenation. It is about changing outmoded and outdated attitudes about aging that hold us back and prevent us from learning more about the biology of aging. Fulfilling the promise is about breaking free of perceptions and stereotypes that hamper our ability to live longer, better lives.

WILLIAM REGELSON, M.D.
August 1996

Resources

IDEALLY, WHEN YOU begin your superhormone regimen you will be able to work with the doctor you already have, who knows your medical history, and with whom you have a good relationship. If, however, you don't have a doctor, or need to find a new one, several of the major compounding pharmacies will provide a list of doctors in your area who routinely prescribe superhormones. (These compounding pharmacies are listed below.) As with any physician referral, however, it is best if you do some legwork yourself to find the doctor who is right for you.

It is essential that you check the physician's credentials with your county medical society (your doctor should be an M.D. or a D.O.— doctors of osteopathy undergo the same rigorous training as M.D.s), and you should interview the physician ahead of time to see if he or she is someone with whom you will have good rapport.

What is most important is that you find a primary-care physician who is concerned about you as an individual and who will be willing to work closely with you. If possible, this should be someone who is a generalist, that is, a physician who treats the whole body and not just one small part of it. I recommend that you look for a physician who is either a family practitioner or an internist. In some cases, a family practitioner or an internist may have a subspecialty in any number of fields including gynecology, gerontology, endocrinology, or neurology. Depending on your particular needs, you may select a primary-care physician with the appropriate subspecialty.

There are hundreds of independent compounding pharmacies in the United States that fill prescriptions for superhormones, and many will fill prescriptions by mail from anywhere in the country. The International Academy of Compounding Pharmacists (IACP), a non-profit organization of independent pharmacists, will help you locate a compounding pharmacist in your area.

For a list of compounding pharmacies in your area, you can either call or write:

The International Academy of Compounding Pharmacists
P.O. Box 1365
Sugar Land, TX 77487
800-927-4227

A partial list of compounding pharmacies is provided below. An asterisk designates that the pharmacist will also provide you with a list of doctors in your area who prescribe superhormones.

The Apothecary
35 Main St.
Keene, NH 03431
617-566-4080

Apothecure, Inc.
13720 Midway Rd.
Dallas, TX 75244
800-969-6601

Bajamar Women's Healthcare Pharmacy*
9609 Dielman Rock Island
St. Louis, MO 63132
800-255-8025
Fax 314-997-2948

For those who have access to the internet (World Wide Web), Bajamar offers an "Ask the Pharmacist" service on their own website. Bajamar's on-line address is:
http://walden.mo.net/~bmizes/hormones.html

California Pharmacy and Compounding Center*
307 Placentia Ave., #0102
Newport Beach, CA 92663
800-575-7776
Fax 714-642-0725

College Pharmacy*
833 North Tejon
Colorado Springs, CO 80903
800-888-9358

Homelink Pharmacy
2650 Elm Ave., Suite 104
Long Beach, CA 90806
800-272-4767

Hopewell Pharmacy
1 West Broad St.
Hopewell, NJ 08525
800-792-6670

Medical Center Pharmacy
10721 Main St.
Fairfax, VA 22030
703-273-7311
Fax 800-238-8239

Pierce Apothecary
1180 Beacon St.
Brookline, MA 02146
617-566-4080

Women's International
  Pharmacy *
5708 Monoma Dr.
Madison, WI 53716-3152
800-279-5708

Wellness Health and
  Pharmaceuticals
2800 South 18th St.
Birmingham, AL 35209
800-227-2627

A Note to Women

For women interested in finding a physician who works with natural hormones, the North American Menopause Society will provide a list of physicians in your area who are knowledgeable in the various forms of hormone replacement therapy. The address and phone number is:

The North American Menopause Society
c/o University Hospitals Department of OB/GYN
11100 Euclid Ave.
Cleveland, OH 44106
216-844-8748
Fax 216-844-8708

Mail Order

For those who want to order superhormones by mail, a partial list of mail order providers are listed below.

To purchase pharmaceutical grade DHEA (25 mg.)
FreeLife International™
354 Woodmount Rd., Suite 5
Milford, CT 06460
800-414-DHEA

To purchase natural progesterone cream
Transitions for Health™
621 S.W. Alder, Suite 900
Portland, OR 97205-3627
800-888-6814

To purchase pharmaceutical grade DHEA (25 mg.) and
pregnenolone (50 mg.)
Life Extension Foundation
P.O. Box 229120
Hollywood, FL 33022
800-841-5433

Diagnostic Tests

Your doctor may be interested in contacting a laboratory that performs salivary hormonal assay tests. A partial list of laboratories is given below.

Aeron Lifecycles
1933 Davis St.
Suite 310
San Leandro, CA 94577
800-631-7900

Diagnos-Techs, Inc.
Clinical and Research Laboratory
6620 South 192nd Pl., J-104
Kent, WA 98032
800-878-3787

Great Smokies Diagnostic Laboratory
18 A. Regent Park Blvd.
Asheville, NC 28806
704-253-0621

National Biotech Laboratory
13758 Lake City Way, N.E.
Seattle, WA 98125
800-846-6285
Fax 206-363-2025

Useful information can be obtained from

The Life Extension Foundation
995 Southwest 24th St.
Ft. Lauderdale, FL 33315
800-841-5433
http://www.lef.org

The American Academy of Anti-Aging Medicine (4M)
401 N. Michigan Ave.
Chicago, IL 60611-427
312-527-6733
Fax 312-321-6869
Internet World Health Network
http://www.worldhealth.net
or call 312-528-4333

DHEA (Dehydroepiandrosterone)— A Pleiotropic Steroid. How Can One Steroid Do So Much?

WILLIAM REGELSON, M.D., AND
MOHAMMED Y. KALIMI, PH.D.*

Introduction

DEHYDROEPIANDROSTERONE (DHEA) is the most abundant steroid in humans secreted primarily by the adrenal cortex, but also synthesized by the brain and skin. Up to recently, this hormone was considered to be important only as an intermediate in the synthesis of the sex steroids. It is now apparent that DHEA has significant physiologic and biologic action on its own, or its effects may be mediated by moderating the action of the glucocorticoids.[1-7]

DHEA declines with progressive age, so that an individual in his or her eighties may produce only 10–20% of what was made in their second decade.[8-10] Moreover, as reported in the epidemiological studies of Barrett-Connors et al. and others,[10-12] higher levels of DHEA in the circulation protect men from coronary mortality.

DHEA stimulates immune responsiveness,[2,13] affects CNS function,[14] inhibits carcinogenesis,[3,15,16] and alters cell energetics and fat metabolism.[5,17,18]

DHEA is a neurosteroid synthesized by oligodendroglial cells in

* Departments of Medicine and Physiology, Medical College of Virginia, Virginia Commonwealth University, Richmond, Virginia

the brain,[19,20] and in addition to hepatic processing, can be metabolized by skin, chromaffin cells, the pregnant cervix, and other tissues
responsive to sex steroids.[6,21] In humans, DHEA, for most individuals, is rapidly sulfated, and the sulfated derivative (DHEA-S)* is the
usual predominant form in the circulation.[22]

It is evident that this hormone is not just a simple intermediate in
the metabolic pathway of the sex hormones, and cannot be dismissed
as a "weak androgen." DHEA has pleiotropic† effects dependent on
its mode of delivery, metabolism, age, sex, and tissue interaction,
and in this manner it is important to a broad range of physiologic
responses.[1-7] We have likened DHEA to a "buffer hormone," whose
actions are governed by "state dependency."[3,21,22] "State dependency"
describes hormone action based upon its expression only within particular physiologic settings independent of a specific end organ targeted effect.

Since 1966, more than 5500 papers on DHEA have appeared. This
extensive literature has suggested a role for DHEA in diabetes, gout,
obesity, atherosclerosis, carcinogenesis, tumor growth, neurite outgrowth, pregnancy, hypertension, collagenolysis, hair growth, skin
integrity, fatigue, depression, memory, virus and bacterial infection,
immune responses, and stress.[1-4] In addition, DHEA has digitalis-like
activity and can affect enzyme systems which include glucose-6-
phosphate dehydrogenase,[3] and protein isoprenylation involved in
cell division.[23]

With the diverse physiological, biological, and biochemical effects
encompassing various cell types, tissues, and organs,[1-7] we must ask
how this one steroid can have such profound effects on such a wide
variety of physiologic or pathophysiologic events ranging from carcinogenesis to memory. We have to study whether DHEA replacement,
to restore youthful values, can counteract its age-related decline to
see whether it can modulate the character of age-related disease.
To better understand DHEA's functional role, we have to see it as
para-endocrine, distinct from its action as a targeted excitatory hormone in the classical sense.

It is important to note that in all DHEA research, one must distin-

---

* Except as indicated, DHEA and DHEA-S (its sulfated form) will be referred to as
DHEA.

† Pleiotropic—the quality of having affinity for several different types of tissue.
Genetics: to manifest in a multiplicity of ways, to produce many effects in the
phenotype. (*Dorland's Medical Dictionary,* 25th edition).

guish studies involving physiologic replacement dosage versus pharmacologic effects produced by dosage of DHEA far above physiologic norms. One must also recognize that women respond to DHEA in a manner that is distinct from clinical response in men. DHEA, which is a prime feature of human and primate physiology, is not a key metabolite in other mammalian species.

Recently, Etienne-Emile Baulieu, the steroid chemist who was the first to identify DHEA,[24] and who demonstrated its brain synthesis, was embraced by the popular press when he reported that DHEA was "a key to the reversal of the symptoms of aging." This was based on a recent paper by Yen's group[9] reporting on the antifatigue effect of DHEA in the elderly. This observation should not have been surprising as DHEA, called "prasterone," or, when combined with estrogen, "astenile," has been available in Europe for fatigue and depression in postmenopasual women, for more than 15 years.[1-3]

In terms of its mechanism of action, DHEA may be an "antihormone" which "cannot serve to 'excite' in the true classical sense of hormone action, but 'de-excites' metabolic processes which overproduce when DHEA is in short supply."[21] In this regard, DHEA acts by buffering or antagonizing the action of corticosteroids (GCS) to modify stress-mediated injury to tissue, an action which we feel is critical to the expression of the degenerative diseases of aging.[3,7] In further support for this, DHEA modulates insulin output,[25-28] and DHEA has been shown to be our most potent peroxisomal inducer, a key organelle that metabolizes lipids, which stimulates catalase formation, and can neutralize peroxides contributing to free radical formation involved in tissue injury or aging.[29] DHEA stimulates liver catalase activity, and high catalase levels are among those free radical scavenging enzymes whose high levels distinguish between long-lived versus short-lived species.[30]

DHEA not only antagonizes GCS inhibition of the immune response,[2] but blocks GCS action on liver and brown fat function.[31,32] In immunologic studies, we have suggested that the anticorticoid or stress-alleviating action of DHEA may be important to inhibition of the clinical expression of viral or infection-mediated degenerative disease.[1-4] However, clinically DHEA and its sulfated metabolite, DHEA-S, levels do not always correlate with elevations of cortisol stress-related response,[6,20,21] but there are significant correlations between the severity of illness, chronic stress, and depressed levels of DHEA.[3,6]

Recent broad reviews of DHEA action and more specific presentations of its effects on immunity,[2] cardiovascular diseases,[3,11,12] obesity,[17,18] androgen secretion,[6] carcinogenesis,[15,16] hepatic function,[3,15,16,33,34] mitochondrial metabolism,[5,35,36] insulin action,[25–28] and receptor availability[1,2] have been published, many of them in our text[1] and in our recent New York Academy of Sciences review.[2,4]

DHEA: Structure and Metabolic Fate (Figure 1)

Pregnenolone derived from cholesterol is the source of DHEA. DHEA is an ACTH-regulated C-19 steroid classified with the adrenal androgens, androstenedione and testosterone.[5,6] It should be noted that in stress, or serious illness, there is a shift in pregnenolone metabolism, of the DHEA precursor, away from DHEA and its sulfate production[35] to that of the glucocorticoids[5,7,35,36] (GCS) or stress steroids.[7,37] This has been related to THy 1 versus THy 2 effects on the immune response,[38] as a thymus related event.

In summary, DHEA Δ 5-androsten-3b-ol-17-one, MW 288.41m is a naturally occurring adrenal steroid in humans and primates. DHEA-S, as the sulfated form, circulates in plasma and represents the major secretory product of the human adrenal gland.[20,24,39] DHEA is converted primarily by the adrenal DHEA-sulfotransferase to DHEA-S in humans (and to a lesser extent in rodents) prior to its export into the plasma.[33,34] Humans rapidly transform DHEA to the water soluble DHEA-S, but significant clinical differences in DHEA to DHEA-S ratios are now being observed. There is an age-related decline and change in DHEA/DHEA-S ratios in both the rhesus monkey and chimpanzee, but this alteration in ratios has not been reported in humans. DHEA can also be glucuronidized and bile excreted,[3] and recent 7α-hydroxy dehydroepiandrosterone has been found to also be a major metabolite particularly as a result of fat stromal action.[40]

Both DHEA and DHEA-S can be equally effective when administered in vivo, but only DHEA is capable of inducing the lymphokine IL-2 when added to certain cell cultures in vitro.[41] DHEA is the precursor for Δ 4-androstenedione, Δ 5-androstenediol (AED), estradiol, testosterone, dihydrotestosterone, estrogen, and etiocholanolone.[35–37,40]

The concentration of DHEA in human adult plasma is about 0.01 μM to 0.02 μM (160–700 ng/dl) while that of DHEA-S is 5 μM to 7 μM (800-5600 μg/L).[42,43] However, in hyperandrogenism, DHEA levels may go as high as 28 µM as seen in polycystic ovaries and hypertrichosis.[1,6] DHEA-S has been used as a biomarker for fetal death[4] and at term very high plasma levels are found, provided transplacentally, which decreases postpartum.[4]

DHEA(-S) levels remain very low for the first 7 years of life, after which they start to rise[43] with a peak at the age of 20–24 years. After the second decade, there is a decline of about 20% for every decade, diminishing linearly by 95% of the second decade values by age 85–90, which is not seen for other steroids.[9] There is one nonpublished report of DHEA values being lower in age matched Downs Syndrome patients[44] supporting the progeric nature of that disease.

DHEA-S is secreted by the liver in bile along with the DHEA glucuronide.[3] We are accumulating collaborative evidence[45] that the capacity of patients to sulfate DHEA can vary remarkably. There appears to be a subpopulation of patients that have difficulty sulfating DHEA,[33,34] but what this means clinically has not yet been determined. DHEA can be metabolized by two completely different pathways, either via the hepatic circulation and/or via a second cutaneous pathway where DHEA is converted to androstenediol (AED) or triol.[2,35,38,46] In the skin, DHEA can be redistributed and sulfated to appear in the circulation as androstenediol sulfate.[46]

There is controversial evidence for an androgenic pituitary trophic hormone that can influence DHEA production,[6] but this has not been established. In young females, the ovaries are responsible for 50% of DHEA production with the remainder coming from peripheral synthesis, i.e., the brain and skin. With aging, clinical estrogen substitution does nothing to restore DHEA levels, suggesting a nonestrogen dependent role for ovarian function in the regulation of DHEA production.[47,48] However, ovariectomy[49] can enhance the age-related decline and an age-related attenuation of circadian pulses of DHEA production has been described.[50,51]

As reported by Milewich,[46] DHEA can be metabolized by platelets, vascular endothelium, and macrophages which mark the sites of its local activity pertinent to its action.[3] DHEA is metabolized by the skin where it can promote hirsutism and sebaceous secretion. The latter declines with age, while hair, with age, can be both lost and gained,[3] depending on the site.

DHEA: Biological Effects

EFFECTS ON IMMUNE AND STRESS RESPONSE

DHEA, given subcutaneously (s.c.), at pharmacologic high dosage, enhances resistance to viral and bacterial infection in mice.[2,38,52] In this regard, systemically, DHEA stimulates monocytosis and can protect the host against lethal viral coxsackie B enterovirus or herpes type 2, and *Enterococcus/faecalis* infection.[2,38,52,53] In support of these observations, Ben Nathan and Feuerstein[54] showed that DHEA protects mice infected with West Nile virus (WNV), Sinbis virus (neurovirulent), and Semliki Forest virus. The above DHEA immunostimulatory action requires an intact immune system to exert its protective effect as enhanced host resistance is not seen in the hairless immunodeficient (Hr/Hr) mouse.[51]

The s.c. injection of DHEA can prevent the development of West Nile virus (WNV) lethality in cold stressed mice.[55] In these cold stress studies, only the control stressed virus infected mice die, which is associated with significant increases in GCS levels. Injection of DHEA to these mice results in protection with a concomitant reduction in GCS levels. These findings are of particular relevance to the role of stress factors in virus expression and support Riley's early studies showing a DHEA protective effect against corticosteroid or stress mediated thymic involution.[56]

To review: elevated GCS levels following viral infection cause immunosuppression responsible for higher viral titers, involution of the spleen and thymus, and increased mortality.[54-57] This may be a factor in HIV infection, as in this regard, DHEA can lower HIV viral titers in vitro,[58] and can supplement azidothymidine inhibition of the HIV virus. However, Loria and Padgett[53] have shown with coxsackie B enterovirus, that in vivo androstendiol (AED) and DHEA do not reduce the titer of infectious virus, but instead limit infection-mediated pathology. DHEA and its AED metabolite protect the host by limiting infection-mediated damage, thus resulting in host protection based on the alleviation of toxic host responses.

Of particular importance to DHEA's place in clinical HIV infection, Rasmussen et al.[60] have reported that in rats, immunosuppressed by dexamethasone, Cryptosporidium parvum gastrointestinal infection was inhibited by DHEA treatment with a decrease in infecting organisms. DHEA enhanced T and B cell immunity in these infected animals. DHEA also enhances resistance to pneumococcal infection.[61]

In further support of its in vivo immunostimulatory action, DHEA has been shown to stimulate T-cell proliferation and IL-2 cytokine production.[41] Daynes et al. report that DHEA is a potent enhancer of IL-2 production by antigen or mitogen-activated T cells.[60] Suzuki et al.[63] demonstrated enhanced transcription of the IL-2 gene and stabilization of IL-2 mRNA. DHEA up-regulates IL-2 secretion which in turn can augment lymphocyte effector function by regulating the number of CD-8 + cytotoxic T cells.[62,64,65]

Araneo et al.[66] have shown that DHEA or its sulfate given together with a hepatitis B antigen restored immune vaccine responsiveness in aged mice, suggesting that DHEA may have value in reversing the impaired immunologic responsiveness of aging. Similar responses resulting in an enhanced vaccine effect in aging mice were seen for a pneumococcus vaccine.[61]

This improvement in immune response has been induced in post-menopausal women.[67] However, immune adjuvancy and vaccine enhancement in immunologically normal young mice is not seen. Aging or infection or stress are the factors making the difference governing the protective effects of DHEA. Szakal[68] has shown that subcutaneous DHEA supplementation can enhance the return of follicular dendritic cells, long-term memory cells which decline in the skin of aging mice.

Suppression of IL-2 production and augmentation of IL-4 production in mice treated with GCS is reversed coincident to in vivo treatment with DHEA or DHEA-S.[62-65] DHEA treatment of GCS-exposed T-cells can effectively overcome the depressive influences exerted by GCS on IL-2 production.[65] DHEA, although incapable of enhancing the production of interferon gamma (IFN-gamma) from T-cells, totally reversed GCS-induced depression of the synthesis and secretion of interferon.[64] This report suggested that DHEA antagonizes GCS immunosuppression at the level of IL-4 and IFN-gamma production which may explain one mechanism of an in vivo antiviral activity, i.e., DHEA prevents stress (GCS) mediated inhibition of interferon production.

Based on the early work of Riley's laboratory in the field of neuroimmunomodulation,[56] Fitzmaurice[69] has reviewed the action of stress as a factor enhancing virus expression and cancer induction and proliferation. In that regard, GCS action modulated by DHEA could clearly play a role as confirmed by Ben Nathan et al.[54,55] in mouse virus infected animals. Stress is clinically pertinent to susceptibility to infection as seen in the sensitivity to influenza in emotionally depressed patients as well as those subject to the common cold (rhinovirus).[70]

In another area, Araneo and Daynes[71] have shown that DHEA given to burned mice can preserve immunocompetence and protect them from L monocytogenes lethality. This relates to preservation of T-cell function. DHEA in vivo, in this model, permitted burned mice to control the increase in IL-6 which can result from GCS induction. Continued elevations of IL-6 are associated with poor prognosis and DHEA administration can normalize IL-6 levels with recovery. However, RU 486, which is a corticosteroid blocking agent with similar action to DHEA, did not protect these mice. On this basis, they claim that the antiglucocorticoid action of DHEA does not completely explain its protective effect.

Despite this, Blauer et al.[72] have reported that in vivo DHEA, in mice, antagonized dexamethasone (DEX) suppression of B and T lymphocyte blastogenesis as well as DEX mediated thymus and spleen atrophy. In addition, Weidmeier et al.[73] showed that thymic function regulates IL-2 and IL-4 production in radiated mice that was restored by DHEA.

We have shown that with DHEA we can reverse dexamethasone induced hypertension in rats in similar fashion to RU 486.[74] We believe that the actions of DHEA are due to its buffering stress mediated GCS action. The effect of DHEA in blocking GCS action is clearly defined. We have reviewed this in our recent paper,[4] and believe it is the most effective explanation for DHEA's broad effectiveness in stimulating host resistance. However, it may be that there are other aspects of DHEA's action that may also be pertinent to its protection against thermal injury, trauma, or endotoxic shock. Dannenberg et al.[75] have shown that DHEA protects mice from endotoxin and tumor necrosis factor lethality, an observation that has been recently confirmed in pigs.[76]

In another area, the decline of DHEA levels with age correlates with a general decline in cell-mediated immune response, and in an increased incidence of cancer.[77] In HIV infection corticosteroid levels are elevated,[78,79] and DHEA values are suppressed,[80,81] which may relate to the previous observation.

Other immunological effects associated with DHEA include the enhanced survival of New Zealand black mice (NZB/W FI). These mice develop an autoimmune disorder similar to human systemic lupus erythematosus (SLE) that is characterized by synthesis of antibodies to double-stranded DNA. DHEA[82] prevents the dramatic increase in antibodies to double-stranded DNA in this disease and thus reduces immune complex formation and its deposition.

These observations have been extended clinically to chronic illness such as rheumatoid arthritis[81] where DHEA values are low. In SLE, DHEA levels are low particularly in patients on corticosteroid therapy,[84] and recent clinical trials have shown DHEA to produce remission in that disease.[85] Clinically, significant remissions in SLE[79] show the potential value for DHEA in polymyalgia and other rheumatoid related syndromes which are under study.[86]

DHEA has also been shown to be effective in the prevention of autoimmune hemolytic anemia[87] in NZB mice and can prolong cardiac allograft survival[88] in rabbits. Of interest to DHEA effects on immune response is our observation in dogs and cats that DHEA produced rapid regression of spontaneous mastosarcomas,[1,4,21] the most common malignancy in pets. Based on this, we believe that DHEA should have a place in the treatment of chronic asthma, allergic rhinitis, colitis, and cutaneous hypersensitivity, which have large mast cell mediated inflammatory components.

Additonal immunological effects of DHEA are seen in its Clinh up-regulation of specific complement components: The deficiency of functionally active Clinh is the most common isolated genetic defect of the complement system[89] which leads to improperly controlled complement activation noted in diseases such as Hereditary Angioneurotic Edema,[90] which responds to DHEA.[3]

It should be emphasized that the in vivo effects of DHEA may be distinct from what is seen in vitro. In vitro, DHEA can be lymphocytotoxic, in similar fashion to corticosteroids, but this has not been clearly demonstrable on systemic administration.[38] Pertinent to this, Ennas et al.[91] reported that DHEA inhibits in vitro lymphocyte proliferation independent of G-6-PD enzyme inhibition. In that regard, the DHEA Br-EPI analogue, which inhibits in vivo carcinogenesis, prevents Epstein-Barr virus-induced lymphoblastic proliferation in vitro.[92]

Again, despite the absence of virus suppression in Loria's models, there may be a direct effect of DHEA on viral replication as Henderson et al.[93] have shown that DHEA and related analogues depress HIV replication in vitro, and similar in vitro effects have been reported by Schinasi et al.[58] and Yang et al.[59] Based on these observations, DHEA should be clinically tested in AIDS patients along with reverse transcriptase inhibitors.

As mentioned earlier, clinically, DHEA levels are low in patients with burn injury or chronic and acute disease.[1] In view of this, DHEA has been given clinically by us to AIDS patients with anecdotal improvement in energy status, and improvement in CNS AIDS-related symptoms, although other therapeutic effects were not seen. Dyner et al.[94] in a phase 1 study of DHEA tolerance, in AIDS, showed neopterin changes, but no effect on AIDS immune status.

Again, one should keep in mind our observation in dogs and cats that DHEA treatment (10 mg/kg/day) produced rapid regression of mastosarcomas.[3,21] In view of IL-4 concentration in mast cells, again, this could be pertinent to the effects of DHEA on modulation of IL-4 levels and appropriate to considering DHEA's use in asthmatic bronchitis or intestinal and cutaneous inflammatory disease.

EFFECTS ON CELL PROLIFERATION

The anticarcinogenic action of DHEA was first clinically related to an inverse DHEA relationship to the incidence of breast cancer.[1,95] This observation is no longer consistent with many studies,[4] but recent evidence supports an association with increased bladder cancer associated with low DHEA levels unrelated to age level decline.[4,96] Paradoxically, smokers at higher risk for cancer may have higher DHEA values,[97] but these values do not stay up in bronchogenic cancer.

Interest in the antitumor action of DHEA may relate to the blocking action of DHEA on GCS responses,[3] as both tumor growth and tumor viral carcinogenesis are subject to neuroimmunomodulation[69] which can alter malignant expression. DHEA, apart from its effects on inhibiting carcinogenesis, may be our best agent for blocking stress mediated support of tumor growth.[56,57]

DHEA, in contrast to DHEA-S, inhibits glucose 6-PO4 dehydrogenase, a key enzyme of the pentose shunt responsible for nucleic acid synthesis.[1,15] DHEA effects on tumor induction and growth are blocked by exogenous mixtures of deoxyribonucleosides and ribonucleosides which Gordon et al.[98] believe is mediated by nucleoside bypass to the DHEA induced decline in ribose-5-phosphate following DHEA inhibition of the pentose shunt.

Based on this, we studied the action of DHEA on spontaneous mastosarcomas in dogs and cats.[21] We saw regression in 6 of 7 animals in a short-term study at 10 mg/kg/day. Following animal studies, in a clinical phase 1 study in 19 advanced cancer patients, we established daily, long-term tolerance at 40 mg/kg/day. Dose above that to 80 mg/kg/day produced nausea and vomiting. No clinical tumor regression was seen, but two patients with renal cancer had stabilization of their disease, and tolerated DHEA oral treatment for as long as 2½ years.[21]

Schultz and Nyce[23] have shown that the DHEA mechanism for the prevention of spontaneous and clinically induced tumors may be mediated by inhibition of mevalonate synthesis. Depletion of mevalonate pools reduces not only cholesterol synthesis, but inhibits isoprenylation of proteins and oncogene expression governing tumor growth. Enhanced antitumor activity was achieved by combining DHEA with a fluoropyrimidine.[99]

DHEA blocks carcinogenic promotion.[14,15] DHEA and related steroids can block initiation or promotion of cancer depending on the model selected and can be thought of as chemopreventatives.[98–100] Effects on remodeling preneoplastic hepatic nodules suggest that the DHEA mechanisms observed may relate to both cytokine mediated differentiating effects or to direct effects on cell multiplication.[101] The hepatic anticarcinogenic effects of DHEA are mediated by a differentiating effect on preneoplastic nodules associated with marked peroxisome and catalase induction, or by effecting carcinogen binding to DHEA.[1,15,16,98,100] However, paradoxically, peroxisome induction by DHEA can be associated with hepatic tumors with high dose dietary intake in the rat.[29]

Pertinent to its anticancer effects, DHEA may act via its action on diverse steroid receptors. DHEA reduced hepatic glucocorticoid receptors in the rat by 50% over 5 days of DHEA administration. Utilizing specific DHEA binding in rat liver, we have identified a DHEA binding macromolecule in Sprague-Dawley rat liver cytosol. The specific binding was highest in the liver and prevented by trypsin and chymotrypsin. The hepatic binding of DHEA was associated with inhibition of proliferation in both normal liver and hepatocarcinoma.[102] Wayne-Meikle et al.[103] have found similar binding affinity in T cells that respond to DHEA.

DHEA can retransform or differentiate cells in an in vitro system: the 3T3-L mouse embryo fibroblast can be differentiated to form typical adipocytes. This process is accelerated by the addition of dexamethasone and inhibited by DHEA. In the process of differentiation from fibroblasts to adipocytes, 3T3-L cells undergo a number of processes, i.e., cell proliferation, lipid biosynthesis, and irreversible morphological alterations, all of which are blocked by DHEA.[104] This, again, is evidence of an anticorticoid action of DHEA despite its GCS-like in vitro inhibition of lymphoblastic response.

In contrast to antitumor action, there are reports that DHEA fed to rats can induce primary cancer of the liver through chronic peroxisomal stimulation.[29,105] In these animals, DHEA induces hepatomegaly, something we have not observed in our patients on doses as high as 40 mg/kg/day for periods ranging from 3 months to several years. Prolonged use of peroxisomal stimulating drugs, which stimulate fatty acid utilization and lowers cholesterol synthesis, have been shown to stimulate hepatic tumor induction in rodents.[102]

In prolonged clinical study involving some 25 of our male patients with cancer or multiple sclerosis, we have not seen stimulation of prostatic hypertrophy and its symptomatology or the appearance of prostatic cancer although this was closely looked for. These studies antedated PSA as a study indicator of prostate neoplasia. However, DHEA levels are reported to be elevated in patients with benign prostatic hypertrophy.[106,107] In contrast, we believe that DHEA should be looked at for possible inhibition of prostate cancer, but it is risky in view of the conversion of DHEA to androgens. However, there are reports that DHEA may lower prostatic testosterone receptors, and IL-6, which may be DHEA inhibited, and may be a growth promoting influence on prostatic tissue.

DHEA's anti-osteoporotic action is not clear.[4,108] However, IL-6 levels which can be depressed by DHEA in other systems,[65,71] are elevated during osteoclastic stimulation or inflammation,[109] and DHEA should be logically considered along with estrogen or testosterone in the treatment of osteoporotic disease as part of hormone replacement therapy.

In regard to the above, Kishimoto et al.[110] have found IL-6 elevations in cardiac myxomas and myelomas which suggest a possible therapeutic place for DHEA in these malignancies. The role of DHEA in the prevention of carcinogenesis and in inhibition of tumor growth has been reviewed extensively in our 1990 text.[1,15,16]

A DHEA analogue (16α-fluoro-5-androsten-17-one [DHEA 8354]) has been considered for clinical trial as a cancer preventative in bowel polyposis. DHEA 8354 has no sex steroid action, and has been shown to be effective against a variety of experimental tumor models, including bowel cancer.[99,100] Its clinical testing is long overdue.

Combination studies using DHEA with chemotherapeutic agents that block nucleic acid synthesis should be undertaken with reference to possible antitumor synergism because of DHEA's ability to inhibit ribose-5-P synthesis, as well as to effect membrane formation and isoprenylation of proteins.[4] Again, it was this action of DHEA on G-6-PD enzyme inhibition that led to our Phase 1 clinical study in advanced cancer patients.[21]

Epidemiologically, observations have been made relative to low clinical DHEA values in bronchogenic[111] and gastric cancer.[112] How relevant this is to cancer incidence and prevention deserves broader evaluation.

In another area of activity, pertinent to cancer, the combined use of DHEA and dexamethasone has been reported to inhibit sponge induced angiogenesis in the rat without causing immunosuppression.[113] Perhaps this combination is worth clinical trial to see if it can inhibit tumor vascularization responsible for cancer growth.

THE CNS AND BEHAVIOR

As mentioned earlier, DHEA is a neurosteroid found in the brain.[19,20] Historically, DHEA-S has been used as early as 1952 in both the treatment of neurasthenia and in selected schizophrenics where DHEA values were reported to be depressed.[4] DHEA-S cortisol ratios were found to be higher in individuals with panic disorders and in individuals on anticonvulsants, DHEA values are depressed.[4]

Roberts et al.[14] have shown that DHEA and DHEA-S in tissue culture maintained the integrity and growth of isolated 14-day-old mouse embryonic brain tissue. This was associated with enhanced concentration of neurofilaments and glial fibrillary acidic protein. This in vitro work has supported observations that DHEA possesses memory enhancing effects in mice when given intracerebrally, by mouth or subcutaneously.[14,114,115]

Based on the work of Roberts' group showing DHEA stimulation of neurite formation and our own observation of the antiviral protective activity of DHEA, our own group[116] and, independently, Roberts and Fauble[117] clinically studied DHEA administration in advanced multiple sclerosis (MS) patients. In our study, we gave DHEA at a pharmacologic dose of 40 mg/kg/day, while Roberts and Fauble[117] administered a low dose, 90 mg/day, and in both nonrandomized studies, involving 38 MS patients, improvement in mood, motor function, heat resistance, and energy was seen in one-third of patients in 90 day studies. These functional improvements, while anecdotal, disappeared on cessation of DHEA administration.

Pertinent to the above, but paradoxically, we have shown, in vitro, that DHEA blocks GCS stimulation of oligodendroglial myelination of nerves[118] in tissue culture. We have to ask if the presence of neurosteroids like DHEA, in the central nervous system, affect neural regeneration. In this case, a fall in DHEA may result in stimulation of GCS myelinating effect.

DHEA and DHEA-S show anxiolytic effects in mice.[119,120] Neurosteroids in the brain[121] like DHEA are derived from pregnenolone which is synthesized by the outer mitochondrial membrane under the influence of benzodiazapam receptors.[122] There is a possible close connection between neurotransmitter GABA mediated behavioral effects and the action of DHEA related steroids.[123] This action on GABA mediated CNS sedating behavior suggests that the antifatigue or memory enhancing action of DHEA may relate to these effects.

Again, DHEA has shown a memory enhancing effect in mice along with stimulation of neuroglial interconnections[113,115] and Bonnet and Brown[124] have provided a detailed single case report of a DHEA induced improvement in a 42-year-old patient with a posttraumatic long-term memory deficiency associated with low clinical values for DHEA.

The studies of Roberts et al.[14,115] and the observations of a DHEA related decline in Alzheimer's disease (AD), unrelated to age,[125,126] is of particular interest in view of Bonnet and Brown's[124] experience in achieving a clinical DHEA treatment improvement in memory. DHEA studies in AD are in progress based on Sunderland et al.'s[125] observations of a 48% greater decrease in age related DHEA levels in AD patients.

Based on the above, Svec and Lopez[126] have suggested that AD patients show a greater age-related loss in DHEA values which they feel is a factor facilitating GCS hippocampal stress related injury, memory loss, and depression.[127,128] Of additional interest to AD, the serum amyloid component in aged rats is decreased by DHEA administration suggesting another role for DHEA,[129] although systemic amyloidosis does not correlate with AD. A trial using pregnenolone, the DHEA precursor, is also warranted[115] because of its similar action to DHEA.

In regard to DHEA stimulation of neural cell interconnection and enhancement of memory, Roberts postulated that DHEA works through activation of cyclic GMP.[14] He suggested that the levels of GMP may be the final common pathway for DHEA action on varied cellular responses.

DHEA synthesis in the brain is independent of systemic endocrine sources and appears to be produced via an oligodendroglial pathway.[19,20] DHEA and related metabolites have been found in all regions of the brain with no specific regional concentrations. However, the highest exogenous concentration of DHEA uptake was found in the rat pineal within one hour of its administration, and significant uptake was also found in the amygdala, hippocampus, thalamus, midbrain, and frontal cortex.[4] Its pineal affinity is most important in view of melatonin and the pineal gland as key factors in the neuroendocrine clock controlling aging.[130]

DHEA or DHEA-S levels may be inversely correlated with type A high coronary risk populations, and high catechol stress personalities.[131] DHEA and DHEA-S have effects on prolactin metabolism in similar fashion to melatonin. As prolactin mediates dopaminergic stimulation of C19 delta 5 adrenal steroid synthesis, DHEA, as a neurosteroid, may play a role in Parkinson's disease. This may involve prolactin as it can reverse Parkinson-like injury in rodents.[4]

Direct intracranial injection of DHEA can prevent audiogenic seizure activity in the rat, probably through a block to glucocorticoid stress mediated effects.[132] This is pertinent to stress and its emotional effects leading to depression.[133] Again, it should be noted that susceptibility to the common cold[70] as well as tumor induction, and other virus infections are enhanced by stress.[69]

One has to take into account the route of DHEA administration as well as its species specificity.[131] DHEA, as a neurosteroid,[14,19,20] can be synthesized via cholesterol and pregnenolone by the brain. Of possible clinical importance, it is to be noted that DHEA, when combined with other androgens in castrated rats, does not produce enhanced sexual performance.[134] If combinations involving DHEA, testosterone, or other sex steroids are utilized concomitantly, their action will not necessarily be complementary,[135] although there are anecdotal reports of DHEA's clinical libido enhancing effects.

VASCULAR EFFECTS

DHEA effects on vascular endothelium, involving both atherosclerosis, fat metabolism, and morphology have been reviewed elsewhere in detail[1,3,4] which may be pertinent to the role of DHEA in the epidemiology of coronary disease.[11,12] DHEA inhibits accelerated coronary disease in the heterotopic rabbit heart model.[135] Weidmeier et al.[136] have related platelet derived growth factor to lymphokine

IL-6 production, suggesting a relationship between aging and immune response that could also involve thrombotic events as IL-6 is elevated as part of normal aging.[37]

Pertinent to this, Milewich and Whisnant[138] have shown human platelets to metabolize androstenedione to DHEA and other more potent androgens and DHEA can prevent platelet aggregation[139] suggesting, as has been seen for lymphocytes and macrophages,[140] that the formed elements of blood can metabolize DHEA. In addition, Milewich et al. have shown that vascular endothelium can metabolize DHEA[141] which may be significant to the increase in lipid containing lysosomes following pharmacologic in vitro exposure of endothelial cells to DHEA[142] which we have observed.

DHEA given subcutaneously to rats prevents, in a dose-related fashion, a DEX induced hypertension; in contrast DHEA failed to reverse DEX weight loss and decline in food intake and muscle mass.[7,72] DHEA also had no effect on deoxycorticosterone (DOCA) induced hypertension. It is difficult to identify a specific mechanism by which DHEA or its metabolites can modulate blood pressure, and it may be that DHEA lowers blood pressure via a block to GCS receptors as has been seen for RU486.[72]

The relationship of DHEA or DHEA-S maintenance levels to coronary disease, although seen as protective in the Barrett-Connor study in males,[11,12] has been controversial as a protective factor in other studies.[143,144] In contrast to Barrett-Connor in the Hautanen Helsinki et al.[145] study and Cincinnati study,[146] DHEA-S elevation was predictive for a higher coronary risk!

In other studies, Eich, Jesse et al.[88,139] showed that DHEA inhibited the accelerated atherosclerosis of heterotypic rabbit heart transplants. Ishihara et al.[147] have found a clinical correlation between low DHEA levels and aortic calcification. It must be emphasized that there is a sex difference relative to coronary disease, where testosterone appears to protect men and estrogen protects women. How DHEA fits into this is not clear.

Again, DHEA has been shown to inhibit angiogenesis in a rat sponge model when given with dexamethasone[113] and DHEA's effects on microcirculation remain to be established.

Metabolism (Obesity, Thyromimetic Action, Diabetes, etc.)

DHEA prevents obesity in mouse models and in dogs,[1,18,149] and there is a correlation between diabetes and obesity that can be DHEA reversed, dependent on the species or mouse strains studied. In adult dogs feeding DHEA mobilizes fat, but there is a subset of obese dogs who are resistant.[148] Although DHEA appears to have clinical anti-obesity values in dogs, minimal effects on obesity have so far been seen in humans, although muscle mass was increased in young men.[25] Of interest, there is a threshold dose of DHEA in the diet which decreases both caloric intake and increases serotonin hypothalamic levels which decreases appetite in the rat.[149]

Reviews dealing with the subject of DHEA effects on energy levels and fat metabolism by Cleary,[17] Berdanier and McIntosh, Prough et al.[1] are pertinent as is the text edited by Lardy and Stratman.[5] DHEA effects on cell respiration, food and fat intake may depend on the species and strain of animal studied, as well as on the nutritional state: fasting, nonfasting, lean or obese condition of the animals studied.[150,151] McIntosh et al.[151] have suggested that DHEA and glucocorticoids may have antagonistic effects to each other in lipogenic models. Of interest, DHEA does not reverse dexamethasone muscle wasting.[74,101]

DHEA induces malic enzyme activity[152-155] and thus behaves in similar fashion to thyroid hormone. McIntosh and Berdanier[153] indicate that DHEA may cause weight loss via energy loss through potentiation of thyroid hormone action. Lardy's group feels this mechanism relates to turning on the futile cycle wherein DHEA also increases cytosolic 3-P dehydrogenase resulting in enhanced thermogenesis and decreased mitochondrial metabolic efficacy.[5,36]

In advanced HIV infection, there is a decline in thyroid T3 function.[156] It would be of interest to see if DHEA can alter the energy status of such patients via an effect mediated through DHEA's thyromimetic action. Perhaps this can explain its reputed anti-fatigue effect in patients[9] and its alerting action in CNS, compromised AIDS patients.

DHEA is a peroxisomal stimulator and also induces hepatic and microsomal P450 drug metabolizing enzymes.[29,157,158] In that regard, DHEA, like other peroxisomal stimulators, can induce hepatomegaly and liver tumors in rodents.[29] As a peroxisomal stimulus, DHEA enhances fatty acid oxidation, and catalase induction. The latter enzyme is important as it functions as a peroxide or free radical scavenging agent, and catalase levels are related to species longevity in comparative animal systems.[30] In this regard, most importantly, DHEA protects the liver from carbon tetrachloride, free radical related injury,[159] and protects tracheal epithelium from paraquat damage[160] suggesting that by itself, or as a catalase inducer, DHEA may be a protective factor against free radical mediated injury.

DHEA, like other peroxisomal inducers, can lower cholesterol levels[4,17,18,25,26,148,149] and its chronic administration can alter patterns of hepatic protein phosphorylation.[161] DHEA can also stimulate hepatic gluco-neogenesis providing glucose from protein or peptide sources.[1,28]

Most importantly, DHEA was found to prevent diabetes in the db/db mouse.[28] Insulin resistance and body fat distribution have been studied in relation to androgenic hormone levels and insulin action.[26,27] Nestler et al.[26] believe that DHEA may be protective against atherosclerosis because it may counteract the hyperinsulinemia of aging that plays a role in the generation of that disease. There is evidence that high insulin levels speed up the metabolism of DHEA, which may explain DHEA's age-related decline.[25,26,162] Most recently, Morales et al.[9] have described a rise in insulin-like growth factor I in older men and women receiving DHEA as a long-term physiologic maintenance dose. They have ascribed possible anabolic and glucose insulin-like effects to this rise in IGF1.

Mechanism of Action of DHEA

The protean nature of DHEA's physiologic activity offers a variety of theoretical explanations which we believe are best explained by its antiglucocorticoid action[3,4] or effects on stress modulation: In general, it is difficult to assess whether the actions of DHEA are due to DHEA itself, to its metabolites, or a combination of both. In this regard, it seems likely that DHEA might act directly on targeted cells,[101,102,157,158] and also indirectly through systemically buffering other steroids.[3] The evidence for the second hypothesis is the observed varied responses to DHEA depending on the route of administration, the sex of the animal, and its distinct in vitro action, which suggests that DHEA is converted to other active metabolites.[1,4] More direct evidence in regard to the importance of DHEA metabolites is that it is not only DHEA but other androgenic steroids which have antidiabetic effects in mouse models.[26,27]

At the present time, it has not been possible to ascertain whether the molecular mechanisms by which DHEA exerts its many beneficial therapeutic effects are the same or even related. Most steroids known so far exert their actions by binding to specific receptors present in the cytosol, nuclei, or both. Whether DHEA follows the same pattern is not clear.[101,102] What is known is that DHEA can modulate behavior by interacting with androgens in ways that are distinct from the action of DHEA as a testosterone precursor.[6,26,27,134]

We have attempted to explain the mechanisms involved in the pleiotropic actions of DHEA by proposing the following eight major foci of action.

1. Direct interactions of DHEA on target cells through a receptor-linked mechanism: This hypothesis is supported by the observations of transcription and induction of IL-2 production in activated murine T-cells[62-65] which are directly regulated by DHEA.[65,70,71] This involves cytokine interactions which include IL-2, IL-4, interferon and IL-6. The action of neurosteroids on GABA receptors may also provide an example of this direct mechanism for DHEA action.[13,112,113,123,164]

   Also, we[101,102] and others[103] have identified DHEA binder macromolecules in rat liver cytosol and in murine T-cells. Beamer et al.[165] have seen gene activation to DHEA in ovarian granulosa cells.

2. Mitochondrial Effects: This may also involve thyroid and other metabolic effects: Berdanier and others[1,151-154] have reviewed the action of DHEA on mitochondrial function, and as we have mentioned, there is a key relationship between thyroid action and DHEA in that both stimulate thermogenesis and liver malic enzyme.[5,153-155] Song et al.[154] have shown DHEA to play a role in transcriptional activation of thyroid mediated malic enzyme.

   DHEA may interfere with state 3 mitochondrial function[153,154] and McIntosh, Lardy and Stratman[5] link the action of thyroxin, catechols, and DHEA through a common stimulation of mitochondrial G-3-P dehydrogenase.[1] In support of this, Williams et al.[166] find similar androgenic and DHEA relationships to fat distribution. In this regard, we must think of the role of sympathetic innervation governing both brown fat and systemic fat distribution that may be influenced by DHEA.

3. Indirect action through modulation of other receptors: In support of this hypothesis both our group and others have found that 5 days of DHEA administration in vivo can reduce the GCS receptors in the rat liver by 50%. This down regulation, as shown by Kalimi et al.[101,102] of the glucocorticoid liver recep-

tor by DHEA may in part explain the observed antiglucocorticoid effects of DHEA, particularly if this phenomenon is systemic in nature. Aspects of the role of DHEA and its precursor pregnenolone as neurosteroids may relate to this type of action.[167]

4. Direct interactions of DHEA via G-6-PD inhibition: Inhibition of mammalian G-6-PD, the rate-limiting enzyme in the pentose phosphate pathway by DHEA can be explained by this hypothesis.[1,15] This inhibition of G-6-PD is believed to mediate the anticancer or anticarcinogenic property of DHEA, and possibly its antiatherogenic effects through inhibition of vascular smooth muscle proliferation or the effect of G-6-PD on inhibiting lipid metabolism. DHEA-S does not have this activity!

5. Antidiabetogenic effects and effects on growth hormone-insulin-like growth factor (IGF 1): The antidiabetogenic action of DHEA in diabetic mutant ob/ob and db/db mice may also be due to blocking of GCS effects. Coleman et al.[28] observed that adrenal cortical hypertrophy secondary to obesity is characteristic of both ob and db obese mutants, and that adrenalectomy results in potentiation of the antidiabetogenic effects of DHEA. Based on this, one can think of diabetes as representing a stress (GCS) related disease for which DHEA can help. Again, DHEA's effects on insulin production and diabetes have been thoroughly reviewed by Nestler.[25–27]

   Morales et al.[9] have recently reported in their clinical 12 week study of DHEA that IGF I values are elevated with respect to its carrier blood protein. IGF I is an insulin-like growth factor produced by the liver which may have an anabolic effect related to growth hormone action. Acute intravenous IGF I studies have shown a glucose lowering protein sparing effect in adult men.[9]

6. Effects on other enzyme responses: Other examples of DHEA cellular enzyme modulating effects are stimulation of mitochondrial respiration, turning on the "futile cycle" involving fatty acyl-CoA hydrolase/synthetase,[4] and 3-P-dehydrogenase,[32,36] peroxidase induction,[29,157,158] reduction of protein isoprenylation via effects on mevalonate synthesis[23] and inhibition of hepatic carbamyl synthetase.[168] DHEA has also been reported to inhibit ornithine decarboxylase,[169] a key to polyamine metabolism and cell division. Roberts[14] believes that the key to

its CNS effects resides in cyclic GMP activation,[170] which is an androgenic hormonal effect.

7. Inhibition of GCS responses: DHEA has been shown to systemically, and in the CNS, induce tyrosine amino transferase, and effect serotonin accumulation in the hippocampus which can relate to GCS stress action.[136]

In cold stress studies, only the stressed virus infected mice die, an event which is associated with significant increases in GCS levels. Giving DHEA to these mice results in protection with a concomitant reduction of GCS levels.[54,55] These findings are of particular relevance to the role of stress factors in virus expression and support Riley's early studies showing a DHEA protective effect against corticosteroid or stress mediated thymic involution.[56]

The DHEA-S/cortisol ratio falls remarkably in normal older subjects (60 years and above) compared with young subjects.[171] As discussed earlier, a very low ratio has been found in patients with Alzheimer's disease compared with age and sex matched controls.[37,125,126] Based on this, it has been proposed that the DHEA/cortisol ratios may serve as an appropriate marker for DHEA as an antiglucocorticoid, through which individuals at risk for the neurotoxic effects of glucocorticoids may be identified. In stressed gynecologic patients, there was a decline in DHEA levels, and this also related to the terminal state of the patient.[172]

As mentioned previously, we have shown[7,74] that administration of a subcutaneous dose of dexamethasone on alternate days to Sprague-Dawley rats results in a marked increase in systolic blood pressure, and that DHEA prevents this dexamethasone-induced hypertension in a dose-dependent manner. DHEA has no effect on the DOCA-salt model of hypertension, again, suggesting an anti-glucocorticoid specificity.

DHEA reduces weight gain in the hypercortisol anemic Zucker fatty rat (an animal model of genetic obesity).[173] DHEA administered i.p. with dexamethasone blocks the activation of the enzymes tyrosine amino transferase (TAT) and ornithine decarboxylase (ODC) induced by i.p. injection of dexamethasone alone. They proposed that the rodent anti-obesity effect of DHEA may represent, at least in part, chronic antiglucocorticoid activity. Similar inhibition of the GCS responding enzyme

TAT by DHEA was observed in male Swiss Webster mice.[174] Most recently, Araneo and Daynes[71] have found DHEA-S to reverse the rise in the cytokine IL-6 secondary to burn injury, a response governed by a block to GCS.

8. Cytokine effects inhibition: e.g., IL-6: One all encompassing explanation for the protective action of DHEA involves its inhibiting responses to IL-6 action.[65,71,137] In that regard, IL-6 levels are lowered by DHEA with improvement in immunologic responses that decline in normal aging.[61,137] There is an associated age-related decline in DHEA with an associated rise in IL-6.

IL-6 is also elevated in endotoxic shock, burn injury and a variety of physiologic events involving both immunity and the response to environmental stress. IL-6 is upregulated by stress, and GCS action and IL-6 values fall on DHEA administration.[65,71,137] This might represent a common path for DHEA's broad input into its control of the pathophysiology of infection, endotoxic shock, tumor growth, and bone resorption.

In summary, we anticipate that the next few years will provide a better understanding of the various mechanisms by which DHEA exerts its pleiotropic effects. It will be of no surprise if we find that additional response may be due to ion channel effects[4] and effects on signal transduction pathways. We will also find multiple effects involving phospholipids, glycolipids, oncogenes, gonadotrophins, and other cytokine factors perhaps influenced by the steroid super family of genes involved in the molecular mechanism of DHEA's multiplicity of action.

Clinical Concerns

DHEA has had a long European history, although it has an unestablished clinical history in the U.S. It has been used as a postmenopausal antidepressant, and has had reported value in psoriasis, gout, and porphyria.[4] Corticosteroid elevation accompanies depression and the action of DHEA as a buffer to corticosteroid action is in trial for the treatment of endogenous depression, where it has had long-term use in treatment of menopausal symptoms.[4]

Recent clinical reports from compounding pharmacies attest to DHEA's popularity among physicians for its antifatigue action, but this subjective improvement is difficult to substantiate although significant anecdotes abound.[9] Our group[116] and Roberts and Fauble[117] have seen functional improvements in multiple sclerosis, but numbers are small, for evidence to be convincing enough for neurologists to establish a major study. Roberts has postulated that DHEA's CNS action could relate to its effects on GABA aminergic function.[14]

In regard to CNS action, it should be remembered that DHEA is metabolized to testosterone which can enhance muscle strength as well as improve subjective well-being. Although not reported in the recent La Jolla study by Yen's groups,[9] DHEA can improve libido in men, when given at dosage to restore blood levels to age 20 values.

Other than at pharmacologic dosage in dogs, DHEA does not appear to alter weight or dietary intake. However, DHEA clinical intake can lower blood cholesterol.[4,25,176] The fall in cholesterol levels may be equal to that seen with Lovestatin (Merck), but definitive studies involving numbers are not available. The relation of DHEA to the prevention of atherosclerosis in laboratory or clinical models can also relate to its effects in decreasing platelet adhesiveness.[88,139] This reaffirms the evidence of Barrett-Connor's[11] epidemiological study which should justify DHEA supplementation to restore second decade levels of DHEA to aging men.

Why is the difference between men and women in the Barrett-Connor[11,12] coronary survival study not clear? There are other studies which support a nonsexual difference for DHEA's anticoronary effects.[143,144,147] However, we are only now beginning to accumulate evidence that individuals differ remarkably in their capacity to sulfate DHEA. We also know little about DHEA's glucuronidization or 7-hydroxylation and bile recirculation as factors making for clinical differences.

In monkeys, DHEA-S infusions suppressed estrogen production and altered ovarian function, suggesting that its androgenic action could inhibit fertility,[176] something that has to be considered if one would use DHEA in fertile women. The naturally high levels in pregnancy would suggest that its action on the fetus would not necessarily be toxic; however, above a certain threshold of dosage, it is possible that its androgenic metabolites might interfere with normal fetal sexual development. Its use in Japan to efface the cervix to institute labor induction must be kept in mind as a contraindication during pregnancy.[3,4]

Of striking clinical importance, DHEA has been shown to be useful in producing remission in SLE.[84] There is also evidence of DHEA low values in polymyalgia [86] and rheumatoid arthritis with anecdotal reports of symptomatic improvement with DHEA use in myositis. Of interest to rheumatoid arthritis, pregnancy, which is associated with remission in that disease, produces the highest levels of systemic DHEA.

Although DHEA is not an anti-inflammatory agent, it does suppress mast cell proliferation [21] which has possible value in asthma, rhinitis, and other allergic or parasitic diseases. It may also modulate cytokine responses responsible for fever and prostration. Its anticomplement effect also suggests a place for its trial in certain hypersensitivity states, involving hemolysis and angioneurotic edema. [89] Morales et al. [9] report symptomatic improvement in some patients with joint pain, as part of their 12-week study in older subjects.

Based on animal studies, DHEA's action in preventing lethal virus or bacterial expression suggest that it be looked at for use in sepsis, or simply be tested as an agent to attenuate the expression of local or systemic herpes infection. DHEA certainly deserves clinical trial in the treatment of endotoxic shock, where it has been clearly shown to aid survival [76] and attenuate tumor necrosis factor production. [2] Recent work has shown it to protect hemorrhaged and traumatized pigs from endotoxic shock and the acute shock lung syndrome. [76]

The evidence that stress can influence the expression of the common cold or influenza suggests that DHEA may be of value in attenuating or preventing the onset of upper respiratory symptoms of the common cold independent of antibody titers. Based on Loria's mouse data, [2] this would be particularly true for coxsackie B enterovirus infection as it can account for 30% of "common colds." In this regard, DHEA in the elderly may help safeguard them from susceptibility to influenza. Similar value for DHEA may apply to its use in attenuating or blocking herpes virus infections.

The Japanese use of DHEA to promote cervical ripening and accelerate delivery [4] suggests that we need to look at DHEA as to other effects on collagen vascular thickening, keloid formation, or wound healing.

DHEA has value in restoring lubrication to the dry skin of older patients, where this androgenic effect may be of manifest value. [44]

Overall, except for reports in rats related to peroxisomal stimulation, [29] DHEA has potent anticarcinogenic activity. [1] DHEA deserves adequate phase II study, testing in advanced cancer patients in combination with antinucleic acid chemotherapy because of its inhibition of glucose-6-PO4, ornithine decarboxylase, and effects on isoprenylation.[1,4]

Its place in immune depleted cancer patients also deserves evaluation. In view of the reported incidence of IL-6 elevation in myxosarcomas, plasmacytomas and myeloma, its antitumor clinical trial in these malignancies[110] is warranted.

The action of DHEA in blocking GCS stimulation of Schwann cell proliferation[118] suggests that DHEA be looked at in the treatment of neurofibromatosis and malignant Schwannomas. Similarly, in view of pregnenolone synthesis, the precursor to DHEA, by glial cells[167] and in view of the nontoxic nature of DHEA, it would be worthwhile, clinically, testing DHEA for antitumor action in glioblastoma.

DHEA's action in breast cancer also requires special study, although no clinical antitumor effects in breast cancer have been seen.[4] Interest in DHEA levels and breast cancer have been said to be inversely related, but DHEA levels are high in the cystic fluid of patients with cystic mastitis.[4]

The decline of DHEA with acute and chronic illness suggest it may be useful as a maintenance or adjuvant therapy in those patients,[3,4,177,178] except we must bear in mind that a DHEA fall could represent a necessary accompaniment of stress under some circumstances where corticosteroid action could be lifesaving.

The energy boost observed in advanced AIDS patients on DHEA administration has not been associated with improvement in CD_4/CD_8 lymphocyte return. However, the high cortisol, low DHEA levels in AIDS patients suggests that DHEA, or related congeners, could have value in perhaps blocking corticosteroid mediated lympholysis, which has been related to HIV-induced serum factors such as free fatty acids.[179] DHEA deserves clinical trial early in HIV-infected patients, who, as yet, show no evidence of immunosuppression, particularly, in view of reports of its action inhibiting HIV replication alone and synergistically with azathymidine.[58,59,93]

The action of DHEA in enhancing insulin activity and affecting insulin blood levels or IGF I deserves study in the treatment of those patients with insulin resistance and early type I and II diabetes.[9,25-28] Is there a pro-oxidant element in clinical islet cell injury that DHEA can protect against as may be true for streptozotocin diabetogenic action which is reversed by DHEA?[28]

DHEA's digitalis-like action deserves special review.[4] DHEA has actually been used to treat congestive failure.[180] Is this related to

effects on sympathetic tone or does DHEA have direct cardiac ino-
tropic effects? There is one report of DHEA's inducing pulsus bigem-
iny in a noncardiac patient at 0.5 gm/day. Finally, a trial of DHEA in
malignant hypertension is warranted in view of its block to dexamethasone mediated hypertension in rats.[7,72]

Dosage

In phase 1 study, at pharmacologic dosage, DHEA has been administered at dosage up to 80 mg/kg/day in cancer patients. It is well
tolerated in cancer and MS patients at 40 mg/kg/day. The only side-
effects are reversible hirsutism in women, although concern must be
expressed for anecdotal reports of enhanced sedation seen in patients
on benzodiazepines and related CNS active drugs. No hemolysis was
seen[116,117] although concern must be taken in patients who might
have a genetically related glucose-6-PO4 deficiency.[1,4,21]

In patients on oral micronized DHEA at 150–300 mg/day, there
was an overproduction of testosterone by 300% in postmenopausal
women.[181] As an androgen precursor, one must be concerned with
the possibility of DHEA stimulating prostatic growth or cancer.
However, DHEA inhibits prostatic cancer in the Copenhagen rat,[4]
and no stimulus to prostatic hypertrophy has been observed, although looked for in our patients receiving high dosage.[21,116]

It must be emphasized that the action of DHEA is distinctly different in men as compared to women. In the latter case, trunkal obesity
in women is associated with higher DHEA-S levels. DHEA governs
androgenic steroid levels, which controls fat metabolism and fat distribution. Data suggests that this can benefit males, but may have an
adverse effect in women.[166] Androgenicity in women, in contrast
to men, is associated with insulin resistance and insulinemia[27] and
enhanced coronary risk. Does the possible libido enhancing and energizing action of DHEA balance coronary risk in women? What
would be the results of combined DHEA and estrogen replacement in
women relative to coronary risk, osteoporosis, and broad anti-aging
effects?

Another caveat has been evidence for hepatic carcinoma in rats
treated with high pharmacologic doses of dietary DHEA, associated
with the effect of DHEA on peroxisomal liver stimulation.[29] In this
regard, the use of vitamin E supplementation in rats treated with

DHEA avoids enzyme changes associated with oxidative stress injury to the liver.[182]

DHEA, as replacement therapy for aging, is rational[9] along with estrogen, testosterone, growth hormone, and melatonin replacement. However, in Canada, DHEA has been given an anabolic steroid schedule III (U.S.) classification, and while it is a mild androgen, it does not have the muscle building clout of testosterone and other more potent anabolic steroids. However, this designation will discourage use by some physicians and patients.

Numerous use patents abound for the clinical application of DHEA or its sulfate, but it would be unusual for any drug company to invest in DHEA's clinical availability based on unique usage with current FDA requirements that entail large patient numbers and millions of dollars for clinical testing. We hope its clinical value in lupus erythematosus[85] might prompt orphan drug status that would stimulate early clinical approval because of FDA interest in this disease which has limited therapeutic options. However, drug companies are looking for DHEA analogues that could provide composition of matter patent control. This means that available DHEA analogues are still years away.

Right now, physicians must depend on compounding pharmacies to provide DHEA, by prescription, without FDA approval. The decision for using DHEA is up to those physicians and their patients who see its virtues despite lack of broad studies affirming its clinical value.

In the study by Yen's group,[9] 50 mg. was given daily HS QN for 12 weeks with improvement in energy and mood. Our recommended dose is 50 mg. QOD, to restore blood values to the second decade. This is empirical, and dose has to be tailor made for the individual. Our dosage concept is based on DHEA replacement to achieve a youthful level (second decade), despite one's chronologic age. Our use of alternating daily morning p.o. treatment is again empiric as there is no evidence available suggesting endogenous depression of DHEA receptors or inhibition of DHEA production on daily exogenous administration. There is no data as to whether an AM schedule is superior to HS QN. We need kinetic studies to determine patterns of metabolism based on dosage schedules attuned to different age groups and time of administration.

We see no virtue to administering DHEA versus DHEA-S, but clinical studies are needed with defined endpoints to determine differences in the metabolism of sulfated metabolics versus DHEA as relates to clinical endpoints. There is both rodent and clinical evidence of biliary excretion of DHEA-S and DHEA gastrointestinal reabsorption.[183]

It must be stressed that there is no clear evidence that DHEA can prolong life in any model system yet available. A recent study in the Netherlands showed no correlation with the functional state of the old-old (those over 85) with their DHEA-S levels.[184] DHEA values were not looked at in these studies. However, the decline of DHEA with aging suggests that, as a biomarker, DHEA along with growth hormone, melatonin, and the sex steroids may represent a key to our understanding the physiology of aging.

Whether replacement of DHEA and other hormones to restore age 20 levels to our older population will make a difference to the quality of their lives remains an individual decision. For medical validity, study requires objective and subjective evaluation in large numbers of patients with a broad variety of complaints. Testing is now related to clinical efforts that are focused on individual patients, and it is hoped that the public enthusiasm for DHEA will result in NIA support and drug company interest for major clinical studies providing numbers that will define, once and for all, the value of DHEA replacement.

Summary

In this paper we have attempted to present an overview of some major actions of DHEA-S. We have focused primarily on immune response, corticosteroid action, and CNS effects. We have briefly focused on metabolic and vascular effects and on antiproliferative action, but have not elaborated on its metabolic (diabetic) and anti-carcinogenic effects which can be seen in appropriate reviews. The observation that DHEA protects mice from a wide variety of infectious agents suggests that DHEA regulates the host immune response, with infection as its stimulus. This is apparently achieved by counteracting the immunosuppressive effects of glucocorticosteroids and is possibly mediated by blocking IL-6 action, or inhibiting complement or mast cell activity. DHEA may also have value in endoxtemia or septic shock.

Clearly, the widespread, sometimes paradoxical, influence of DHEA upon many immune effector functions implicates this steroid as a central control element in maintaining the homeostatic functions of the immune system, and it has a growing place in the treatment of AIDS, lupus and/or other autoimmune related diseases.

The role of DHEA as a neurosteroid may provide for its place in depression, (fatigue), neural repair, or neuro-immunomodulation. Clinical studies and the potential clinical value of DHEA in cancer, hypertension, lupus, atherosclerosis, diabetes and infection have been summarized in our recent reviews,[2-4] those of Nestler et al.[25,27] and others.[9,85,184]

Whether DHEA's actions are receptor or state dependent, the focus of all DHEA studies must involve detailed attention to its precursor, pregnenolone, and the role of its metabolism to produce DHEA and DHEA's intermediate metabolites in the synthesis of the sex steroids and etiocholanolone. (See Figure 1.) Studies must distinguish not only between the species, strain, sex, and test animal used, the targeted cells involved, but also pharmacologic versus physiologic dosage, the route and time of administration, and the effect of age, obesity, or other underlying modulating pathology.

Whatever DHEA's mechanism of action, it is our belief that DHEA and its congeners will rival the glucocorticoid and sex steroids in their physiologic versatility, and DHEA or its analogues or metabolites will be used for both physiologic replacement, i.e., to replace age or disease related decline, or for focused pharmacologic effects. The latter, unfortunately, must await the development of unique delivery systems or commercially available synthetic analogues to meet the competitive needs of the marketplace.

References

1. Kalimi, M., Regelson, W., Eds. *The Biologic Role of Dehydroepiandrosterone (DHEA)*. New York: Walter de Gruyter, 1990.
2. Regelson, W., Loria, R., Kalimi, M. Dehydroepiandrosterone (DHEA) The "Mother Steroid" I: Immunologic Action. *Ann NY Acad Sci* 719: 553–563, 1994.
3. Regelson, W., Kalimi, M., Loria, R. DHEA: Some thoughts as to its biologic and clinical action. In: *The Biologic Role of Dehydroepiandrosterone (DHEA)*. Kalimi, M., Regelson, W., Eds., New York: Walter de Gruyter, pp. 405–445, 1990.
4. Regelson, W., Kalimi, M. Dehydroepiandrosterone (DHEA)— The Multifunctional Steroid II. Effects on the CNS, cell proliferation, metabolic and vascular, clinical and other effects. Mechanism of Action? *Ann NY Acad Sci* 719: 564–575, 1994.

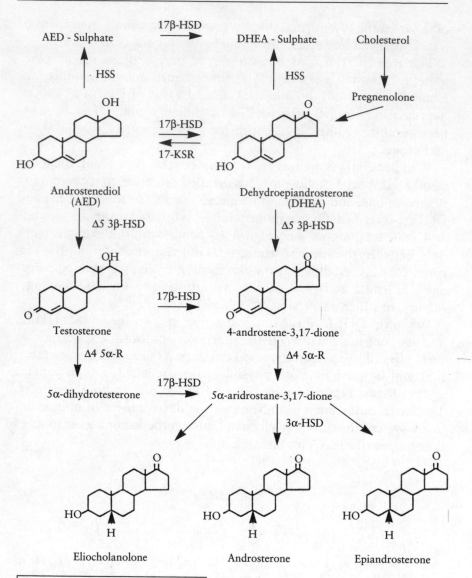

AED - Sulphate

17β-HSD

DHEA - Sulphate   Cholesterol

HSS

HSS

Pregnenolone

17β-HSD

17-KSR

Androstenediol
(AED)

Dehydroepiandrosterone
(DHEA)

Δ5 3β-HSD

Δ5 3β-HSD

Testosterone

17β-HSD

4-androstene-3,17-dione

Δ4 5α-R

Δ4 5α-R

5α-dihydrotesterone

17β-HSD

5α-aridrostane-3,17-dione

3α-HSD

Eliocholanolone

Androsterone

Epiandrosterone

KSR	= Ketosteroid Reductase
HSD	= Hydrosteroid Dehydrogenase
R	= Reductase
H	= Hydrolase
HSS	= Hydrosteroid Sulphatase

5. Lardy, H., Stratman, F., Eds. *Hormones, Thermogenesis and Obesity.* New York: Elsevier, 1989.

6. Parker, L.N. *Adrenal Androgens in Clinical Medicine.* San Diego, CA: Academic Press, pp. 118–134, 1989.

7. Kalimi, M., Shafagoj, Y., Loria, R., et al. Anti-glucocorticoid effects of dehydroepiandrosterone (DHEA). *Mol Cell Biochem* 131: 99–104, 1994.

8. Birkennager-Gillesse, E.G., Derksen, J., Lagady. A.M. Dehydroepiandrosterone sulphate (DHEAS) in the oldest old—aged 85 and over. *Ann NY Acad Sci* 719: 543, 552, 1994.

9. Morales, A.J., Nolan, J.N., Nelson, J.C., Yen, S.S. Effect of replacement dose of dehydroepiandrosterone in men and women of advancing age. *J Clin Endocrinol Metab* 78: 1360–1367, 1994.

10. Belanger, A., Candas, B., DuPont, A., et al. Changes in serum concentrations of conjugated and unconjugated steroids in 40- to 80-year-old men. *J Clin Endocrinol Metab* 79: 1086–1090, 1994.

11. Barrett-Connor, E., Khaw, K.T., Yen, S.S.C. A prospective study of dehydroepiandrosterone sulfate, mortality and cardiovascular disease. *N Engl J Med* 315: 1519–1524, 1986.

12. Barrett-Connor, E., Khaw, K. The epidemiology of DHEAS with particular reference to cardiovascular disease: The Rancho Bernado study. In: *The Biologic Role of Dehydroepiandrosterone (DHEA).* Kalimi, M., Regelson, W., Eds., New York: Walter de Gruyter, pp. 281–298, 1990.

13. Loria, R.M., Regelson, W., Padgett, D.A. Immune response facilitation and resistance to viral and bacterial infections with DHEA. In: *The Biologic Role of Dehydroepiandrosterone (DHEA).* Kalimi, M., Regelson, W., Eds., New York: Walter de Gruyter, pp. 107–130, 1990.

14. Roberts, G. Dehydroepiandrosterone (DHEA) and its sulfate (DHEAS) as neural facilitators: Effects on brain tissue in culture and on memory in young and old mice. Acyclic GMP hypothesis of action of DHEA and DHEAS in nervous system and other tissues. In: *The Biologic Role of Dehydroepiandrosterone (DHEA).* Kalimi, M., Regelson, W., Eds., New York: Walter de Gruyter, pp. 13–42, 1990.

15. Feo, F., Pastale, R. Glucose-6-phosphate dehydrogenase and the relation of dehydroepiandrosterone to carcinogenesis. In: *The Biologic Role of Dehydroepiandrosterone (DHEA).* Kalimi, M., Regelson, W., Eds., New York: Walter de Gruyter, pp. 331–360, 1990.

16. Mayor, D., Weber, F., Bannasch, P. Modulation of liver carcinogenesis by dehydroepiandrosterone. In: *The Biologic Role of Dehydroepiandrosterone (DHEA).* Kalimi, M., Regelson, W., Eds., New York: Walter de Gruyter, pp. 361–385, 1990.

17. Cleary, M.P. The role of DHEA in obesity. In: *The Biologic Role of*

Dehydroepiandrosterone (DHEA). Kalimi, M., Regelson, W., Eds., New York: Walter de Gruyter, pp. 281–298, 1990.

18. MacEwen, E.G., Maki-Haffa, A.L., Kurzman, I.D. DHEA effects on cholesterol and lipoproteins. In: *The Biologic Role of Dehydroepiandrosterone (DHEA).* Kalimi, M., Regelson, W., Eds., New York: Walter de Gruyter, pp. 299–316, 1990.

19. Baulieu, E.F., Robel, P. Neurosteroids: A new brain function? *J Steroid Biochem Mol Biol* 37: 305–403, 1990.

20. Robel, P., Baulieu, E.E., Corpechot, C., et al. Neurosteroids: 3b-Hydroxy-5 derivatives in rat and monkey brain. *J Steroid Biochem Mol Biol* 27: 649–655, 1982.

21. Regelson, W., Loria, R., Kalimi, M. Hormonal Intervention: "buffer hormones" or "state dependency." The role of dehydroepiandrosterone (DHEA), thyroid hormone, estrogen and hypophysectomy in aging. *Ann NY Acad Sci* 521: 260–273, 1988.

22. Regelson, W., Kalimi, M., Loria, R. Dehydroepiandrosterone (DHEA): the precursor steroid: introductory remarks. In: *The Biologic Role of Dehydroepiandrosterone (DHEA).* Kalimi, M., Regelson, W., Eds., New York: Walter de Gruyter, pp. 1–6, 1990.

23. Schultz, S., Nyce, J.W. Inhibition of isoprenylation and p21 membrane association by dehydroepiandrosterone in human colonic adenocarcinoma cells *in vitro. Cancer Res* 51: 6563–6567, 1991.

24. Baulieu, E.E., Corpechot, C., Dray, F., Emiolozzi, R., et al. An adrenal secreted "Androgen": Dehydroepiandrosterone sulfate. Its metabolism, and a tentative generalization on the metabolism of other steroid conjugates in man. *Rec Progr Horm Res* 21: 411–500, 1965.

25. Nestler, J.E., Clore, J.N., Blackard, W.G. Regulation of dehydroepiandrosterone (DHEA) metabolism by insulin and metabolic effects of dehydroepiandrosterone in man. In: *The Biologic Role of Dehydroepiandrosterone (DHEA).* Kalimi, M., Regelson, W., Eds., New York: Walter de Gruyter, pp. 189–205, 1990.

26. Nestler, J.E., Clore, J.N., Blackard, W.G. Dehydroepiandrosterone: the "missing link" between hyperinsulinemia and atherosclerosis. *FASEB J* 6: 3073–3075, 1992.

27. Nestler, J.E. Insulin and adrenal androgens. *Seminar in Reproductive Endocrinol* 12: 1–5, 1994.

28. Coleman, D.C. Dehydroepiandrosterone (DHEA) and diabetic syndromes in mice. In: *The Biologic Role of Dehydroepiandrosterone (DHEA).* Kalimi, M., Regelson, W., Eds., New York: Walter de Gruyter, pp. 179–180, 1990.

29. Rao, M.D., Reid, B., Ide, T. T., et al. Dehydroepiandrosterone induced peroxisome proliferation in the rat. Evaluation of sex differences. *Proc Soc Exp Biol Med* 207: 186–190, 1994.

30. Sohal, R.S., Agarwal, S., Orr, W. C. Oxidative stress as a causal factor

in senescence. Report 13th Ross Conference on Medical Res., Abbott Labs, Columbus, Ohio, pp. 6–10, 1994.

31. Berdanier, C.D., McIntosh, M.D. DHEA and mitochondrial respiration. In: *The Biologic Role of Dehydroepiandrosterone (DHEA)*. Kalimi, M., Regelson, W., Eds., New York: Walter de Gruyter, pp. 231–252, 1990.

32. Lardy, H., Su, C.Y., Kneer, N., Wieglus, S. Dehydroepiandrosterone induces enzymes that permit thermogenesis and decrease metabolic efficiency. In *Hormones, Thermogenesis and Obesity*. Lardy, H.A., Stratman, F., Eds. New York: Elsevier, pp. 415–426, 1989.

33. Weinshilboum, R., Aksoy, I. Sulfation pharmacogenetics in humans. *Chem Biol Interact* 92: 233–246, 1994.

34. Hobkirk, R. Steroid sulfotransferases and steroid sulfate sulfatases: characteristics and biological roles. *Can J Biochem Cell Biol* 63: 1127–1144, 1985.

35. Prough, R.A., Wu, H.Q., Milewich, C. Effect of DHEA on rodent liver microsomal mitochondrial and peroxisomal proteins. In: *The Biologic Role of Dehydroepiandrosterone (DHEA)*. Kalimi, M., Regelson, W., Eds., New York: Walter de Gruyter, pp. 253–279, 1990.

36. Bobyleva, V., Kneer, N., Bellei, M., et al. Concerning the mechanism of increased thermogenesis in rats treated with dehydroepiandrosterone. *J Bioenergetics Biomembranes* 25: 313–321, 1993.

37. Roberts, E., Fitten, J. Serum steroid levels in two old men with Alzheimer's disease (AD) before, during and after oral administration of dehydroepiandrosterone (DHEA). Pregnenolone synthesis may become rate-limiting in aging. In: *The Biologic Role of Dehydroepiandrosterone (DHEA)*. Kalimi, M., Regelson, W., Eds., New York: Walter de Gruyter, pp. 43–63, 1990.

38. Padgett, D.A., Loria, R.M. In vitro potentiation of lymphocyte activation by DHEA, andostenediol and andostenetriol. *J Immunol* 153: 1544–1552, 1994.

39. Leiter, E., Beamer, W., Coleman, D., Longcope, C. Androgenic and estrogenic metabolites in serum of mice fed dehydroepiandrosterone: Relationship to antihyperglycemic effects. *Metabolism* 36: 863–869, 1987.

40. Khalil, M.W., Strutt, L.B., Vachon, D., et al. Metabolism of dehydroepiandrosterone by cultured human adipose stromal cells. Identification of 7α hydroxydehydroepiandrosterone. *J Steroid Biochem Mol Biol* 46: 505–595, 1993.

41. Daynes, R. A., Dudley, D.J., Aranco, B.A. Regulation of murine lymphokine production in vivo. II. Dehydroepiandrosterone is a natural enhancer of IL-2 synthesis by helper T-cells. *Europ J Immunol* 20: 793–801, 1990.

42. De Peretti, E., Forest, M.G. Pattern of plasma dehydroepiandroster-

one sulfate levels in human from birth to adulthood: Evidence for testicular production. *J Clin Endocrinol Metab* 47: 572–577, 1978.

43. Orentreich, N., Brind, J.L., Rizer, R.L., et al. Age changes and sex differences in serum dehydroepiandrosterone sulfate concentrations throughout adulthood. *J Clin Endocrinol Metab* 59: 551–555, 1984.

44. Orentreich, N. Personal communication, 1984.

45. Braverman, E., Regelson, W. Work in progress, 1995.

46. Milewich, L., Shaw, C.B. Sondheimer, R.D. Steroid metabolism by epidermal keratinocytes. *Ann NY Acad Sci* 548: 66–89, 1988.

47. Purifoy, F.E., Koopmans, L.H., Tatum, R.W. Steroid hormones and aging: Free testosterone and androstendione in normal females aged 20–87 years. *Human Biol* 52: 181–191, 1980.

48. Cumming, D.C., Rebar, R.W., Hopper, B.R., Yen, S.S. Evidence for an influence of the ovary on circulating dehydroepiandrosterone sulfate levels. *J Endocrinol Metab* 54: 1069–1071, 1982.

49. Lu, C.H., Lauglin, C.A., Fisher, V.G., Yen, S.S. Marked attenuation of ultradian and circadian rhythms of DHEA in post-menstrual women. Evidence for a reduced 17, 20 desmolase enzymatic activity. *J Clin Endocrinol Metab* 71: 900–906, 1990.

50. Del Ponte, A., DiMonte, M.G., Grazianni, D., et al. Changes in plasma DHEAS circadian rhythm in elderly men. *Prog Clin Biol Res* 341 A, 791–796, 1990.

51. Mann, D., Castracane, D., McLaughlin, F., et al. Developmental patterns of serum luteinizing hormone, gonadal and adrenal steroids in the sooty mangabey (Cercocebus atys.). *Biol Repro* 28: 279–284, 1983.

52. Loria, R.M., Inge, T.H., Cook, S., Szakal, A., Regelson, W. Protection against acute lethal viral infections with the native steroid dehydroepiandrosterone (DHEA). *J Med Virology* 26: 301–314, 1988.

53. Loria, R.M., Padgett, D.A. Androstenediol regulates systemic resistance against lethal infections in mice. *Arch Virology* 127: 103–115, 1992.

54. Ben-Nathan, D., Feuerstein, G. The influence of cold and isolation stress on resistance of mice to West Nile virus encephalitis. *Experientia* 46: 285–290, 1990.

55. Ben-Nathan, D., Lachmi, B., Lustig, S., Feuerstein, G. Protection of dehydroepiandrosterone (DHEA) in mice infected with viral encephalitis. *Arch Virology* 120: 263–271, 1991.

56. Riley, V., Fitzmaurice, M.A., Regelson, W. DHEA and thymus integrity in the mouse. In: *The Biologic Role of Dehydroepiandrosterone (DHEA)*. Kalimi, M., Regelson, W., Eds., New York: Walter de Gruyter, pp. 131–155, 1990.

57. May, M., Hollmes, E., Rogers, W., et al. Protection from glucocorticoid induced thymic involution by dehydroepiandrosterone. *Life Sci* 46: 1627–1631, 1990.

58. Schinazi, R.F., Eriksson, B.F.H., Arnold, B.H., et al. Effects of dehydroepiandrosterone in lymphocytes and macrophages infected with human immunodeficiency virus. In: *The Biologic Role of Dehydroepiandrosterone (DHEA)*. Kalimi, M., Regelson, W., Eds., New York: Walter de Gruyter, pp. 155–177, 1990.

59. Yang, J.Y., Schwartz, A., Henderson, E.E. Inhibition of 3'azido-3' deoxythymidine resistant HIV-I infection by dehydroepiandrosterone in vitro. *Biochem Biophys Res Commun* 201: 1424–1432, 1994.

60. Rasmussen, K.R., Martin, L.E.G., Arrowood, M.J., et al. Effect of dexamethasone and dehydroepiandrosterone in immunosuppressed rats infected with Crytosporidium parvum. *J Protozool* 38: 157–159, 1991.

61. Garg, M., Bondada, S. Reversal of age assoicated decline in immune response in PNU immune vaccine by supplementation with the steroid hormone DHEA. *Infect Immun* 61: 2238–2241, 1993.

62. Daynes, R.A., Araneo, B.A. Contrasting effects of glucocorticoids on the capacity of T cells to produce the growth factor interleukin 2 and interleukin 4. *Europ J Immunol* 19: 2319–2325, 1990.

63. Suzuki, T., Suzuki, N., Daynes, R.A., Engleman, E.G. Dehydroepiandrosterone enhances IL-2 production and cytotoxic effector function of human T-cells. *Clin Immunol Immunopathol* 61: 202–211, 1991.

64. Daynes, R.A., Araneo, B.A., Dowel, T.A., et al. Regulation of murine lymphokine production in vivo III. The lymphoid microenvironment exerts regulatory influences over T helper function. *J Exp Med* 171: 979–996, 1990.

65. Daynes, R.A. Araneo, B.A. Natural regulators of T cell lymphokine production in vivo. *J Immunother* 12: 174–179, 1992.

66. Araneo, B.A., Woods, M.L.H., Daynes, R.A. Reversal of the immunosenescent phenotype by dehydroepiandrosterone: hormone treatment provides an adjuvant effect on the immunization of aged mice with recombinant hepatitis B surface antigen. *J Infect Dis* 167: 830–840, 1993.

67. Casson, P.R., Andersen, R.N., Herrod, H.G. Oral dehydroepiandrosterone modulates immune function in post-menopausal women. *Am J Obstet Gynecol* 169: 1536–1539, 1993.

68. Szakal, A.K. Personal communication, 1994.

69. Fitzmaurice, M.A. Physiological relationships among stress, viruses and cancer in experimental animals. *Intern J Neurosci* 39: 307–324, 1988.

70. Cohen, S., Tyrrell, D.A.J., Smith, A.P. Psychological stress and susceptibility to the common cold. *N Engl J Med* 325: 606–612, 1991.

71. Araneo, B., Daynes, R. Dehydroepiandrosterone functions as more than an antiglucocorticoid in preserving immunocompetence after thermal injury. *Endocrinol* 136: 393–401, 1995.

72. Blauer, K.L., Rogers, W.M., Bernton, E.W. Dehydroepiandrosterone antagonizes the suppressive effects of dexamethasone on lymphocyte proliferation. *Endocrinol* 129: 3174–3179, 1991.

73. Wiedmeier, S.E., Araneo, B.A., Huang, K., Daynes, R.A. Thymic modulation of IL-2 and IL-4 synthesis by peripheral T cells. *Cell Immunol* 135: 501–518, 1991.

74. Shafagoj, Y., Opoku, J., Quereshi, D., et al. Dehydroepiandrosterone prevents dexamethasone-induced hypertension in rats. *Am J Physiol* 263: 210–213, 1992.

75. Dannenberg, H.D., Alpert, G., Lustig, S., et al. DHEA protects mice from endotoxin toxicity and reduces tumor necrosis factor production. *Antimicrob Agents Chemother* 36: 2275–2279, 1992.

76. Proctor, K. Personal communication, 1995.

77. Schwartz, A.G., Fairinan, K.K. Pashko, L.L. The biologic significance of dehydroepiandrosterone. In: *The Biologic Role of Dehydroepiandrosterone (DHEA)*. Kalimi, M., Regelson, W., Eds., New York: Walter de Gruyter, pp. 7–12, 1990.

78. Malone, J., Oldfield III, E.G., Wagner, K.F., et al. Abnormalities of morning serum cortisol levels and circadian rhythms of CD4 + lymphocyte counts in human immunodeficiency virus type I infected adult patients. *J Infect Dis* 165: 185–186, 1992.

79. Merril, C.R., Harrington, M.G., Sunderland, T. Reduced plasma dehydroepiandrosterone concentration in HIV infection and Alzheimer's disease. In: *The Biologic Role of Dehydroepiandrosterone (DHEA)*. Kalimi, M., Regelson, W., Eds., New York: Walter de Gruyter, pp. 101–106, 1990.

80. Jacobson, M.A., Fusaro, R.E., Galmarini, M., Lang, W. Decreased serum dehydroepiandrosterone is associated with an increased progression of human immunodeficiency virus infection in men with CD4 cell counts of 200–499. *J Infect Dis* 164: 864–868, 1991.

81. Findling, J.W., Buggy, B.P., Gilson, I.H., et al. Longitudinal evaluation of adrenocortical function in patients infected with the human immunodeficiency virus. *J Clin Endocrinol Metab* 79: 1091–1096, 1994.

82. Matsunaga, A., Miller, B.C., Cottam, G.L. Dehydroepiandrosterone prevention of autoimmune disease in NZB/WF$_1$ mice: Lack of an effect on associated immunological abnormalities. *Biochimica Biophysica Acta* 992: 265–271, 1989.

83. de la Torre, B., Hedman, M., Nilsson, E., et al. Relationship between blood and joint tissue DHEAS levels in rheumatoid arthritis and osteoarthritis. *Clin Exp Rheumatol* 11: 597–601, 1993.

84. Hedman, M., Nilsson, E., de la Torre, B. Low sulpho-conjugated steroid hormone levels in systemic lupus erythematosus (SLE). *Clin Exp Rheumatol* 7: 583–588, 1989.

85. Van Vollenhaven, R.F., Engelman, E.G., McGuire, J.L. An open study

of DHEA in systemic lupus erythematosis. *Arthritis Rheum* 37: 1305–1310, 1994.

86. Nilsson, E., de la Torre, B., Hedman, M., et al. Blood DHEA-S levels in polymyalgia rheumatica/giant cell arteritis and primary fibromyalgia. *Clin Exp Rheumatol* 12: 415–417, 1994.

87. Tannen, R.H., Schwartz, A.G. Reduced weight gain and delay of Coomb's positive hemolytic anemia in NZB mice treated with dehydroepiandrosterone (DHEA). *Fed Proc* 41: 463 (Abstract), 1982.

88. Eich, D.M., Johnson, D.E., Nestler, J.E., et al. Inhibition of cardiac allograft atherosclerosis by dehydroepiandrosterone. *Clin Res* 38: 2A (Abstract), 1990.

89. Falus, A., Feher, K.G., Walez, E., et al. Hormonal regulation of complement biosynthesis in human cell lines. I. Androgens and gamma-interferon stimulate the biosynthesis and gene expression of C1 inhibitor in human cell line U937 and HepG2. *Mol Immunol* 27: 191–195, 1990.

90. Colton, H.R. Hereditary angioneurotic edema, 1887–1987. *N Engl J Med* 317: 43–45, 1987.

91. Ennas, M.G., Lanconi, S., Dessai, S., et al. Influence of dehydroepiandrosterone on G-6-PD activity and ^{3}H-thymidine uptake on human lymphocytes in vitro. *Toxicol Pathol* 15: 241–244, 1987.

92. Henderson, E.A., Schwartz, A., Pashko, L., et al. Dehydroepiandrosterone and 16α-bromoepiandrosterone: inhibition of Epstein-Barr virus induced transformation of human lymphocytes. *Carcinogenesis* 2: 683–686, 1981.

93. Henderson, E., Yang, J.Y., Schwartz, A. Dehydroepiandrosterone (DHEA) and synthetic DHEA analogs are modest inhibitors of HIV IIIB replication. *AIDS Res Hum Retroviruses* 8: 625–631, 1992.

94. Dyner, T.S., Lang, W., Geaga, J., et al., An open label dose escalation trial of oral DHEA tolerance and pharmacokinetics in patients with HIV disease. *J Acquir Immune Defic Syndr* 6: 459–465, 1993.

95. Schwartz, A.G., Whitcomb, J.M., Nyce, J.W., et al. Dehydroepiandrosterone and structural analogs: A new class of cancer chemopreventive agents. *Adv Cancer Res* 51: 391–423, 1988.

96. Gordon, G.B., Helzlsover, K.J., Comstock, G.W. Serum levels of DHEA and its sulfate, and the risk of developing bladder cancer. *Cancer Res* 51: 1366–1369, 1991.

97. Field, A.E.R., Colditz, G.A., Willett, W.C., et al. The relation of smoking, age, relative weight, and dietary intake to serum adrenal steroids, sex hormones, and sex hormone-binding globulin in middle aged men. *J Clin Endocrinol Metab* 79: 1310–1316, 1994.

98. Gordon, G. B., Shantz, L.M., Talalay, P. Modulation of growth, differentiation, and carcinogenesis by dehydroepiandrosterone. *Adv Enzymology Regulation* 26: 355–382, 1987.

99. Boone, C.W., Kelloff, G.J., Malone, W.C. Identification of candidate cancer preventative agents and their evaluation in animal models and human clinical trials. A review. *Cancer Res* 50: 2–9, 1990.

100. Hastings, L.A., Pashko, L.L., Lewbart, M.L., Schwartz, A.G. Dehydroepiandrosterone and two structural analogs inhibit 12-O-tetradecanoylphorba-13-acetate stimulation of prostaglandin G2 content in mouse skin. *Carcinogenesis* 9: 1099–1102, 1988.

101. Kalimi, M., Opoku, J., Sheng Lu, Q., et al. Studies of the biochemical action and mechanism of dehydroepiandrosterone. In: *The Biologic Role of Dehydroepiandrosterone* (DHEA). Kalimi, M., Regelson, W., Eds., New York: Walter de Gruyter, pp. 397–404, 1990.

102. Kalimi, M., Regelson, W. Physicochemical characterization of (^{3}H)DHEA binding in rat liver. *Biochem Biophys Res Comm* 156: 22–29, 1988.

103. Wayne-Meikle, A., Dorchuck, R., Araneo, B., et al. The presence of a dehydroepiandrosterone-specific receptor binding complex in murine T cells. *J Steroid Biochem Mol Biol* 42: 293–304, 1992.

104. Shantz, L.M., Talalay, P., Gordon, G.B. Mechanism of inhibition of growth of 3T3-LI fibroblasts and their differentiation to adipocytes by DHEA and related steroids. Role of glucose-6-phosphate dehydrogenase. *Proc Natl Acad Sci* 86: 3852–3856, 1989.

105. Rao, C.V., Tokumo, K., Rigotti, J., et al. Chemoprevention of colon cancer by dietary administration of peroxicam, difluoromethylornithine, 16-fluoro-5-androsten-17-one, and ellagic acid individually and in combination. *Cancer Res* 51: 4528–4534, 1991.

106. Brochu, M., Belanger, A. Comparative study of plasma steroid and steroid glucuronide levels in normal men and men with benign prostatic hyperplasia. *Prostate* 11: 33–40, 1987.

107. Stege, R., Carlstrom, K. Testicular and adrenocortical function in healthy men and in men with benign prostatic hyperplasia. *J Steroid Biochem Mol Biol* 42: 357–362, 1992.

108. Spector, T.D., Thompson, P.W., Perryl, A., Grunnos, A.C. The relationship between sex steroids and bone mineral content in women soon after menopause. *Clin Endocrinol* 34: 37–41, 1991.

109. Jilka, R.L., Hangoc, G., Girasole, G., et al. Increased osteoclast development after estrogen loss. Mediated by interleukin-6. *Science* 257: 88–91, 1992.

110. Kishimoto, T., Akira, S., Taga, T. Interleukin 6 and its receptor and paradigm for cytokines. *Science* 258: 593–597, 1992.

111. Taggart, D.P., Gray, C.E., Bowman, A., et al. Serum androgens and gonadotrophins in bronchial carcinoma. *Respir Med* 87: 455–460, 1993.

112. Gordon, G.B., Helzlsover, K.J., Alberg, A.J., et al. Serum levels of

dehydroepiandrosterone and DHEAS and the risk of developing gastric cancer. *Cancer Epidemiol Biomarkers Prev* 2: 33–35, 1993.

113. Hu, D.E., Fan, T.P.D. The combined use of DHEA and dexamethasone inhibits angiogenesis in the rat without causing immunosuppression. *Br J Pharmacol* 107: 260, 1992.

114. Melchoir, C.L., Glasky, A., Ritzmann, R.F. Dehydroepiandrosterone (DHEA) improves memory in normal mice and mice with age induced memory deficits. *Neuroscience Abs* 487:2, 1992.

115. Flood, J.F., Morley, J.E., Roberts, E. Memory enhancing effects in male mice of pregnenolone and steroids metabolically derived from it. *Proc Natl Acad Sci USA* 89: 1567–1571, 1992.

116. Calabrese, V.P., Isaacs, E.R., Regelson, W. Dehydroepiandrosterone in multiple sclerosis: Positive effects on the fatigue syndrome in a non-randomized study. In: *The Biologic Role of Dehydroepiandrosterone (DHEA)*. Kalimi, M., Regelson, W., Eds., New York: Walter de Gruyter, pp. 65–79, 1990.

117. Roberts, E., Fauble, T. Oral dehydroepiandrosterone in multiple sclerosis. Result of a phase one, open study. In: *The Biologic Role of Dehydroepiandrosterone (DHEA)*. Kalimi, M., Regelson, W., Eds., New York: Walter de Gruyter, pp. 81–93, 1990.

118. Neuberger, T.J., Kalimi, M., Regelson, W., et al. Glucocorticoids enhance the potency of Schwann cell mitogens. *J Neurosci Res* 38: 300–313, 1994.

119. Melchoir, C.L, Ritzmann, R. F. Dehydroepiandrosterone is an anxiolytic in mice on the plus maze. *Pharmacol Biochem Behavior* 47: 437–441, 1994.

120. Demirgoren, S., Majewska, M.D., Spivak, C.E., et al. Receptor binding and electrophysiological effects of dehydroepiandrosterone sulfate, an antagonist to the GABAA receptor. *Neuroscience* 45: 127–135, 1991.

121. Mather, C., Prasad, V.V.K. Raju, S., et al. Steroids and their conjugates in the mammalian brain. *Proc Natl Acad Sci USA* 90: 85–88, 1993.

122. Papadopoulos, W., Berkovich, A., Kreuger, K.E., et al. Diazepam binding inhibitor and its processing products stimulate mitochondrial steroid biosynthesis via an interaction with mitochondrial benzodiazepine receptors. *Endocrinol* 129: 1481–1488, 1991.

123. French-Mullen, J.M.H., Spence, T.K. Neurosteroids block Ca2 + channel current in freshly isolated hippocampal Cal neurons. *Euro J Pharmacol* 202: 269–272, 1991.

124. Bonnet, K.A., Brown, R.P. Cognitive effects of DHEA replacement therapy. In: *The Biologic Role of Dehydroepiandrosterone (DHEA)*. Kalimi, M., Regelson, W., Eds., New York: Walter de Gruyter, pp. 65–79, 1990.

125. Sunderland, T., Merrill, C.R., Harrington, M.G., et al. Reduced plasma dehydroepiandrosterone concentrations in Alzheimer's disease (Letter). *Lancet* 2: 570, 1989.

126. Svec, F., Lopez, A. Antiglucocorticoid actions of dehydroepiandrosterone and low concentrations in Alzheimer's disease (Letter). *Lancet* 2: 570, 1989.

127. Leblhuber, F.E., Windhager, E., Neubauer, C., et al. Antiglucocorticoid effects of DHEAS in Alzheimer's disease. *Am J Psychiatry* 149: 1125–1126, 1992.

128. Wolkowitz, O.M., Reus, V.I., Manfredi, F., Roberts, E. Letters to editor. *Am J Psychiatry* 149: 8, 1992.

129. Hashimoto, S., Migita, S. Serum amyloid P component regulation by sex steroids in rat. *Nippon-Ketsueki-Gakkai-Zasshi* 53: 89–97, 1990.

130. Pierpaoli, W., Regelson, W. Pineal control of aging effect of melatonin and pineal grafting on aging mice. *Proc Natl Acad Sci USA* 91: 787–792, 1994.

131. Taylor, G.T., Scherrer, J., Weiss, J., Pitha, J. Endocrine interactions: Adrenal steroids and precursors. *Am J Physiol* 266: E676–E681, 1994.

132. Shugh, V., Kalimi, M., Phan, T-H, Biber, M.C. Intra-cranial dehydroepiandrosterone blocks the activation of tryptophane hydroxylase in response to acute sound stress. *Mol Cell Neurosci* 5: 176–181, 1994.

133. Murphy, B.E.P. Steroids and depression. *J Steroid Biochem Mol Biol* 28: 537–559, 1991.

134. Canonaco, M., Ando, S., Valenti, A., et al. The in vitro transformation of [H^3] DHEA into its principal metabolites in the adrenal cortex of adult castrated male rats and following steroid treatment. *J Endocrinol* 121: 419–424, 1989.

135. Eich, D.M., Nestler, J.E., Johnson, D.E., et al. Inhibition of accelerated coronary atherosclerosis with dehydroepiandrosterone in the heterotopic rabbit model of cardiac transplantation. *Circulation* 87: 261–269, 1993.

136. Wiedmeier, S.E., Mu, H.H., Araneo, B.A., Daynes, R.A. Age and micro environment associated influences by platelet derived growth factor on T cell function. *J Immunol* 152: 3417–3426, 1994.

137. Daynes, R.A., Araneo, B.A., Ershler, W.B., et al. Altered regulation of IL-6 production with normal aging. *J Immunol* 150: 5219–5230, 1993.

138. Milewich, L., Whisnant, M.G. Metabolism of androstendione by human platelets: A source of potent androgens. *J Clin Endocrin Metab* 54: 919–974, 1982.

139. Jesse, R., Nestler, J., Eich, D., et al. Dehydroepiandrosterone in vivo and in vitro inhibits platelet aggregation. *J Am Coll Cardiol* 17: 376A (Abstract), 1991.

140. Milewich, L., Whisnant, M.G., Sawyer, M.K. Androstenedione metabolism by human lymphocytes. *J Steroid Biochem* 16: 81–85, 1982.

141. Milewich, L., Hendricks, T.S., Johnson, A. R. Metabolism of Dehydroepiandrosterone and androstenedione in human pulmonary endothelial cells in culture. *J Clin Endocrin Metab* 56: 930–935, 1983.

142. Sholley, M.M., Gudas, S.A., Schwartz, C.C., Kalimi, M.Y. Dehydroepiandrosterone and related steroids induce multilamellar lipid structures in cultured human endothelial cells. *Am J Pathol* 136: 1187–1199, 1990.

143. La Croix, A.Z., Yano, K., Reed, D.M. Dehydroepiandrosterone sulfate, incidence of myocardial infarction and extent of atherosclerosis in men. *Circulation* 86: 1529–1535, 1992.

144. Fava, M., Littman, A., Lamon-Fava, S., et al. Psychological behavioral and biochemical risk factors for coronary artery disease. *Am J Cardiol* 70: 1412–1416, 1992.

145. Hautanen, A., Manttar, I.M., Manninen, V., et al. Adrenal androgens and testosterone as coronary risk factors in the Helsinki heart study. *Atherosclerosis* 105: 191–200, 1994.

146. Rice, T., Sprecher, D.L., Borecki, I.B., et al. The Cincinnati myocardial infarction and hormone family study. Family resemblance for DHEAS in control and myocardial infarct patients. *Metabolism* 42: 1284–1290, 1993.

147. Ishihara, F., Hiramatsu, K., Shigematsu, S., et al. Role of adrenal androgens in the development of arteriosclerosis as judged by pulse wave velocity and calcification of the aorta. *Cardiol* 80: 332–338, 1992.

148. MacEwen, E.G., Kurzman, I.D. Obesity in the dog: Role of the adrenal steroid dehydroepiandrosterone (DHEA). *J Nutr* 121: 551–555, 1991.

149. Kurzman, I.D., MacEwen, E.G., Haffa, A.L.M. Reduction in body weight and cholesterol in spontaneously obese dogs by dehydroepiandrosterone. *Int J Obesity* 14: 95–104, 1990.

150. Abadie, J.E., Wright, B., Correa, G., et al. Effect of DHEA on neurotransmitter levels and appetite regulation of the obese Zucker rat. *Diabetes* 42: 662–669, 1993.

151. McIntosh, M.K., Pan, J.S., Berdanier, C.D. In vitro studies on the effects of dehydroepiandrosterone and corticosterone on hepatic steroid receptor binding and mitochondrial respiration. *Biochem Physiol A* 104: 147–153, 1993.

152. Wright, B.E., Brown, F.S., Svec, F., Porter, J.R. Divergent effect of dehydroepiandrosterone on energy intakes of Zucker rats. *Physiol Behav* 53: 39–43, 1993.

153. McIntosh, M.K., Berdanier, C.D. Influence of DHEA on the thyroid hormone status of BHE/cdb rats. *J Nutr Biochem* 3: 194–199, 1992.

154. Song, M.K., Grieco, D., Rall, J.E., Nikodem, V.M. Thyroid hormone-mediated transcriptional activation of the rat liver malic enzyme gene by dehydroepiandrosterone. *J Biol Chem* 264, 18981–18985, 1989.

155. Mohan, P., Cleary, M. Effect of short term DHEA administration on liver metabolism of lean and obese rats. *Am J Physiology* 255: 1–8, 1988.

156. Olivieri, A., Soricini, M., Battisti, P., et al., Thyroid hypofunction related with the progression of human immunodeficiency virus infection. *J Endocrinol Invest* 16: 407–413, 1993.

157. Prough, R.A., Webb, S.J., Wu, H.O., et al. Induction of microsomal and peroxisomal enzymes by dehydroepiandrosterone and its reduced metabolite in rats. *Cancer Res* 54: 2878–2886, 1994.

158. Sakuma, M., Yamada, J., Suga, T. Induction of peroxisomal B oxidation by structural analogues of DHEA in cultural rat hepatocytes. Structure activity relationships. *Biochem Biophys Acta* 1169: 66–72, 1993.

159. Aragno, M., Tamagno, E., Boccuzzi, G. DHEA pretreatment protects rats against the pro-oxidant and necrogenic effects of carbon tetrachloride. *Biochem Pharm* 46: 1689–1694, 1993.

160. Lee, T.C., Lai, G.J., Kao, S.L. Protection of rat tracheal epithelial cell line from paraquat toxicity by inhibition of glucose-6-phosphate dehydrogenase. *Biochem Pharm* 45: 1143–1147, 1993.

161. Marreno, M., Prough, R.A., Frenkel, R.A., Milewich, L. DHEA feeding and protein phosphorylation, phosphatases and liposinil enzymes in mouse liver. *Proc Soc Exp Biol Med* 193: 110–117, 1989.

162. Haffner, S.M., Valdez, R.A., Mykkanen, L., et al. Decreased testosterone and DHEAS concentrations are associated with increased insulin and glucose concentrations in non-diabetic men. *Metabolism* 43: 599–603, 1994.

163. McEwen, B. An overview of novel action of steroids within and upon cells. Presented at Novel Action of Steroids Conference. Anaheim, CA, Oct. 24, 1992.

164. Gee, K.W. Neurosteroid actions at the GABA A receptors. Presented at Novel Action of Steroids Conference. Anaheim, CA, Oct. 24, 1992.

165. Beamer, W.G., Tennet, B.J., Schulz, K.L., et al. Gene for ovarian granulosa susceptibility, et: in SWXJ recombinant inbred strains revealed by dehydroepiandrosterone. *Cancer Res* 48: 5092–5095, 1989.

166. Williams, D.P., Boyden, T.W., Pamenter, R.W., et al. Relationship of body fat percentage and fat distribution with DHEAS in premenopausal females. *J Clin Endocrinol Metab* 77: 80–85, 1993.

167. Jung-Testas, I., Hu, Z.Y., Baulieu, E.E., Robel, P. Neurosteroids—Biosynthesis of pregnenolone and progesterone in primary cultures of rat glial cells. *Endocrinol* 125: 2083–2091, 1989.

168. Marrero, M., Prough, R.A., Putnam, R.S., et al. Inhibition of carbamyl phosphate synthetase-I by dietary dehydroepiandrosterone. *J Steroid Biochem Mol Biol* 38: 599–609, 1991.

169. Merriman, R.L., Tanzer, L.R., Stamm, N.B. Chemoprevention of malignant transformation by dehydroepiandrosterone (DHEA) in C3H10T1/2 cells. *13th Int Cancer Congress Proc* Seattle, WA. abs. 3102 (Abstract), p. 543, 1982.

170. Vesely, D.L. Testosterone and its precursors and metabolites enhance guanylate cyclase activity. *Proc Natl Acad Sci USA* 76: 3491–3494, 1979.

171. Ozasa, H., Kita, M., Inove, T., Mori, T. Plasma dehydroepiandrosterone to cortisol ratios as an indicator of stress to gynecologic patients. *Gynecol Oncol* 37: 178–182, 1990.

172. Spratt, D.I., Longcope, C., Cox, P.M., et al. Differential changes in serum concentrations of androgens and estrogens (in relation with cortisol) in postmenopausal women with acute illness. *J Clin Endocrinol Metab* 76: 1542–1547, 1993.

173. Wright, B.E., Porter, J.R., Browne, E.S., Svec, F. Anti-glucocorticoid action of DHEA in young obese Zucker rats. *Int J Obesity* 16: 579–583, 1992.

174. Browne, E., Wright, B., Porter, J., Svec, F. Dehydroepiandrosterone: Antiglucocorticoids action in mice. *Am J Med Res* 303(6): 366–371, 1992.

175. El Rashidy, R. Personal communication, 1991.

176. Kowalski, W., Chatterton, R.T., Jr. Effects of subchronic infusion of dehydroepiandrosterone sulfate on serum gonadotropin levels and ovarian function in the cynomolgus monkey. *Fertil Steril* 57: 912–920, 1992.

177. Ruiz-Salmeron, R.J., del Arbol, J.L., Raya-Munoz, J., et al. Dehydroepiandrosterone sulfate, cortisol and their precursors in severely ill (acute and chronic) patients. *Rev Clin Exp* 187: 389–394, 1990.

178. Parker, C.R., Schuster, M.W. Effects of syphilis infection on adrenocortical function in man. *Proc Soc Exp Biol Med* 197: 165–167, 1991.

179. Christeff, N., Michon, C., Goertz, G., et al. Abnormal free fatty acids and cortisol concentrations in the serum of AIDS patients. *Eur J Cancer Clin Oncol* 24: 1179–1183, 1988.

180. Sonka, J. Dehydroepiandrosterone metabolic effects. *ACTA Univ Carol* 71: 9–137, 1976.

181. Buster, J.E., Casson, R.R., Straughn, A.B., et al. Postmenopausal steroid replacement with micronized dehydroepiandrosterone. Preliminary oral availability and dose proportionality studies. *Am J Obstet Gynecol* 166: 1163–1170, 1992.

182. McIntosh, M.K., Goldfarb, A.H., Curtis, L.N., Cote, P.S. Vitamin E alters hepatic antioxidant enzymes in rats treated with dehydroepiandrosterone (DHEA). *J Nutr* 123: 216–224, 1993.

183. Radominska, A., Comer, K.A., Zimmak, P., et al. Human liver steroid sulphotransferase sulfates and bile salts. *Biochem J* 272: 507–804, 1990.

184. Birkenhager-Gillesse, E.G., Derksen, J., Lagany, A.M. DHEA-S in the oldest old, aged 85 and over. *Ann NY Acad Sci* 719: 543–552, 1994.

Bibliography

DHEA (Dehydroepiandrosterone)

Please refer to Appendix 1: DHEA by W. Regelson and M. Kalimi: "Dehydroepiandrosterone (DHEA)—A Pleiotropic Steroid. How Can One Steroid Do So Much?" In *Adv. in Anti-Aging Medicine*, v. 1; edited by Ronald M. Klatz, 287–317. New York: Mary Ann Liebert, Inc., 1996. This summarizes the literature to June 1995.

A more recent conference review: Bellino, F. L.; Daynes, R. A.; Hornsby, P. J.; Lavrin, D.H.; and Nestler, J., eds. "Dehydroepiandrosterone (DHEA) and Aging," *Ann. N.Y. Acad. of Sciences* v. 74, 1995.

Regelson, W.; Loria, R.; Kalimi, M. "Dehydroepiandrosterone (DHEA)— The 'MotherSteroid.' I Immunologic Action," *Ann. N.Y. Acad. of Sciences* 719/553–63, 1994.

Regelson, W., and Kalimi, M. "Dehydroepiandrosterone (DHEA)—The Multifunctional Steroid. II Effects on the CNS, Cell Proliferation, Metabolic and Vascular, Clinical; and other Effects." *Ann. N.Y. Acad. of Sciences* 564–75, 1994.

Kalimi, M., and Regelson, W., eds. "The Biologic Role of Dehydroepiandrosterone (DHEA)." Berlin-New York: Walter de Gruyter, 1990.

The above provide a broad review of DHEA's place as a superhormone.

Belanger, A.; Candas, B.; Dupont, A.; et al. "Changes in Serum Concentration of Conjugated and Unconjugated Steroids in 40- to 80-Year-Old Men," *J. Clin. Endocrin. Metab.* 79:1086–90, 1994.

Bradley, W. G.; Kraus, L. A.; Good, R. A.; Day, N. K. "Dehydroepiandrosterone inhibits replication of feline immunodeficiency virus in chronically infected cells," *Vet. Immunol. Immunopathol.* 46:159–68, 1995.

Dandona, P.; Thusu, K.; Cook, S.; Snyder, B.; et al.: "Oxidative damage to DNA in diabetes mellitus." *The Lancet* 237:444–46, 1996.

Friess, E.; Trachsel, L.; Guldner, J.; et al. "DHEA Administration Increases Rapid Eye Movement Sleep and EEG Power in the Sigma Frequency Range," *Am. J. Physiol.* 268:E107–E113, 1995.

Haffner, S. M.; Newcomb, P. A.; Marcus, P. M.; et al.: "Relation of sex hormones and dehydroepiandrosterone sulfate (DHEA-SO4) to cardiovascular risk factors in postmenopausal women," *Am. J. Epidemiol.* 142:925–34, 1995.

Haffner, S. M.; Valdez, R. A.; Mykkanen, L.; et al. "Decreased Testosterone and DHEA Sulfate Concentrations Are Associated with Increased Insulin and Glucose Concentrations in Nondiabetic Men," *Metabolism* 43:599–603, 1994.

Hedman, M.; Nilsson, E.; De La Torre, B.: "Low blood and synovial fluid levels of sulpho-conjugated steroids in rheumatoid arthritis," *Clin. Exper. Rheuma.* 10:25–30, 1992.

Herrington, D. M. "DHEA and Coronary Atherosclerosis," *Ann. N.Y. Acad. of Sciences* 774:259–70, 1995.

Hess, V.; Jahreis, G.; Schambach, H.; Vogel, H.; et al. "Insulinlike growth factor I changes of the hormonal status in puberty and age," *Exp. Clin. Endocrinol.* 102:289–98, 1994.

Holsboer, F.; Grasser, A.; Friess, E.; Wiedemann, K. "Steroid Effects on Central Neurons and Implications for Psychiatric and Neurological Disorders," *Ann. N.Y. Acad. of Sci.* 746:345–59, 1994.

Jakubowicz, D. J.; Beer, N. A.; Nestler, J.: "Disparate Effects of Weight Reduction by Diet on Serum DHEAS Levels in Obese Men and Women," *J. Clin. Endocrin. Metab.* 80:3373–76, 1995.

Kawai, S.; Yahata, N.; Nishida, S.; et al.: "Dehydroepiandrosterone inhibits B16 mouse melanoma cell growth by induction of differentiation," *Anticancer Res.* 15:427–31, 1995.

Khorram, O. A.; Vu, L.; Yen, S. S. C. "Activation of Immune Function by Dehydroepiandrosterone (DHEA) in Age Advanced Men," *J. Gerontol.* in press, 1996.

Kim, H. R.; Ryu, S. Y.; Kim H. S.; et al.: "Administration of Dehydroepiandrosterone Reverses the Immune Suppression Induced by High Dose Antigen in Mice." *Immunol. Invest.* 24:583–93, 1995.

Majewska, M. "Neuronal Actions of DHEA. Possible Role in Brain Development, Aging and Memory," *Ann. N.Y. Acad. of Sci.* 774:111–20, 1995.

Masi, A. T.; Feigenbaum, S. L.; Chatterton, R. T. "Hormonal and Pregnancy (Relationships to Rheumatoid Arthritis: Convergent Effects with Immunologic and Microvascular Systems," *Semin. Arthritis Rheum.* 25:1–27, 1995.

Morales, A. J.; Nolan, J. J.; Nelson, J. C.; Yen, S. S. C. "Effect of Replacement Dose of DHEA in Men and Women of Advancing Age," *J. Clin. Endocrin. Metab.* 78:1360–67, 1994.

Nilsson, E.; De La Torre, B.; Hedman, M.; et al. "Blood DHEAS Levels in Polymyalgia Rheumatica/Giant Cell Arteritis and Primary Fibromyalgia," *Clin. Exp. Rheumatol.* 12:415–17, 1994.

Okabe, T.; Haji, M.; Takayanagi, R.; et al. "Up-Regulation of High Affinity DHEA Binding Activity by DHEA in Activated T Lymphocytes," *J. Clin. Endocrin. Metab.* 80:2993–96, 1995.

Orentreich, N.; Brind, J. L.; Vogelman, J. II.; et al. "Long-Term Measurements of Plasma Dehydroepiandrosterone Sulfate in Normal Men," *J. Clin. Endocrin. Metab.* 75:1002–1005, 1992.

Paul, S. M.; Purdy, R. H. "Neuroactive Steroids, *FASEB J.* 6:2311–22, 1992.

Porter, J. R.; Svec, F. "DHEA Diminishes Fat Food Intake in Lean and Obese Zucker Rats," *Ann. N.Y. Acad. of Sci.* 774:329–31, 1995.

Ravaglia, G.; Forti, P.; Maioli, F.; et al. "The Relationship of DHEA Sulfate (DHEAS) to Endocrine-Metabolic Parameters and Functional Status in the Oldest Old. Results from an Italian Study on Healthy Free-Living Over-Ninety-Year-Olds," *J. Clin. Endocrin. Metab.* 81:1173–78, 1996.

Schwartz, A. G.; Pashko, L. L.: "Cancer Prevention with Dehydroepiandrosterone and Nonandrogenic Structural Analogs," *J. Cell Biochem.* Suppl. 22:210, 1995.

Svec, F.; Porter, J. R. "Synergistic Anorectic Effect of DHEA and Fenfluramine on Zucker Rat Food Intake and Selection," *Ann. N.Y. Acad. of Sci.* 774:332–34, 1995.

Thomas, G.; Frenoy, N.; Legrain, S.; et al. "Serum DHEAS Levels as an Individual Marker," *J. Clin. Endocrin. Metab.* 79:1273–76, 1994.

Van Vollenhoven, R. F., et al.: "An open study of dehydroepiandrosterone in systemic lupus erythematosus," *Arthritis Rheum.* 37:1305–10, 1994.

Wolkowitz, O. M.; Reus, V. I.; Roberts, E.; et al. "Antidepressant and Cognition-Enhancing Effects of DHEA in Major Depression," *Ann. N.Y. Acad. of Sci.* 774:337–39, 1995.

Pregnenolone

Akwa, Y.; Schumacher, M.; Jung-Testas, I.; Baulieu, E.-E. "Neurosteroids in Rat Sciatic Nerves and Schwann Cells," *CR Acad. Sci. Paris, Life Sciences* 316:410–14, 1993.

Baulieu, E.-E. "Neurosteroids: A New Function in the Brain," *Bio. Cell.* 71:3–10, 1991.

Davison, R.; Koets, P.; Snow, W. G.; Gabrielson, L. G. "Effects of delta 5 Pregnenolone in Rheumatoid Arthritis," *Arch. Int. Medicine* 85:365–88, 1950.

Flood, J. F.; Morley, J. F.; Roberts, E. "Memory Enhancing Effects in Male Mice of Pregnenolone and Steroids Metabolically Derived from It," *Proc. Nat. Acad. Sci. USA* 89:1567–71, 1992.

Freeman, H.; Pincus, G.; Bachrach, S.; et al. "Steroid Medication in Rheumatoid Arthritis," in *Symposium on Steroids in Experimental and Clinical Practice,* edited by A. White, 181–98, Blakiston, New York, 1951.

Freeman, H.; Pincus, G.; Bachrach, S.; et al. "Therapeutic Efficacy of delta 5 Pregnenolone in Rheumatoid Arthritis," *JAMA* 143:338–44, 1950.

George, M. S.; Gudotti, A.; Rubinow, D.; et al. "CSF Neuroactive Steroids in Affective Disorders: Pregnenolone, Progesterone, and DBI." *Biol. Psychiatry* 35:775–80, 1994.

Guest, C. M.; Kammerer, W. H.; Cedil, R. L.; Berson, S. A. "Epinephrine, Pregnenolone, and Testosterone in Rheumatoid Arthritis," *JAMA* 143:338–44, 1950.

Guth, L.; Zhang, Z.; Roberts, E. "Key Role for Pregnenolone in Combination Therapy That Promotes Recovery After Spinal Cord Injury," *Proc. Natl. Acad. Sci. USA* 91:12308–12, 1994.

Isaacson, R. L.; Yoder, P. E.; Varner, J. "The Effects of Pregnenolone on Acquisition and Retention of a Food Search Task," *Behav. Neurol. Biol.* 61:170–76, 1994.

Ishmael, W. K.; Heilbaum, A.; Kuhn, J. F.; Duffy, M. "Effects of Certain Steroid Compounds on Various Manifestations of Rheumatoid Arthritis," *J. Okla. State Med. Assoc.* 42:434–37, 1949.

McCauley, L. D.; Park, C. H.; Lan, N. C.; et al. "Benzodiazepines and Peptides Stimulate Pregnenolone Synthesis in Brain Mitochondria," *Eur. J. Pharmacol.* 276:145–53, 1995.

McGavack, T. H.; Chevally, J.; Weissberg, J. "The Use of delta 5 Pregnenolone in Various Clinical Disorders," *J. Clin. Endocrinol.* 11:559–77, 1951.

Madhu, C.; Klassen, C. D. "Protective Effect of Pregnenolone 16 alpha Carbonitrile on Acetaminophen-induced Hepatotoxicity in Hamsters," *Toxicol. Appl. Pharmacol.* 109:305–13, 1991.

Mathis, C.; Paul, S. M.; Crawley, J. N. "The Neurosteroid Pregnenolone Sulfate Blocks NMDA-induced Deficits in a Passive Avoidance Memory Task," *Psychopharm.* 116:201–6, 1994.

Mayo, W.; Dedhu, F.; Robel, P.; et al. "Infusion of Neurosteroids into the Nucleus Basalis Magnocellularis Affects Cognitive Processes in the Rat," *Brain Res.* 607: 324–28, 1993.

Melchoir, C. L.; Allen, P. M. "Interaction of Pregnenolone and Pregnenolone Sulfate with Ethanol and Pentobarbital," *Pharmacol. Biochem. Behav.* 42:605–11, 1992.

Melchoir, C. L.; Ritzmann, R. F. "Pregnenolone and Pregnenolone Sulfate, Alone and with Ethanol, in Mice on the Plus Maze," *Pharmacol. Biochem. Behav.* 48:893–97, 1994.

Morfin, R.; Courchay, G. "Pregnenolone and DHEA as Precursors of Native Hydroxylated Metabolites Which Increase the Immune Response in Mice," *J. Steroid. Biochem. Mol. Biol.* 50:91–100, 1994.

Pincus, G.; Hoagland, H. "Effects of Administered Pregnenolone on Fatiguing Psychomotor Performance," *J. Aviat. Med.* 15:98–115, 1944.

Pincus, G.; Hoagland, H. "Effects on Industrial Production of the Administration of delta 5 Pregnenolone to Factory Workers," *I. Psychosomatic Med.* 7:342–46, 1945.

Pincus, G.; Hoagland, H.; Wilson, C. H.; Fay, N. J. Ibid. II. *Psychosomatic Med.* 7:347–52, 1945.

Robel, P.; Young, J.; Corpechot, C.; et al. "Biosynthesis and Assay of Neurosteroids in Rats and Mice: Functional Correlates," *J. Steroid Biochem. Mol. Biol.* 53:355–60, 1995.

Roberts, E. "Pregnenolone—From Selye to Alzheimer and a Model of the Pregnenolone Sulfate Binding Site on the GABAA Receptor," *Biochem. Pharmacol.* 49:1–16, 1995.

Steiger, A.; Trachsel, L.; Guldner, J.; et al. "Neurosteroid Pregnenolone Induces Sleep EEG Changes in Man Compatible with Inverse Agonistic GABAA-Receptor Modulation," *Brain Res.* 615:267–74, 1993.

Testosterone

Ashton, W. S.; Degnan, B. M.; Daniel, A.; Francis, G. L. "Testosterone Increases Insulinlike Growth Factor 1 and Insulinlike Growth Factor Binding Protein," *Ann. Clin. Lab. Sci.* 25:381–88, 1995.

Bagatelli, C. J.; Bremner, W. J. "Androgens in Men—Uses and Abuses," *Drug Therapy* 334:707–14, 1996.

Barrett-Connor, E. L. "Testosterone and Risk Factors for Cardiovascular Disease in Men," *Diabetes and Metab.* 21:156–61, 1995.

Bhasin, S.; Storer, T. W.; Berman, N.; et al. "The Effects of Supraphysiologic Doses of Testosterone on Muscle Size and Strength in Normal Men," *N. Eng. J. Med.* 335:1–7, 1996.

Davidson, J. M.; Camargo, C. A.; Smith, E. R. "Effects of androgen on sexual behavior in hypogonadal men," *J. Clin. Endo. & Metab.* 48:955–58, 1979.

Davidson, J. M.; Chen, J. J.; Crapo, L.; Gray, G. "Hormonal changes and sexual function in aging men," *J. Clin. Endo. & Metab.* 57:71–79, 1983.

Flood, J. F.; Farr, S. A.; Kaiser, F. E.; et al., "Age Related Decrease of Plasma Testosterone in Samp8 Mice; Replacement Improves Age Related Impairment of Learning and Memory," *Physiol. and Behavior* 57:669–73, 1995.

Gouchie, C.; Kimura, D. "The relationship between testosterone levels and cognitive ability patterns," *Psychoneuroendocrinology* 16:323–34, 1991.

Hakkinen, K.; Pakerinen, A. "Serum Hormones and Strength Development During Strength Training in Middle-Aged and Elderly Males and Females," *Acta Physiol. Scandinav.* 150:211, 1994.

Kaiser, F.; Morley, J. E. "Gonadotropins, Testosterone and the Aging Male," *Neuro. of Aging* 15:559–63, 1994.

Kasra, M.; Grynpas, M. D. "The Effects of Androgens on the Mechanical Properties of Primate Bone," *Bone* 17:265–70, 1995.

McLure, R. D.; Oses, R.; Ernst, M. L. "Hypogonadal Impotence Treated by Transdermal Testosterone," *Urology* 37:224–28, 1991.

Marin, P. "Testosterone and Regional Fat Distribution," *Obesity Res.* 3 Suppl 4:609S–12S, 1995.

Mateo, L.; Nolla, J. M.; Bonnin, M. R., et al. "Sex Hormone Status and Bone Mineral Density in Men with Rheumatoid Arthritis," *J. Rheumatol.* 22:1455–60, 1995.

Meriggiola, M. C.; Marcovina, S.; Paulsen, C. A.; Bremner, W. J. "Testosterone Enanthate at a Dose of 200mg/week Decreases HDL Cholesterol Levels in Healthy Men," *Int. J. Androl.*, 18:237–42, 1995.

Mermall, J.; Southern, R. B.; Kanabrocki, E. L.; et al. "Temporal (circadian) and functional relationship between prostate-specific antigen and testosterone in healthy men," Urology 46:45–52, 1995.

Monath, J. R.; McCullough, D. K. L.; Hart, L. J.; Jarow, J. P. "Physiologic variations of serum testosterone within the normal range do not affect serum prostate-specific antigen," *Urology* 46:58–61, 1995.

Morley, J. E.; Kaiser, F. E. "Hypogonadism in the Elderly Man," *Adv. Endocrin.* 4:241–62, 1993.

Naessens, G.; De Slypere, J. P.; Dijs, H.; Driessens, M. "Hypogonadism as a Cause of Recurrent Muscle Injury in a High Level Soccer Player," *Int. J. Sports Medicine* 16:413–17, 1995.

Nicklas, B. J.; Ryan, A. J.; Treuth, M. M.; et al. "Testosterone, Growth Hormone and IGF-1 responses to Acute and Chronic Resistive Exercise in Men Aged 55–70 Years," *Int. J. Sports Med.* 16:445–50, 1995.

Phillips, G. B.; Pinkernell, B. H. "The Association of Hypotestosteronemia with Coronary Artery Disease in Men," *Arterioscler. Thromb.* 14:701–6, 1994.

Ravaglia, G.; Forti, P.; Maioli, F.; et al. "Hormonal Changes in Male Subjects Over Ninety," *Boll. Soc. Ital. Biol. Exper.* 71:133–39, 1995.

Rudman, D.; Drinka, P. J.; Wilson, C. R.; et al. "Relations of Endogenous Anabolic Hormones and Physical Activity to Bone Mineral Density and Body Mass in Elderly Men," *Clin. Endocrinol. Oxf.* 40:653–61, 1994.

Salehian, B.; Wang, C.; Alexander, G.; et al. "Parmacokinetics, Bioefficiency, and Safety of Sublingual Testosterone Cyclodextrin," *J. Clin. Endocrinol. Metab.* 80:3567–75, 1995.

Silver, J. J.; Einhorn, T. A. "Osteoporosis and Aging," *Clin. Orthoped. and Related Res.* 316:10–20, 1995.

Sprinivasan, G.; Campbell, E.; Bashirelahi, N. "Androgen, Estrogen, and Progesterone Receptors in Normal and Aging Prostates," *Microsc. Res. Tech.* 30:293–304, 1995.

Tenover, J. S. "Androgen Administration to Aging Men," *Endocrinol. and Metab. Clinics of North America* 23:877–88, 1994.

Tenover, J. S. "Effects of Testosterone Supplementation in the Aging Male," *J. Clin. Endocrinol. Metab.* 75:1092–98, 1992.

Tsitouras, P. D.; Bulat, T. "The Aging Male Reproductive System," *Endocrinol. Metab. Clinics of North America* 24:297–315, 1995.

Urban, R. J.; Bodenburg, Y. H.; Gilikson, C.; et al. "Testosterone Administration to Elderly Men Increases Muscle Strength and Protein Synthesis," *Am. J. Physiol. (Endocr.)* 269:E820–26, 1995.

Young, R. L. "Androgens in Postmenopausal Therapy?" *Menopause Management,* May 1993, pp. 21–24.

Estrogen-Progesterone

Baker, V. L. "Alternatives to Oral Estrogen Replacement," *Obs. and Gyn. Clin. of North America* 21:297–99, 1994.

Don Gambrell, R.; Maier, R. C.; Sanders, B. I. "Decreased Incidence of Breast Cancer in Postmenopausal Estrogen-Progestogen Users," *Ob. Gynecol.* 62:435–43, 1983.

Fonda, D. "Local Oestrogen Replacement for Local Symptoms in Older Community Dwelling Women," *Gerontology* 40 Suppl. 3:9–13, 1994.

Garcia-Segura, L. M.; Chowen, J. A.; Duenes, M.; et al. "Gonadal Steroids as Promoters of Neuro-Glial Plasticity," *Psychoneuroendocrinol.* 19:445–53, 1994.

Gibbs, R. B. "Estrogen and Nerve Growth Factor Related Systems in Brain," *Ann. N.Y. Acad. of Sci.* 743:165–96, 1994.

Hargrove, J. T.; Maxson, W. S.; Wentz, A. C.; et al. "Menopausal Hormone Replacement Therapy with Continuous Daily Oral Micronized Estradiol and Progesterone," *Ob. Gyn.* 73:606–12, 1989.

Koenig, H. L.; Schumacher, M.; Fewrzaz, B.; et al. "Progesterone Synthesis and Myelin Formation by Schwann Cells," *Science* 268:1500–1502, 1995.

Lee, J. R. "Osteoporosis Reversal: The Role of Progesterone," *Int. Clin. Nutr. Rev.* 10:384–91, 1990.

Martorano, J. T.; Ahlgrimm, M.; Meyers, D. "Differentiating Between Natural Progesterone and Synthetic Progestogens: Clinical Implications for Premenstrual Syndrome Management," *Comprehensive Therapy* 19:96–98, 1993.

Moldofsky, H. "Central Nervous System and Peripheral Immune Functions and the Sleep-Wake System," *J. Psychiatry-Neurosci.* 19:368–74, 1994.

Nachtigall, L. E. "Emerging Delivery Systems for Estrogen Replacement: Aspects of Transdermal and Oral Delivery," *Am. J. Obstet. Gynecol.* 173:993–97, 1995.

Nelson, J. F.; Felicio, L. S. "Reproductive Aging in the Female: An Etiological Perspective," *Rev. Biol. Res. in Aging* 2:251–314, 1985.

Nordbo, I.; Berge, L.; Bonaa, K. H.; Nordoy, A. "Serum Ferritin, Sex Hormones and Cardiovascular Risk Factors in Healthy Women," *Arterioscler. and Thromb.* 14:857–61, 1994.

PEPI Trial "Effects of Estrogen or Estrogen/Progestin Regimens on Heart Disease Risk Factors in Postmenopausal Women," *JAMA* 273:199–208, 1995.

Picazo, O.; Fernandez-Guasti, A. "Anti-Anxiety Effects of Progesterone and Some of Its Reduced Metabolites: An Evaluation Using the Burying Behavior Test," *Brain Res.* 680:135–41, 1995.

Prior, J. C. "Progesterone as a Bone-Trophic Hormone," *Endocrine Revs.* 11:386–98, 1990.

Ross, J. L.; McCauley, E.; Roeltgen, D.; et al. "Self Concept and Behavior in Adolescent Girls with Turners Syndrome: Potential Estrogen Effects," *J. Clin. Endocrinol. Metab.* 81:926–31, 1996.

Savvas, M.; Studd, J. W. W.; Norman, S.; et al. "Increase in Bone Mass After One Year of Percutaneous Oestradiol and Testosterone Implants in Post-menopausal Women Who Have Previously Received Long-term Oral Oestrogens," *Br. J. Ob. Gyn.* 99:757–60, 1992.

Sherwin, B. B. "Sex Hormones and Psychological Functioning in Postmenopausal Women," *Exp. Gerontol.* 29:423–30, 1994.

Shiraki, M.; Orimo, H. "The Effect of Estrogen and Sex Steroids and Thyroid Hormone Preparation on Bone Mineral Density in Senile Osteoporosis," *Folia endocrinol.* 67:84–95, 1991.

Simpkin, J. W.; Singh, M.; Bishop, J. "The Potential Role for Estrogen Replacement Therapy in the Treatment of the Cognitive Decline and Neurodegeneration Associated with Alzheimer's Disease," *Neurobiol. Aging* 15 suppl 2:S195–97, 1994.

Stevenson, J. C.; Cust, M. P.; Gangar, K. F. "Effects of Transdermal versus Oral Replacement Therapy on Bone Density in Spine and Proximal Femur in Postmenopausal Women," *Lancet* 336:265–69, 1990.

Tranquilli, A. L.; Mazzani, L.; Cugini, A. M.; et al. "Transdermal Estradiol and Medroxyprogesterone Acetate in Hormone Replacement Therapy Are Both Antioxidants," *Gynecol. Endocrinol.* 9:137–41, 1995.

Vogel, W.; Klaiber, E.; Broverman, D. "Roles of the Gonadal Steroid Hormones in Psychiatric Depression in Men and Women," *Prog. Neuro-Psychopharm.* 2:487–503, 1978.

Whitehead, M. I.; Fraser, D.; Schenkel, L.; et al. "Transdermal Administration of Oestrogen/progestagen Hormone Replacement Therapy," *Lancet* 335:310–12, 1990.

Thyroid

Antipenko, A.; Antipenko, T. N. "Thyroid Hormones and Regulation of Cell Reliability Systems," *Advan. Enzyme Regul.* 34:173–98, 1994.

Babenko, N. A.; Filonenko, N. S. "Effect of Thyroid hormones and diacylglycerols on sphingomyelin metabolism in liver cell nuclei in rats of various ages," *Biokhimica* 57(3):371–77, 1991.

Barnes, B.; Galton, L. *Hypo-thyroidism: The Unsuspected Illness.* New York: Harper & Row Publishers, 1976.

Danese, M. D.; Powe, N. R.; Sawin, T.; Ladenson, P. W. "Screening for Mild Thyroid Failure at the Periodic Health Examination," *JAMA* 276:285–92, 1996.

Divino, C. M.; Schussler, G. C. "Transthyretin Receptors on Human Astrocytoma Cells," *J. Clin. Endocrinol. Metab.* 71:1265–68, 1990.

Engler, S.; Burger, A. G. "Deiodination of the Iodothyronines and of Their Derivatives in Man," *Endocrinol. Rev.* 5:151–83, 1984.

Felicetta, J. V.; Sowers, J. R. "The Thyroid and Aging," in *The Thyroid Gland,* edited by L. Van Middlesworth, Chicago, London: Year Book Med Pub., 1986, pp. 131–47.

Felzen, B.; Lotan, R.; Binah, O. "Role of Thyroid state in age-dependent cardiac effects of ouabain in guinea pigs," *Dev. Pharmacol. Ther.* 17:87–94, 1991.

Galton, V. A.; McCarthy, P. T.; St. Germain, D. L. "The Ontogeny of Iodothyronine Deiodinase Systems in Liver and Intestine of the Rat," *Endocrinology* 128: 1717–22, 1991.

Giannella, R. A.; Orlowski, J.; Jump, M. L.; Lingrel, J. B. "Na,K-ATPase Gene Expression in Rat Intestine and Caco-2 Cells: Response to Thyroid Hormone," *Am. J. Physiol.* 265 (*Gastrointest. Liver Physio.* 28): G775–G782, 1993.

Giustina, A.; Wehrenberg, W. B. "Influence of Thyroid Hormones on the Regulation of Growth Hormone Secretion," *J. Endocrin.* 133:646–53, 1995.

Goiochot, B.; Schlienger, J. L.; Grunenberger, F.; et al. "Thyroid hormone status and nutrient intake in the free-living elderly. Interest of Reverse Triiodothyronine assessment," *Eur. J. Endocrinol.* 130:244–52, 1994.

Greenspan, S. L.; Klibanski, A.; Rowe, J. R.; Elahi, D. "Age Related Alterations in Pulsatile Secretion of TSH: Role of Dopaminergic Regulation," *Am. J. Physiol. (Endocrinol. Metab.)* 260:E486–E491, 1991.

Griffin, J. E. "Review: Hypothyroidism in the Elderly," *Am. J. Med. Sci.* 299:334–45, 1990.

Hatterer, J. A.; Herbert, J.; Hidaka, C.; et al. "CSF Transthyretin in Patients with Depression," *Am. J. Psychiatry* 150:813–15, 1993.

Joffe, R. T.; Levitt, A. J. "Major Depression and Subclinical (Grade 2) Hypothyroidism," *Psychoneuroendocrinology* 17:215–21, 1992.

Klatsky, S. A.; Manson, P. N. "Thyroid Disorders Masquerading as Aging Changes," *Ann. Plastic Surg.* 28:420–26, 1992.

Lenzen, G.; Bailey, C. J. "Thyroid hormones, gonadal and adrenocortical steroids and the function of the islets of Langerhans," *Endocrine Reviews* 5:411–34, 1984.

Lewis, G. F.; Alessi, C. A.; Imperial, J. G.; Refetoff, S. "Low serum free thyroxine index in ambulating elderly is due to a resetting of the threshold of thyrotropin feedback suppression," *J. Clin. Endocrinol. Metab.* 73:843–49, 1991.

Lurie M. B. "Resistance to Tuberculosis: Experimental Studies in Native and Acquired Defensive Mechanisms," Cambridge, Mass.: Harvard Univ. Press, 1964.

McKenzie, J. "Stress and Thyroid Function. A Pathophysiological Approach," in *Clin. Neuroendocrinology* edited by G. Tolis, et al. New York: Raven Press, 1979.

Marcocci, C.; Golia, F.; Bruno-Bossio, G.; et al. "Carefully Monitored Levothyroxine Suppressive Therapy Is Not Associated with Bone Loss in Premenopausal Women," *J. Clin. Endocrinol. Metab.* 78:818–23, 1994.

Mooradian, A. D, "The Hepatic Transcellular Transport of 3,5,3'-triiodothyronine Is Reduced in Aged Rats," *Biochim. Biophys. Acta* 1054:1–7, 1990.

Mooradian, A. D.; Habib, M. P.; Dickerson, F., et al. "Effect of age on L-3,5,3'-triiodothyronine-induced ethane exhalation," *J. Appl. Physiol.* 77:160–64, 1994.

Mooradian, A. D.; Wong, N. C. "Age Related Changes in Thyroid Hormone Action," *Eur. J. Endocrinol.* 131:451–61, 1994.

Muller, M. J. "Thyroid and Ageing," *Eur. J. Endocrinol.* 130:242–43, 1994.

Nogami, H.; Yokose, T.; Tachibana, T. "Regulation of Growth Hormone Expression in Fetal Rat Pituitary Gland by Thyroid or Glucocorticoid Hormone," *Am. J. Physiol. (Endocrinol. Metab.)* 268:E262–E267, 1995.

Oh, J. D.; Butcher, L. L.; Woolf, N. J. "Thyroid Hormone Modulates the Development of Cholinergic Terminal Fields in the Rat Forebrain: Relation to Nerve Growth Factor Receptor," *Dev. Brain Res.* 59:133–42, 1991.

Pasquini, J. M.; Adamo, A. M. "Thyroid Hormones and the Central Nervous System," *Dev. Neurosci,* 16:161–68, 1994.

Penzes, L.; Izsak, J.; Kranz, D.; et al. "Effect of Aging on Cold Tolerance and Thyroid Activity in CBA/CA Inbred Mice," *Exp. Gerontol.* 26:601–8, 1991.

Pinchera, A.; Mariotti, S.; Barbesino, G.; Bechi, R.; et al. "Thyroid Autoimmunity and Ageing," *Horm. Res.* 43:64–68, 1995.

Provinciali, M.; Muziioli, M.; Di Stefano, G.; Fabris, N. "Recovery of Spleen Cell Natural Killer Cell Activity by Thyroid Treatment on Old Mice," *Nat. Immun. Cell Growth Regulation* 10:226–36, 1991.

Regelson, W. "The evidence for pituitary and thyroid control of aging: Is age reversal a myth or reality?! The search for a 'death hormone,' " *Intervention in the Aging Process, part B,* edited by W. Regelson, M. Sinex. New York: Alan R. Liss, 1983, pp. 3–52.

Reymond, F.; Denereaz, N.; Lemarchand-Beraud, T. "Thyrotropin Action Impaired in the Thyroid Gland of Old Rats," *Acta Endocrinologica* 126:55–63, 1992.

Robbins, J.; Lakshmanan, M. "The Movement of Thyroid Hormones in the Central Nervous System," *Acta Med. Austriaca* 19 Suppl. 1:21–25, 1992.

Roti, E.; Gardini, E.; Minelli, R.; et al. "Prevalence of Anti-Thyroid Peroxidase Antibodies in Serum in the Elderly: Comparison with Other Tests for Antithyroid Antibodies," *Cli. Chem.* 38:88–92, 1992.

Runnels, B. L.; Garry, P. J.; Hunt, W. C.; Standefer, J. C. "Thyroid Function in a Healthy Elderly Population: Implications for Clinical Evaluation," *J. Gerontol.* 46:B39–44, 1991.

Sawin, C. T.; Geller, A.; Kaplan, M. M.; et al. "Low Serum Thyrotropin (Thyroid Stimulating Hormone) in Older Persons without Hyperthyroidism," *Arch. Intern. Med.* 151:165–68, 1991.

Schreiber, G.; Aldred, A. R.; Jaworski, A.; et al. "Thyroxine Transport from Blood to Brain via Transthyretin Synthesis in the Choroid Plexus," *Am. J. Physiol.* 258:R338–45, 1990.

Shinder, D. A.; Rakhimov, K. R.; Usmanova, O. D. "Delay in Natural Decline of Lactase Activity in the Small Intestine of Prematurely Weaned Rats as Related to Changes in Their Thyroid Status," *Comp. Biochem. Physiol.* 111A(3):453–59, 1995.

Simons, R. J.; Simon, J. M.; Demers, L. M.; Santen, R. J. "Thyroid Dysfunction in Elderly Hospitalized Patients," *Arch. Intern. Med.* 150:1249–53, 1990.

Stouthard, J. M. L.; Van der Poll, T.; Endert, E. "Effects of Acute and Chronic Interleukin-6 Administration on Thyroid Hormone Metabolism in Humans," *J. Clin. Endocrinol. Metab.* 79:1342–46, 1994.

Sustrova, M.; Strbak, V. "Thyroid function and plasma immunoglobulins in subjects with Down's syndrome (DS) during ontogenesis and zinc therapy." *J. Endocrinol. Invest.* 17:385–90, 1994.

Tan, S. A.; Lewis, J. E.; Berk, L. S.; Wilcox, R. B. "Extrathyroidal Physiology of Monoiodotyrosine in Humans," *Clin. Physiol. Biochem.* 8:109–15, 1990.

Tietz, N. W.; Shuey, D. F.; Wekstein, D. R. "Laboratory Values in Fit Aging Individuals, Sexagenarians through Centenarians," *Clin. Chem.* 38:1167–85, 1992.

Urban, R. J. "Neuroendocrinology of Aging in the Male and Female," *Neuroendocrinology I: Endocrinology and Metabolism Clinics of North America* 21:921–30, 1992.

Viticchi, C.; Grinta, R.; Piantanelli, L. "Influence of Age on the Thyroid Hormone-induced Up-regulation of Beta-adrenoceptors in Mouse Brain Cortex," *Gerontology* 36: 286–92, 1990.

Vos, R. A.; DeJong, M.; Bernard, B. F.; et al. "Impaired Thyroxin and

3,5,3'-Triiodothyronine Handling by Rat Hepatocytes in the Presence of Serum of Patients with Nonthyroidal Illness," *J. Clin. Endocrin. Metab.* 80:2364–68, 1995.

Vranck, R.; Savu, L.; Lambert, N.; et al. "Plasma Proteins as Biomarkers in the Aging Process," *Am. J. Physiol.* 268:R536–48, 1995.

Wiener, R.; Utiger, R. D.; Lew, R.; Emerson, C. H. "Age, Sex, and Serum Thyrotropin Concentration in Primary Hypothyroidism," *Acta Endocrinologica* 124:364–69, 1991.

Wijkhuisen, A.; Djouadi, F.; Vilar, J.; et al. "Thyroid hormones regulate development of energy metabolism enzymes in rat proximal convoluted tubule," *Am. J. Physiol.* (Renal Fluid Electrolyte Physiol. 37) 268:F634–F642, 1995.

Growth Hormone

Agrawal, A. K.; Pampori, N. A.; Shapiro, B. H. "Neonatal phenobarbital induced defects in age and sex specific growth hormone profiles regulating monoxygenases," *Am. J. Physiol.* 268:E439–45, 1995.

Auernhammer, C. J., et al. "Effects of growth hormone and insulinlike growth factor I on the immune system," *Eur. J. Endocrinol.* 133:635–45, 1995.

Burman, P., et al. "Quality of life in adults with growth hormone (GH) deficiency: Response to treatment with recombinant human GH in a placebo-controlled 21 month trial," *J. Clin. Endocrin. Metab.* 80(12): 3585–90, 1995.

Clayden, A. M.; Young, W. G.; Zhang, C. Z.; et al. Ultrastructure of cementogenesis as affected by growth hormone in the molar peridontium of the hypophysectomized rat," *J. Peridontal Res.* 29:166–75, 1994.

Fazui, S.; Sabatini, D.; Capaldo, C.; et al. "A Preliminary Study of Growth Hormone in the Treatment of Dilated Cardiomyopathy," *N. Eng. J. Med.* 334:809–14, 1996.

Gelato, M. C. "Aging and immune function: A possible role for growth hormone," *Horm. Res.* 45:46–49, 1996.

Goya, R. G.; Gagnerault, M. C.; De Moraes, M. C.; et al. "In vivo effects of growth hormone on thymus function in aging mice," *Brain Behav. Immun.* 6:341–54, 1992.

Jeevanandam, M.; Petersen, S. R. "Altered lipid kinetics in adjuvant recombinant human growth hormone treated trauma patients," *Am. J. Physiol.* 267:E560–65, 1994.

Jorgensen, J.; Vahl, N.; Tansen, T.; et al. "Influence of growth hormone and androgens on body composition in adults," *Horm. Res.* 45:94–98, 1996.

Loh, E.; Swain, J. L. "Growth Hormone for Heart Failure—Cautious Optimism," *N. Eng. J. Med.* 334:E856–57, 1996.

Muller, E. E.; Cella, S. G.; Parenti, M.; et al. "Somatotrophic dysregulation in old mammals," *Horm. Res.* 43:39–45, 1995.

Papadeakis, M. A.; Grady, D.; Black, D.; et al. "Growth hormone replacement in healthy older men improves body composition but not functional ability," *Annals of Internal Medicine* 124:708–16, 1996.

Rosen, T.; Eden, S.; Larson, G.; et al. "Cardiovascular risk factors in adult patients with growth hormone deficiency," *Acta Endocrin.* 129:195–200, 1993.

Rosen, T.; Johannsson, G.; Johansson, J.; Bengtsson, B. "Consequences of growth hormone deficienty in adults and the benefits and risks of recombinant human growth hormone," *Horm. Res.* 43:93–99, 1995.

Rudman, D.; Feller, A. G.; Nagraj, A. G.; et al. "Effects of human growth hormone in men over 60 years old," *N. Eng. J. Med.* 323:1–9, 1990.

Rudman, D.; Kutner, M. H.; Rogers, C. M.; et al. "Impaired growth hormone secretion in the adult population: relation to age and adiposity," *J. Clin. Invest.* 67: 1361–69, 1981.

Schmbelan, M. "Studies suggest growth hormone is an effective treatment of wasting syndrome in HIV," *Endocrine News* 21, #2, April 1996.

Stirling, H. F.; Kelner, C. J. "Who needs growth hormone?" (Editorial) *J. R. Soc. Med.* 87:497–98, 1994.

Vermeulen, A.; Kaufman, J. M. "Aging of the hypothalamo-pituitary testicular axis in men," *Horm. Res.* 43:25–28, 1995.

Wolthers, T.; Thorbjorn, G.; Lunde, J. O. "Effects of GH administration on functional hepatic nitrogen clearance: Studies in normal subjects and GH deficient patients," *J. Clin. Endocr. Metab.* 78:1220–24, 1994.

Melatonin

Please refer to our text *The Melatonin Miracle* by Walter Pierpaoli, William Regelson, and Carol Coleman. New York: Simon & Schuster, 1995. There are five other books, designed for a popular audience that have been published discussing the laboratory and clinical potential of melatonin in the past year.

Abe, M.; Reiter, R.; Orhil, P. B.; et al. "Inhibitory Effect of Melatonin on Cataract Formation in Newborn Rats: Evidence for an Antioxidative Role for Melatonin," *J. Pineal Res.* 17:94–100, 1994.

Acuna-Castroviejo, D.; Escames, G.; Macias, M.; et al. "Cell Protective Role of Melatonin in the Brain," *J. Pineal Res.* 19:57–63, 1995.

Benouali-Pellissier, S. "Melatonin Is Involved in Cholecystokinin Induced Changes of Ileal Motility in Rats," *J. Pineal Res.* 17:79–85, 1994.

Brackowski, R.; Zubelewicz, B.; Romanowski, W.; et al. "Preliminary study on modulation of the biological effects of tumor necrosis factor-alpha in advanced cancer patients by the pineal hormone melatonin," *J. Biol. Regulators and Homeostatic Agents* 3:77–80, 1994.

Cagnoli, C. M.; Atabay, C.; Kharlamova, E.; Marney, H. "Melatonin Protects Neurons from Singlet Oxygen Induced Apoptosis," *J. Pineal Res.* 18:222–26, 1995.

Calvo, J. R.; Rafii-El-Idrissi, M.; Pozo, D.; Guerrero, J. M. "Immunomodulatory Role of Melatonin: Specific Binding Sites in Human and Rodent Lymphoid Cells," *J. Pineal Res.* 18:119–26, 1995.

Cardinali, D. P.; DelZar, M. M.; Vacas, M. I. "The effects of melatonin in human platelets," *Apptla* 43:1–13, 1993.

Carneiro, R. C.; Toffoleto, O.; Cipolla-Neto, J.; Markus, R. P. "Modulation of sympathetic neurotransmission by melatonin," *Eur. J. Pharmacol.* 257(1-2):73–77, 1994.

Chardon, S. P.; Degli, F.; Degli, R.; et al. "Parallel Nocturnal Secretion of Melatonin and Testosterone in the Plasma of Normal Men," *J. Pineal Res.* 19:16–22, 1995.

Cos, S.; Blask, D. E. "Melatonin Modulates Growth Factor Activity in MCF-7 Human Breast Cancer Cells," *J. Pineal Res.* 17:25–32, 1994.

Dollins, A. B.; Lynch, H. J.; Wurtman, R. J.; et al. "Effect of Pharmacological Daytime Doses of Melatonin on Human Mood and Performance," *Psychopharmacology* 112:490–96, 1993.

Dollins, A. B.; Zhdanova, I. V.; Wurtman, R. J.; et al. "Effect of Inducing Nocturnal Serum Melatonin Concentrations in Daytime on Sleep, Mood, Body Temperature, and Performance," *Proc. Nat. Acad. of Sci. USA* 91:1824–28, 1994.

Gonzalez, R.; Sanchez, A.; Ferguson, J. A. "Melatonin therapy of advanced human malignant melanoma," *Melanoma Res.* 1:237–43, 1991.

Humbert, W.; Pevet, P. "The Pineal Gland of the Aging Rat," *J. Pineal Res.* 18:32–40, 1995.

Jan, J. E.; Espezel, H. "Melatonin Treatment of Chronic Sleep Disorders" (Letter), *Dev. Med. and Child Neurology* 37:279–81, 1995.

Jan, J. E.; Espezel, H.; Appleton, R. E. "The Treatment of Sleep Disorders with Melatonin," *Dev. Med. and Child Neurology* 36:97–107, 1994.

Kerenyi, N. A.; Pandula, E.; Feuer, G. M. "Oncostatic Effects of the Pineal Gland," *Drug Metab. and Drug Interactions* 8:313–90, 1990.

Lerchi, A.; Partsch, C.-J.; Nieschlag. E. "Circadian and Ultradian Variations of Pituitary and Pineal Hormones in Normal Men: Evidence for a Link Between Melatonin, Gonadotrophin, and Prolactin Secretion," *J. Pineal Res.* 18:41–48, 1995.

Lewis, A. J.; Kerenyi, N. A.; Feuer, G. "Neuropharmacology of Pineal Secretions," *Drug Metab. and Drug Interactions* 8, 1990.

Lissoni, P.; Barni, S.; Cazzaniga, M.; et al. "Efficacy of the Concomitant Administration of the Pineal Hormone Melatonin in Cancer Immunotherapy with Low Dose IL-2 in Patients with Advanced Solid Tumors Who Had Progressed on II-2 Alone," *Oncology* 51:344–47, 1994.

Lissoni, P.; Meregalli, S.; Fossati, V.; et al. "A Randomized Study of Low Dose Subcutaneous Interleukin-2 plus Melatonin vs. Chemotherapy for Advanced Non-Small Cell Lung Cancer," *Tumori* 80:464–67, 1994.

Maestroni, G. J. M.; Conti, A.; Lissoni, P. "Colony-Stimulating Activity and Hemapoetic Rescue from Cancer Chemotherapy Compounds by Melatonin via Endogenous Interleukin 4," *Cancer Res.* 54:4740–43, 1994.

Maestroni, G. J. M.; Covacci, V.; Conti, A. "Hematopoietic Rescue via T-Cell Dependent Endogenous Granulocyte Macrophage Colony Stimulating Factor Induced by the Pineal Neurohormone Melatonin in Tumor Bearing Mice," *Cancer Res.* 54:2469, 1994.

Mocchegiani, E.; Bulian, D.; Santarelli, L.; et al. "The immuno-reconstituting effect of melatonin or pineal grafting and its relation to zinc pool in aging mice," *J. Neuroimmunol.* 53:189–201, 1994.

Morgan, P. J.; Barrett, P.; Howell, H. E.; et al. "Melatonin Receptors: Localization, Molecular Pharmacology, and Physiological Significance," 24:101–46, 1994.

Neri, B.; Fiorelli, C.; Moroni, F.; et al. "Modulation of Human Lymphoblastoid Interferon Activity in Metastatic Renal Carcinoma. A Phase II Study," *Cancer* 73:3015–19, 1994.

Oaknin-Bendahan, S.; Anis, U.; Nir, I.; Zisapel, N. "Effects of long-term administration of melatonin and a putative antagonist on the aging rat," *Neuroreport* 6(5):785–88, 1995.

Osborne, N. N. "Serotonin and Melatonin in the Iris/Ciliary Process and Their Involvement in Intraocular Pressure," *Acta Neurobiol. Exp.* 54:57–64, 1994.

Pierpaoli, W.; Bulian, D.; Dall'Ara, A. "Circadian Melatonin and Young-to-Old Grafting Postpone Aging and Maintain Juvenile Conditions of Reproductive Functions in Mice and Rats," *Exp. Gerontology* in press; Abstract: Third Int. Symp. on Neurobiology and Neuroendocrinology of Aging, 1996.

Przybylska, B. K.; Lewczuk, B.; Dusza, L. "Effect of long-term administration of melatonin on ultrastructure of pinealocytes in gilts," *Folia Morphol.* 53,3, 129–36, 1994.

Reiter, R. J. "Pineal Function During Aging: Attenuation of the Melatonin Rhythm and Its Neurobiological Consequences," *Acta Neurobiol. Exp.* 54:31–39, 1994.

Schapel, G. J.; Beran, R. G.; Kennaway, D. L.; et al. "Melatonin Response in Active Epilepsy," *Epilepsia* 36:75–78, 1995.

Schmid, H. A.; Raykhtsaum, G. "Age Related Difference in the Structure of Human Pineal Calcium Deposits: Results of Transmission Electron Microscopy and Mineralographic Microanalysis," *J. Pineal Res.* 18:12–20, 1995.

Sewerynek, E.; Melchiorri, D.; Ortiz, G. G.; et al. "Melatonin Reduces H2O2-induced Lipid Peroxidation in Homogenates of Different Rat Brain Regions," *J. Pineal Res.* 19:51–56, 1995.

Slominski, A.; Pruski, D. "Melatonin Inhibits Proliferation and Melanogenesis in Rodent Melanoma Cells," *Experimental Cell Res.* 206:189–94, 1993.

Slominski, A.; Chassalcvris, M.; Mazurkiewica, J.; et al. "Murine skin as a target for melatonin in bioregulation," *Exp. Dermatol.* 3:45–50, 1994.

Ying, S.-W.; Niles, L. P.; Crocker, C. "Human Malignant Melanoma Cells Express High Affinity Receptors for Melatonin: Antiproliferative Effects of Melatonin and 6-Chloromelatonin," *Eur. J. Pharmacol.* 246:89–96, 1993.

Index